Already published in BRACCO EDUCATION IN DIAGNOSTIC IMAGING

SYLLABUS 1: CLINICAL MRI (Editor: H. Imhof)
11th Annual Scientific Meeting of the
European Society for Magnetic Resonance in Medicine
(Vienna, April 20-24, 1994)

SYLLABUS 2: MUSCULOSKELETAL IMAGING: AN UPDATE
Categorical Course ECR '95
(Eds. A. L. Baert, P. Grenier, U. V. Willi - Invited Ed. J. L. Bloem)
(Vienna, March 5-10, 1995)

SYLLABUS 3: CHEST, MUSCULOSKELETON, G.I. AND ABDOMEN,
URINARY TRACT (Editor: L. Dalla Palma)
5th Radiological Refresher Course
(Budapest-Tihany, May 6-9, 1996)

SYLLABUS 4: FUNCTIONAL MRI (Editors: P. Pavone and P. Rossi)
European Seminars on Diagnostic and Interventional Radiology
(Rome, October 26-28, 1995)

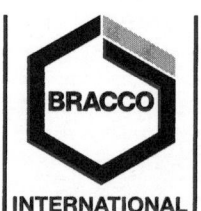
Kindly offered by INTERNATIONAL

Springer
Berlin
Heidelberg
New York
Barcelona
Budapest
Hong Kong
London
Milan
Paris
Santa Clara
Singapore
Tokyo

SYLLABUS

FUNCTIONAL MRI

ESDIR, Seminar No. 24
Rome, October 26-28, 1995

EDITORS: P. PAVONE and P. ROSSI

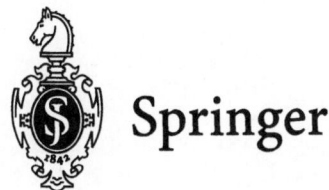 Springer

Dr. Paolo Pavone
Prof. Plinio Rossi
Istituto di Radiologia
Università La Sapienza
Policlinico Umberto I
Viale Regina Elena 4
I-00161 Roma

EAR Teaching Programmes
European Seminars on Diagnostic
and Interventional Radiology (ESDIR)

Committee:
R. Passariello (Chairman)
W.M. Ross (EAR)
C.D.R. Flower, Y. Grumbach
L. Horvath, O.E.S. Pohlenz
H.S. Thomsen, M. Mirtcheva (JRF), C. Catalano (Secretary)

ISBN 978-3-540-75025-3   ISBN 978-88-470-2194-5 (eBook)
DOI 10.1007/978-88-470-2194-5

Die Deutsche Bibliothek - CIP-Einheitsaufnahme

Syllabus functional MRI / ed.: P. Pavone and P. Rossi. - Berlin; Heidelberg; New York; Barcelona;
Budapest; Hong Kong; London; Milano; Paris; Santa Clara; Singapore; Tokyo: Springer, 1996

NE: Pavone, Paolo [Hrsg.]

Library of Congress Cataloguing - in - Pubblication Data: applied for

Typesetting: Compostudio, Cernusco sul Naviglio (Milano)

Functional MRI

Preface

Every day MRI is gaining more and more appreciation by all medical specialists for its impressive quality of anatomical images. This morphological information gives consistent help in terms of earlier diagnosis, lesion characterisation, and definition of the extent of disease. However, morphology is not the only information obtained through MRI.

Recently, a large number of researchers have exploited the possibility of also obtaining functional information with MRI. Results of brain activation studies have been initially performed in Boston and have been confirmed by investigators all over the world. Important functional data can be obtained not only on the brain, but also on the heart and on parenchymal organs.

The diffusion nowadays of commercial MR units used with high field gradient and echo planar techniques allows functional data to be obtained in any routine clinical activity.

This book appears at the right time to provide information on fMRI to all MR users wanting to obtain clinical experience with this new tool. We thank the authors of each paper for their efforts and for the outstanding contribution both to the seminar and on these pages.

We are especially grateful to BRACCO INTERNATIONAL, who generously supported the publication of this Syllabus and the European Seminar on Diagnostic and Interventional Radiology (ESDIR), held in Rome on October 26-28, 1995.

We hope that this editorial work will be valid as a reference collection of papers on this new field of medicine.

The Editors

Table of Contents

BASICS OF FUNCTIONAL MRI

Evaluating Brain Activation: A Methodological Perspective

F. Orzi

I.N.M. Neuromed, Pozzilli (IS) and Dipartimento Scienze Neurologiche, Università "La Sapienza", Rome, Italy

The Kety and Schmidt Method: a Starting Point

Commonly used methods for measuring cerebral blood flow (CBF) stem from the nitrous oxide method. The method developed by Kety and Schmidt [1] first provided a means for measuring CBF and rates of glucose and oxygen consumption in the human brain [2]. The Kety and Schmidt method is based on the Fick Principle. Given a compartment (W) with one entrance and one exit, the relationship among the instantaneous (at any time t) concentration values of a tracer in the in-flowing (Ca) and out-flowing (Cv) liquid (blood), the flow rate of the blood perfusing the compartment, and the concentration of the dye within the compartment (Ci) is expressed by the following equation:

$$dCi / dt = F / W(Ca - Cv)$$

The equation defines the parameters to be measured in order to calculate flow, expressed per unit of mass of tissue (F/W). The principle is applied to the brain, which satisfies the requirements imposed by the model. Assessments of the blood concentrations of a suitable indicator are performed in samples drawn from the in-coming arterial and out-coming jugular blood. The tissue concentrations of the indicator are inferred from the venous concentrations of a freely diffusible tracer according to the blood-tissue exchange theory [1]. Blood flow values, however, refer to the brain as a whole. The Kety and Schmidt method is ineffective in resolving the heterogeneity of the brain.

Local Measurements

Local CBF measurements imply techniques for evaluating local Ci and local Cv. Ca is considered to be equal all over the brain and equal to blood from any large peripheral artery. Ci is measured by autoradiography, tomographic techniques ("in vivo autoradiography"), or by other means of external detection of brain radioactivity. Values of local Cv are obtained from local Ci and knowledge of the blood-brain partition coefficient (λ). For any specific freely diffusible tracer, for any homogenous area of the brain, the ratio Ci/Cv is a constant. Such a constant is the partition coefficient, λ. A basic assumption for most of CBF methods is, therefore, that the tracer is freely diffusible, which is that its uptake by the tissue is limited by blood flow and not by diffusion. Under these conditions, and in absence of arterio-venous shunts, the venous blood draining the tissue is in equilibrium with the tissue. The blood-brain partition coefficient is considered to have the same value throughout the whole brain. This is a reasonable assumption for most of the blood flow tracers commonly used, under physiological conditions. Thus, λ can be measured separately in a different group of subjects. The measured value can be used for the whole brain of the subjects under investigation to compute local values of Cv, according to the following equalities:

$$\lambda = Ci/Cv, \text{ and therefore } Cv = Ci / \lambda$$

Because of the required diffusibility, blood flow tracers are often radioactive gases. However, in order to avoid a number of cumbersome procedures finalized to prevent loss of tracer from the blood and tissues because of its volatility, the use of non-volatile, diffusible ^{14}C-labelled tracers were then introduced [3]. Thus, Ci is measured by autoradiography or any other technique which allows local assessment within the brain tissue. Cv is computed from Ci on the basis of knowledge of λ. Ca is measured in a large peripheral arterial vessel. A number of techniques subserve the theoretical models which describe behavior of the tracer in the system. Models refer to any homogeneous area of the brain with respect to blood flow, solubility of the tracer and a well mixed compartment. Spatial resolution of the methods depends upon the techniques employed for measurements of local tissue tracer concentrations. Techniques include exploitation of hydrogen electrode, tissue sampling, autoradiography, and emission tomography (gamma cameras, single photon emission computed tomography (SPECT), positron emission tomography (PET)) for in vivo evaluations. Theoretical models refer essentially to the tissue equilibration and tissue fractionation approaches [4].

Tissue Equilibration Model

In the tissue equilibration model CBF is the variable which affects blood-brain partition of a freely diffusible tracer in presence of a concentration gradient. The blood-tissue gradient is achieved in the tissue saturation phase during introduction of the tracer into the system according a suitable infusion rate. A reversed gradient also occurs in the wash-out (clearance) phase which follows interruption of the tracer infusion once the saturation had been reached. The autoradiographic antipyrine, or iodoantipyrine [3], method is probably the most commonly used application of the tissue equilibration model. Gamma cameras and clearance methods opened the field of functional imaging in human brain [5, 6]. [133]Xenon clearance techniques following inhalation, or intracarotid injection, of the tracer were used in association with external scintillation detection of gamma radiation from the human brain. Recently, dedicated, rotating gamma cameras were developed which can tomographically monitor the local rates of cerebral xenon wash out and therefore provide regional measurements of CBF. Development of in vivo autoradiography by PET and computed tomography (CT) allowed exploitation of the tissue equilibration model in humans by using [15]0-labelled water [7] and stable xenon as flow tracers, respectively.

Indicator Fractionation Model

The indicator fractionation model deals with tracers which are completely trapped within the brain tissue. The model, therefore, assumes Cv equal to zero. In this case the instantaneous rate of accumulation of the tracer depends upon blood flow and arterial concentration of the tracer. Requirements of the method are met by use of microspheres which are mechanically trapped into capillaries of experimental animals. These are radiopharmaceuticals which are used for extension of the method to humans by means of SPECT. These molecules are claimed to behave as chemical microspheres, since they are trapped within the tissue at their first passage and remain in the tissue for relatively long time. A number of molecules labelled with gamma- emitting isotopes have been developed. Following systemic administration, the tissue concentration of these molecules reaches a quasi steady state which makes feasible the use of relatively slow tomographic instruments, such as general purpose gamma cameras. There are pitfalls with the use of chemical microspheres. First of all, while it is generally recognized that they have a tremendously high partition coefficient, there is not a complete trapping

within the tissue, and Cv > 0. These molecules, therefore, do not meet the basic requirement of the tissue fractionation model. Other difficulties which prevent the obtainment of quantitative evaluation of CBF by SPECT and tissue fractionation model, include uncertainties about the kinetic and metabolic properties of the available molecules [8]. For instance, the partition coefficient may vary throughout the brain. In addition, the molecules are metabolized during the procedure. Breakdown products often carry the label, so that detected radioactivity comprises metabolites which have lost the kinetic properties of the tracer. Measuring radioactivity in the blood, therefore, introduces errors in the computation of the arterial concentration of the tracer. Thus, uncertainties about the metabolic properties of the chemical microspheres cause errors in the measurement of both the input function and the brain concentration of the indicator.

CBF and Brain Activation

Methods for measuring CBF based on the mentioned models provide detailed maps of local perfusion. The methods showed the dynamic response of CBF regulation to focal brain functional activation. Thus, the first demonstration of functional brain imaging was achieved with the antipyrine method. Changes in local CBF, under physiological conditions, were since then interpreted as changes in brain function. Under physiological conditions cerebral blood flow and glucose metabolism are closely correlated to each other. Both flow and metabolism respond quickly to changes in functional activity. The extension of the changes and their intensity are often similar. There are uncertainties as to the mechanisms which regulate cerebral circulation during neuronal activation. Intraparenchymal blood vessels are innervated by intrinsic neuronal terminals and by terminals arising from cranial autonomic ganglia. There are central pathways which include the rat cerebellar fastigial nucleus which also mediate global increase in cerebral blood flow [9]. Different neurotransmitters are present in perivascular terminals, including catecholamines, acetylcholine, serotonin, and a number of neuropeptides. However, lesions or pharmacological blockade of neurotransmission do not attenuate blood flow increases induced by somatosensory stimulation. Local chemical changes often referred to as likely candidates for mediating local vascular regulation in the brain parenchyma may occur later than vascular dilatation itself. There is growing interest in nitric oxide as a key molecule in regulating cerebral circulation during neural activity. Indications in this direction are mostly based on data showing that inhibitors of nitric oxide synthase prevent increases in blood flow associated with neuronal activity. However, data are controversial [10]. Thus, under physiological conditions, blood flow is locally adjusted to energy requirements. Increments in energy metabolism correlate with increments in frequency of stimulation of neuronal pathways [11]. There is evidence that the site of increased metabolism during activation is at the level of axon terminals, and not of cell bodies. An elegant demonstration was provided by Kadekaro et al. [12] who showed increased glucose utilization in the lumbar spinal cord during electrical stimulation of the dorsal root, but not during antidromic stimulation of the ventral root. Thus, the increased metabolic activity probably reflects Na^+/K^+ ATPase needed to restore ionic distribution across the membrane in the synaptic terminal and not in the postsynaptic elements.

References

1. Kety SS and Schmidt CF (1948) The nitrous oxide method for quantitative determination of cerebral blood flow in man: Theory, procedure, and normal values. Clin Invest 27: 476-483
2. Sokoloff L (1960) Quantitative measurement of cerebral blood flow in man. In: Methods in Medical Research, Vol VIII, Bruner HD (ed), 253-261
3. Sakurada O, Kennedy C, Jehle J, Brown JD, Carbin GL, Sokoloff L (1978) Measurement of local cerebral blood flow with ^{14}C-iodoantipyrine. Am J Physiol 239: H59-H66
4. Patlak CS, Blasberg RG, Fenstermacher JD (1994) An evaluation of errors in the determination of blood flow by the Indicator Fractionation and Tissue Equilibration (Kety) Methods. J Cereb Blood Flow Metab 4: 47-60
5. Conn HL (1955) Measurement of organ blood flow without blood sampling. J Clin Invest 34: 916
6. Lassen NA and Ingvar DH (1972) Radioisotopic assessment of regional cerebral blood flow. Prog Nucl Med 1: 376-409
7. Raichle ME, Martin WRW, Herscovitch P, Mintun MA, Markham J (1983) Brain Blood flow measured with intravenous $H_2^{15}O$ II. Implementation and validation. J Nucl Med 24: 790-798
8. Lucignani G, Nehlig A, Blasberg R, Patlak CS, Anderson L, Fieschi C, Fazio F, Sokoloff L (1985) Metabolic and kinetic considerations in the use of [^{125}I] HIPDM for quantitative measurement of regional cerebral blood flow. J Cereb Blood Flow Metab 5: 86-89
9. Iadecola C (1993) Regulation of cerebral circulation during neural activity: is nitric oxide the missing link? Trends Neurosci 16: 206-214
10. Adachi K, Takahashi S, Melzer P, Campos KL, Nelson T, Kennedy C, Sokoloff L (1994) Increases in local cerebral blood flow associated with somatosensory activation are not mediates by NO. Am J Physiol 267: H2155-62
11. Yarowsky P, Kadekaro M, Sokoloff L (1983) Frequency-dependent activation of glucose utilization in the superior cervical ganglion by electrical stimulation of cervical sympathetic trunk. Proc Natl Acad Sci USA 80: 4179-4183
12. Kadekaro M, Hugh Vance W, Lee Terell M, Gary H, Eisenberg MH, Sokoloff L (1987) Effects of antidromic stimulation of the ventral root on glucose utilization in the ventral horn of the spinal cord in the rat. Proc Natl Acad Sci USA 84: 5492-5495

Intrinsic Parameters Measurable with MRI

C. Segebarth

Inserm U438, Centre Hospitalier Universitaire, Pavillon B, BP 217, 38043 Grenoble Cedex 09, France

Introduction

One of the specificities of magnetic resonance imaging (MRI) – and one of its major strengths – lies in the possibility it provides to modulate the image contrasts between various biological tissues. The MR image contrasts, due mainly to differences in intensity of MR signals from water protons from different tissues, depend on the interplay between certain instrumental parameters (radiofrequency (RF) pulse angles, delays between RF pulses, type of RF pulse sequences applied) and a large number of biophysical parameters characterizing the different tissues. Among the latter, water density as well as the longitudinal (T_1) and transverse (T_2) relaxation times of the water protons play an overwhelming role. Other biophysical parameters of particular importance include the magnetic susceptibility (either the bulk magnetic susceptibilities of the tissues or the magnetic susceptibilities of certain microscopic components within, such as the intra- and extracapillary spaces), the self-diffusion properties of water molecules, and the bulk tissue movements.

The prediction – or the interpretation – of the MR signal behaviour from a particular spin system requires a detailed, microscopic understanding of that system. For a particular biological tissue, one needs to know in detail its molecular composition, the way it is compartmentalized, and the exchange processes which occur between compartments. Clearly, the extreme complexity of biological tissues prevents us from describing them in this detail on a microscopic level.

A number of qualitative properties of spin systems from biological tissues can be predicted, however, using more or less simple tissular models. As water is by far the predominant tissular constituent, the simplest model is that of pure water. The aim of this paper is to present the relationships between the relaxation properties of the NMR signal from pure water and certain dynamic features of water molecules. These relationships may constitute a qualitative introduction to the biophysical phenomena underlying relaxation behaviour of the water proton NMR signal in biological tissues.

Water

Oxygen is essentially non-magnetic (the natural abundance of the magnetic isotope ^{17}O of oxygen is about 0.04%). The magnetic interactions of water are therefore those between protons and the external magnetic field (the so-called "Zeeman" interactions which predominate in the usual experimental conditions) and those among protons (the "dipolar" interactions). In what follows, we will concentrate on these dipolar interactions, as they are responsible for the relaxation properties of the spin system. For the sake of simplicity, rather than considering all protons of a water bath, we will focus the discussion initially on the case of two interacting protons within a bath. At the present time, we may consider these protons as being part of the same water molecule or of different water molecules.

The dipolar interaction energy between the magnetic moments μ_1 and μ_2 of two protons represents the interaction energy of one of the magnetic moments with the magnetic field produced by the other. In classical terms, it may be written as:

$$E_d = \frac{1}{r^3}\left\{\mu_1 . \mu_2 - 3\left(\mu_1 . n\right)\left(\mu_2 . n\right)\right\}, \qquad (1)$$

where n represents a unit vector in the internuclear direction, and r the internuclear distance. Translated into quantum mechanical terms, this expression becomes the dipolar Hamiltonian equation H_d of the two interacting protons:

$$H_d = \frac{\hbar^2 \gamma^2}{r^3}\left\{I_1 . I_2 - 3\left(I_1 . n\right)\left(I_2 . n\right)\right\}, \qquad (2)$$

where γ represents the gyromagnetic ratio of the protons, $\hbar$ is the fundamental physical constant of Planck, and I_1 and I_2 are the angular momentum operators of the two protons. The dipolar Hamiltonian may be written conveniently as follows:

$$H_d = \frac{\hbar^2 \gamma^2}{r^3} \sum_m V_m F_m, \qquad (3)$$

where V_m represents bilinear spin operators derived from the individual spin operators I_2 and I_2, and where F_m represents simple angular functions describing the relative orientations of the external magnetic field and the internuclear vector. In this sum, the bilinear spin operators are grouped according to certain quantum mechanical properties they have in common (these are the transitions which they induce between energy levels of the Zeeman Hamiltonian, or, in other terms, their "commutation rules" with the Zeeman Hamiltonian).

Relaxation of Water Protons and Rotational Brownian Motion

Brownian motion in water induces fluctuations in the internuclear distances r between protons (translational motion) as well as in the relative orientations of the internuclear vectors and the external magnetic field (translational as well as rotational motion). Thus, Brownian motion introduces a time-dependency into the dipolar Hamiltonian.

I will, in what follows, neglect the translational motion, as detailed calculations show that the relaxation behaviour of water protons is predominantly due to the rotational Brownian motion. Thus, considering only the molecular reorientation, the time-dependent Hamiltonian $H_d(t)$ describing the intramolecular dipolar couplings can be written as:

$$H_d\left(t\right)=\frac{\hbar^2\gamma^2}{r^3}\sum_m V_m F_m\left(t\right)=\sum_m H_d^m\left(t\right), \qquad (4)$$

where $F_m(t)$ represents fluctuating angular functions.

Two concepts are now of particular importance in discussing the relaxation properties of water protons. The first concept is called the *autocorrelation function* $G_m(\tau)$. The autocorrelation function of a particular term $H_d^m(t)$ of the dipolar Hamiltonian is defined as follows:

$$G_m\left(\tau\right)=\int H_d^m\left(t\right)H_d^m\left(t+\tau\right)\mathrm{dt}. \qquad (5)$$

The autocorrelation function tells us how the dipolar couplings at one particular time are correlated to their value at a later time. Typically, for times shorter than some critical time, τ_c, called *the correlation time*, the effects of the motion may be considered negligible, so that $H_d^m(t) \approx H_d^m(t+\tau)$. For times τ longer than τ_c, the values of $H_d^m(t+\tau)$ become progressively less correlated to $H_d^m(t)$, so that $G_m(\tau)$ goes to zero. Thus, the autocorrelation function exhibits a maximum at $\tau=0$, and falls off progressively for $\tau > \tau_c$.

The second concept is termed the *spectral density function $J_m(\omega)$*. It is defined as the Fourier transform of the autocorrelation function:

$$J_m\left(\omega\right)=\int G_m\left(\tau\right)\exp\left(-i\omega\tau\right)\mathrm{d}\tau. \qquad (6)$$

Calculations show that the relaxation rates (i.e. the inverse of the relaxation times) can be described in terms of the values of the spectral density functions at the particular frequencies $2\omega_0$, ω_0, and 0. These frequencies correspond to the transitions induced by the bilinear spin operators contained in V_m (Eq. 3):

$$\frac{1}{T_1} = \left(\frac{\hbar^2\gamma^2}{r^3}\right)^2 4\left\{J_1\left(\omega_0\right)+4J_2\left(2\omega_0\right)\right\}, \qquad (7)$$

$$\frac{1}{T_2} = \left(\frac{\hbar^2\gamma^2}{r^3}\right)^2 \left\{6J_0\left(0\right)+J_1\left(\omega_0\right)+4J_2\left(2\omega_0\right)\right\}. \qquad (8)$$

It can be shown that rotational Brownian motion leads to exponential correlation functions:

$$G_m\left(\tau\right)\approx \exp-\frac{\tau}{\tau_c}. \qquad (9)$$

The spectral density functions $J_0(0)$, $J_1(\omega_0)$ and $J_2(2\omega_0)$ can in this case be estimated easily ($J_1(\omega_0)$ and $J_2(2\omega_0)$ turn out to be represented by identical expressions), leading to the following expressions for the relaxation rates:

$$\frac{1}{T_1} = \frac{3}{10}\left(\frac{\hbar^2\gamma^2}{r^3}\right)^2\tau_c\left\{\frac{1}{1+\left(\omega_0\tau_c\right)^2}+\frac{4}{1+\left(2\omega_0\tau_c\right)^2}\right\}, \qquad (10)$$

$$\frac{1}{T_2} = \frac{3}{20}\left(\frac{\hbar^2\gamma^2}{r^3}\right)^2\tau_c\left\{3+\frac{5}{1+\left(\omega_0\tau_c\right)^2}+\frac{2}{1+\left(2\omega_0\tau_c\right)^2}\right\}. \qquad (11)$$

Figure 1 shows the angular frequency dependence of the spectral density functions J_1 and J_2. Three curves have been displayed which have been calculated for different values of the correlation time: $\tau_c = 10$ ms, $\tau_c = 1$ μs, and $\tau_c = 1$ ps. In the case of water, the correlation times characterizing rotational tumbling will obviously not span this extended range. In the case of other liquids, such as glycerine, the viscosity may vary considerably with temperature, so that the correlation times might span an extended range. The three curves cross each other because the integral of the spectral density function is independent of the correlation time. (It depends only on the *strength* of the dipolar interactions; this feature may be verified by considering the inverse Fourier relationship of Eq. 6.)

Consider now, as an example, the particular case of measurements performed in a static field of 0.02 Tesla, for which the (angular) resonance frequency of water protons is about 10^6 rad/s. One can easily verify from

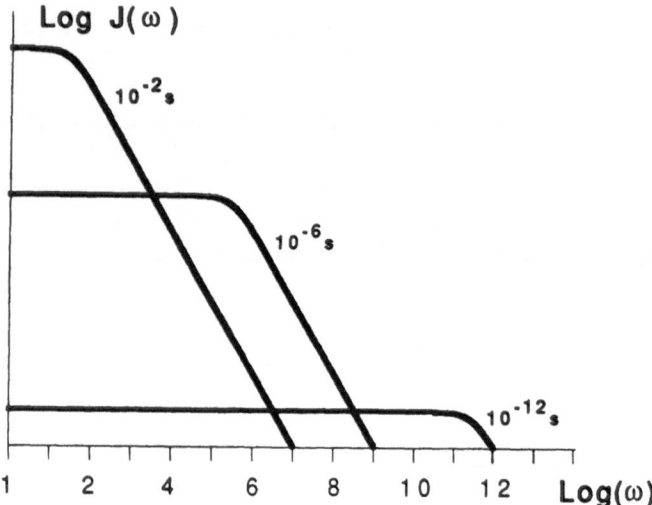

$$\frac{1}{T_1} = \frac{1}{T_2} = \frac{3}{2} \left(\frac{\hbar^2 \gamma^2}{r^3} \right)^2 \tau_c. \qquad (13)$$

Fig. 1. *Spectral density functions of the fluctuating dipolar coupling between protons from a particular water molecule.* The spectral densities have been calculated for rotational correlation times of 10^{-2} s, 10^{-6} s and 10^{-12} s

In the case of water, the usual experimental conditions correspond to the fast regime. At room temperature, the rotational correlation times of water molecules are about 10^{-14} s. Thus, $\omega_0 \tau_c \ll 1$, and Eq. 13 is valid. At room temperature, this corresponds to transverse and longitudinal relaxation times of the water protons of the order of 3.5 s.

Static Field Inhomogeneities and Transverse Relaxation: T_2^* vs. T_2

We know that, in practice, a transverse relaxation time of several seconds is rarely observed. This is due to the imperfections of the static magnetic field applied, and in particular to its lack of homogeneity. The magnetic field inhomogeneity ΔB_0 within the sample under study causes the resonance frequencies to vary continuously in space. The transverse magnetization, which is made up from contributions from all over the sample, will as a consequence decay more or less rapidly due to a loss of phase coherence between transverse magnetization vectors from regions characterized by different resonance frequencies. Thus, rather than observing the mono-exponential transverse relaxation of water protons, one observes a decay predominantly due to imperfections of magnetic field homogeneity. Although this decay is usually not

Fig. 1 that, among the three cases displayed, it is the spectral density function calculated for the correlation time $\tau_c = 1$ μs which provides the largest value at that particular resonance frequency. This example illustrates a general property that, at a particular (angular) resonance frequency ω_0, the spectral density functions J_1 and J_2 are maximum for movements characterized by a correlation time $\tau_c = (\omega_0)^{-1}$. The regime of movements characterized by correlation times approximately equal to the inverse of the resonance frequency is dubbed the *intermediate regime*. Similarly, if the movements are characterized by correlation times much smaller or much larger than the inverse of the resonance frequency, one speaks of the *rapid regime*, or of the *slow regime*, respectively.

As the longitudinal relaxation rates are proportional to the spectral density functions $J_1 (\omega_0)$ and $J_2 (2\omega_0)$ (Eqs. 7, 10), one may anticipate that the longitudinal relaxation time T_1 will provide a minimum in experimental conditions corresponding to the intermediate regime, i.e., when:

$$\omega_0 \tau_c \approx 1. \qquad (12)$$

This property is illustrated in Fig. 2 which represents the variations of T_1 and T_2 with $(\omega_0 \tau_c)^{-1}$. The two curves have been obtained from Eqs. 10 and 11, respectively. The transverse relaxation rate is expressed not only in terms of $J_1 (\omega_0)$ and $J_2 (2\omega_0)$, but also in terms of a spectral density function $J_0 (0)$ calculated at zero frequency (Eqs. 8 and 11). As a result, when the motion is slow ($\omega_0 \tau_c \gg 1$), the transverse relaxation rate is much larger than the longitudinal relaxation rate. It may easily be verified (Eqs. 10-11) that when the motion is rapid ($\omega_0 \tau_c \ll 1$), the transverse and longitudinal relaxation rates are identical, and given by:

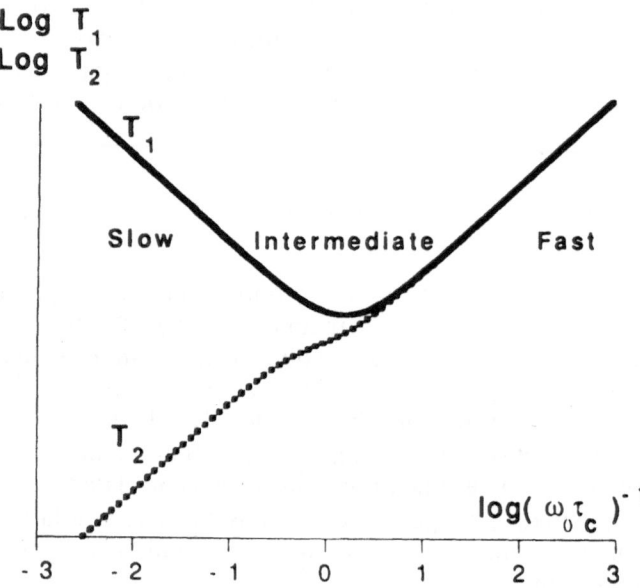

Fig. 2. *T_1 and T_2 as functions of $(\omega_0 \tau_c)^{-1}$.* Conditions of slow, intermediate, and fast motion correspond to $\omega_0 \tau_c$ being much larger than 1, about 1, or much smaller than 1, respectively

mono-exponential, one describes it by the characteristic time T_2^*:

$$\frac{1}{T_2^*} = \frac{1}{T_2} + \frac{1}{2}\,\gamma\Delta B_0. \tag{14}$$

We also know that, if the translational Brownian motion may be neglected (i.e. if the static field inhomogeneities are sufficiently small), the ideal transverse relaxation curve can be assessed, point by point, by generating spin echoes by means of 180 degree RF pulses. These pulses compensate for the loss of phase coherence due to static field inhomogeneities.

In the presence of translational Brownian motion in strong field inhomogeneities, this is no more true, as the displacement of water molecules through regions characterized by different field strengths induces irreversible loss of phase coherence among the components making up the transverse magnetization. In the next paragraphs, we will assess the effects of translational Brownian motion on the transverse relaxation.

Signal Decay of Water Protons and Translational Brownian Motion

1. Self-diffusion

We will describe the translational Brownian motion of water molecules in terms of discrete, instantaneous hops. For simplicity, we will resolve the Brownian motion in a single direction, z. We will call τ the mean time between hops and ζ the root mean square (rms) displacement, i.e. the average step length, in the z-direction. A water molecule has equal probability of hopping in either the positive or negative z-direction. Thus, the position of a particular water molecule after n hops (starting at the origin) is given by:

$$z(n\tau) = \zeta \sum_{i=1}^{n} a_i, \tag{15}$$

where a_i is a random number equal to ± 1. On the average, there is no net displacement of the water molecules (we consider the *ensemble average*, i.e. the average over the total set of water molecules considered. The ensemble average of a particular quantity p is written as $\overline{p}$):

$$\overline{z(n\tau)} = 0. \tag{16}$$

If at time t = 0 all water molecules were concentrated at z = 0, at time t = nτ they would be distributed randomly around the origin, with a mean square displacement $\overline{z^2}(n\tau)$ given by:

$$\overline{z^2(n\tau)} = n\,\zeta^2. \tag{17}$$

The *self-diffusion coefficient D* is now defined as half of the ratio between the mean square displacement per hop and the average time between hops:

$$D = \frac{\zeta^2}{2\tau}. \tag{18}$$

Thus, the mean square displacement (in the z-direction) after some time t is given by the twice the product of the self-diffusion coefficient and the time[1]:

$$\overline{z^2(n\tau)} = 2\,D\,t. \tag{19}$$

How does molecular self-diffusion affect the NMR signal of water? As stated earlier, the rotational Brownian motion predominantly affects the transverse and longitudinal relaxation behaviour of water protons. Thus, in ideal (unrealistic) conditions of perfect static field homogeneity, the translational Brownian motion (self-diffusion) of water molecules does not significantly affect the water proton signal. In realistic experimental conditions, i.e. in a static field presenting significant inhomogeneity over the sample studied, the self-diffusion of the water molecules may affect the intensity of the spin echo, as mentioned earlier. In what follows, we will consider the case of an inhomogeneous static field, and assess the effect of translational Brownian motion on the NMR signal from the water protons. We will show that not only the intensity of the spin echo, but also the free induction decay (FID) is affected by self-diffusion. For the sake of simplicity, we continue resolving the motion in the z-direction only. Also, we will consider a static magnetic field, the intensity of which varies linearly in the z-direction. In other words, the field inhomogeneities considered are due to a linear gradient G_z in the direction of the movement. This linear gradient is superimposed onto the homogeneous field B_0. We will assume that all water molecules are at the isocenter of the magnet at time t = 0 (i.e. at that particular time, they all experience the same field of intensity B_0).

2. Self-diffusion and signal decay from the protons from a particular water molecule

For a particular water molecule, the Larmor frequency after n hops (at time t = nτ) is given by:

$$\omega(n\tau) = \gamma B_0 + \delta\omega(n\tau), \tag{20}$$

where:

$$\delta\omega(n\tau) = \gamma\,G_z z(n\tau). \tag{21}$$

---

[1]Similar expressions would obviously be obtained for the mean square displacement in each of the two other orthogonal directions x and y of space. Thus, if we had taken into account the random displacements in three dimensions, we would have obtained the following expression for the mean square displacement $\overline{r^2}(n\tau)$: $\overline{r^2}(n\tau) = 6\,D\,t$. The self-diffusion coefficient D of pure water is about 3.0×10^{-3} mm²/s at room temperature.

The phase shift $\delta\Phi(n\tau)$ acquired by the transverse magnetization of the water molecule, *while* it resides in $z(n\tau)$, is:

$$\delta\Phi(n\tau) = \tau\delta\omega(n\tau). \qquad (22)$$

Thus, the total phase shift $\Delta\Phi_a(n\tau)$ *accumulated* by the transverse magnetization of the water molecule at time $t = n\tau$ is the sum of the phase shifts acquired during successive hops, from $t = 0$ until $t = n\tau$:

$$\Delta\Phi_a(n\tau) = \delta\Phi(\tau) + \delta\Phi(2\tau) + ... + \delta\Phi((n\text{-}1)\tau) + \delta\Phi(n\tau). \qquad (23)$$

Thus:

$$\Delta\Phi_a(n\tau) = \tau \sum_{m=1}^{n} \delta\omega(m\tau). \qquad (24)$$

From Eqs. 15, 21, and 24, we obtain the following expression for the phase shift accumulated by the protons from one particular water molecule after n hops:

$$\Delta\Phi_a(n\tau) = \gamma G_z \tau \zeta \sum_{m=1}^{n} \sum_{i=1}^{m} a_i. \qquad (25)$$

Thus, *for the protons from a particular water molecule*, self-diffusion results in a *phase-modulation* of the transverse magnetization. This phase modulation is given by:

$$\exp j\Delta\Phi_a(n\tau), \qquad (26)$$

where $\Delta\Phi_a(n\tau)$ is expressed in Eq. 25.

3. Self-diffusion and Signal Decay from the Protons from an Ensemble of Water Molecules

What we are considering, in practice, is not an isolated water molecule, but a large ensemble of water molecules. Thus, what we wish to assess is the ensemble average $\overline{\exp j\Delta\Phi_a(n\tau)}$ of the phase modulation obtained for one particular molecule. As $\Delta\Phi_a(n\tau)$ varies randomly over the ensemble (due to different trajectories followed by the different water molecules), and as we are dealing with an ensemble of many molecules, we may assume (central limit theorem) that the accumulated phase $\Delta\Phi_a(n\tau)$ is described by a Gaussian distribution. Taking this into account, the following relationship may be demonstrated:

$$\overline{\exp j\Delta\Phi_a(n\tau)} = \exp - \frac{1}{2}\overline{\Delta\Phi_a(n\tau)^2}. \qquad (27)$$

In other words, *the ensemble average transforms the phase modulation of the transverse magnetization from one particular molecule into an amplitude attenuation of the transverse magnetization of the ensemble of molecules*. Using Eqs. 25, 27, one may show that the attenuation of the NMR signal from a water bath is given by the following expression:

$$\exp - \frac{1}{2}\overline{\Delta\Phi_a(n\tau)^2} = \exp - \frac{1}{3}\gamma^2 G_z^2 Dt^3. \qquad (28)$$

The exponential decay with a cubic time-dependency is a characteristic feature of a diffusion phenomenon.

The above result indicates that translational Brownian motion through an inhomogeneous magnetic field induces a non-linear exponential signal decay of the water signal, which must be considered in addition to the static dephasing term and the mono-exponential decay due to rotational Brownian motion (Eq. 14).

4. Self-diffusion and Intensity of the Spin Echo from Protons from an Ensemble of Water Molecules

Signal attenuation due to static dephasing may be recovered in the spin echo, as stated earlier. Translational Brownian motion induces irreversible signal attenuation of the spin echo with a cubic dependency on the echo time T_E:

$$\exp - \frac{1}{2}\overline{\Delta\Phi_a^2(T_E)} = \exp - \frac{1}{12}\gamma^2 G_z^2 DT_E^3. \qquad (29)$$

Conclusion

This paper has dealt with the intrinsic parameters determining the MR signal from pure water. Water was considered a simplified model for biological tissue. The paper has discussed the relationships between rotational Brownian motion of the water molecules and the transverse and longitudinal relaxation times of the water protons. It has further discussed translational Brownian motion in the presence of static field inhomogeneities. The effects of self-diffusion on the MR signal decay, as well as on the intensity of the spin echo have been considered.

References

1. Slichter CP (1990) Principles of Magnetic Resonance. Springer, Berlin, Heidelberg, New York (Springer Series in Solid-State Sciences, vol. I pp. 145-215).
2. Goldman M (1992) Quantum Description of High-Resolution NMR in Liquids. Oxford Science Publications, Clarendon Press (International Series of Monographs on Chemistry, vol. 15 pp. 226-259).
3. Callaghan PT (1993) Principles of Nuclear Magnetic Resonance Microscopy. Oxford Science Publications, Clarendon Press, Oxford pp. 157-169.

Assessment of Hemodynamic Function with Phase Contrast Flow Quantitation

J.F. Debatin

Department of Medical Radiology, University Hospital Zürich, 8091 Zürich, Switzerland

Introduction

Magnetic resonance (MR) techniques can reach beyond the morphologic assessment of the cardiovascular system by allowing direct quantitative characterization of flow dynamics. Reflecting the inherent motion sensitivity of the MR imaging experiment with regard to both amplitude and phase, two different MR techniques are available for flow measurements: one is based on the influence of motion on signal amplitude, and the other on the influence of motion on signal phase. They can be combined with various gating schemes to achieve excellent temporal resolution throughout the cardiac cycle [1]. Compared to Doppler ultrasound, both techniques are less operator dependent and do not require the presence of an appropriate acoustic window.

Pioneered by Wehrli et al. [2], the amplitude technique exploits a time-of-flight effect. It is based on the application of a thin saturation band across the vessel of interest and tracking the flow induced displacement of this band. This technique, referred to as bolus tracking, requires in-plane visualization of the vessel. While it has been shown to accurately measure flow velocities in large thoracic vessels as well as in the portal venous system [3, 4], the technique is handicapped by saturation phenomena, volume averaging and insensitivity to slow flow, particularly in small vessels.

The phase technique provides velocity maps that directly determine the spatial mean velocity within each voxel across the lumen of a vessel. By analyzing the vessel of interest in cross section, the technique overcomes many of the limitations inherent to bolus tracking and Doppler ultrasound [1]. This is particularly true with regard to flow volume quantitation. Doppler ultrasound and MRI bolus-tracking sample flow parameters only in a single plane of a vessel's cross section. Quantitation of blood flow volume therefore requires the additional determination of the vessel's diameter as well as assumptions regarding the actual flow pattern within the interrogated vessel. Although the characterization and classification of the frequently complex flow dynamics seen throughout the vascular system have been subject to some controversy, there is general agreement that physiologic velocity profiles usually constitute a mixture of different classic flow profiles [5]. Modeling of in vivo flow is hence rather difficult and can potentially introduce considerable measurement error. Due to the voxel-based flow analysis inherent to MRI phase mapping, the phase contrast (PC) technique remains totally insulated from the ramifications of this discussion. Hence, accurate flow and velocity quantitation is possible throughout virtually all vascular structures with the phase-based flow mapping technique [1]. Following technical refinements in gradient and sequence design, the phase technique has thus emerged as the method of choice for flow quantitation with MRI [6].

As with any new sophisticated technique, achieving good results with PC flow mapping requires a thorough understanding of the physical principles underlying the flow measurements and careful attention to detail in the performance of the method. This chapter will focus on the physical principles of this phase-based flow quantitation technique, referred to as phase contrast (PC) flow mapping, and will define the optimal parameters for phase contrast quantitating sequences.

Principle of Phase

Each MRI raw data set produces an image that is based upon the transverse magnetization within each voxel. This transverse magnetization is a vector quantity defined by both magnitude and direction. The latter represents the phase of a particular spin. Phase contrast flow mapping exploits the fact that the precessing frequency of spins is dependent on the strength of the magnetic field. Spins moving through magnetic field gradients will therefore obtain a different precessing frequency and thus a different phase. In fact, in the presence of a magnetic field gradient, constant velocity motion produces a change in phase (ϕ) proportional to velocity (v):

$$\phi = v\,(\gamma M_1) \qquad (1)$$

where M_1 is the first moment of the gradient wave form $G(t)$ evaluated at the time of the center of the echo and γ is the constant gyromagnetic ratio.

Phase information is not merely affected by velocity, but also by many other processes such as magnetic field inhomogeneities, Eddy currents and pulse sequence tuning. Insensitivity to other sources of phase shift can be achieved by obtaining two measurements with different velocity-induced phase shifts, but with the same phase effects due to other sources. The two data sets with different first moments along one direction are acquired in an interleaved fashion. If two complete data sets are acquired, the difference in phase ($\Delta\phi$) in each voxel is:

$$\Delta\phi = v(\gamma \Delta M_1) \qquad (2)$$

where ΔM_1 is the change in first moment and v is the velocity component traveling in the direction of ΔM_1. The moment change causes spins moving in the encoded direction to acquire a phase shift proportional to velocity [1]. Since static structures exhibit no phase change, the subtraction eliminates undesired phase effects. Hence the resultant phase contrast image merely reflects motion in the direction of ΔM_1. This concept can be generalized for the measurement of flow in any direction [7, 8]. For reasons of measurement accuracy it is crucial, however, that quantitative flow measurements are performed always in the slice select direction.

Flow Quantitation

The phase contrast image depicts pixel values that are dependent only on motion in the slice select direction. By properly scaling the phase shift data, velocity images can be formed. Velocity data are expressed on a gray scale with negative values displayed as dark pixels, positive values as bright ones, and zero velocity as gray. By convention, flow from right to left, anterior to posterior, and superior to inferior is defined as positive, while flow in the opposite direction is considered negative. To suppress noise in regions of low signal, vascular images are frequently "magnitude masked" by multiplying the phase shift with the signal magnitude in each pixel [1].

PC velocity measurements (cm/s) can be used directly, much like Doppler measurements can be. For flow that is oblique to the imaging plane, the velocity values must be corrected by $\cos(\theta)$, where θ is the angle between the flow direction and the slice select direction. For through-plane flow, the flow rate (ml/s) is defined by the product of measured flow velocity (cm/s) and pixel area (cm^2).

$$\text{velocity (cm/s)} \times \text{area (cm}^2) = \text{flow rate (ml/s)} \quad (3)$$

The flow volume rate through any vessel can be obtained by summing the flow rates in all pixels within a region of interest that includes the entire vessel lumen.

Flow Sensitivity Adjustment

The strength of the flow-encoding gradient and hence the sensitivity of the PC technique to flow is controlled by ΔM_1. It can be characterized by the phase change per unit velocity and expressed as rad per cm/s. A more intuitive parameter is the velocity encoding value (VENC), defined as the velocity that produces a phase shift of π rad or 180°. Hence, VENC controls the dynamic range of velocities that can be measured.

Since phase is unique only over 360°, the phase shift computed from different phase reconstructions is forced to lie in the ± 180° range. Any actual phase shift outside this range is erroneously depicted by a multiple of 360°. A velocity of 1.1 VENC will be erroneously depicted as -0.9 VENC. This phenomenon is referred to as velocity aliasing, and must be considered analogous to spatial wrap-around artifacts in MRI. To avoid such aliasing, VENC should always be chosen to exceed the expected maximal velocity within the vessel of interest. VENC should, however, not be chosen too high, since it is inversely proportional to the signal-to-noise ratio (SNR) in phase contrast images [7]. Thus, Evans et al. [9] suggest that VENC should be chosen to exceed the maximal expected velocity by not more than 25%.

Strategies for PC-Synchronization

PC velocity data are temporal averages of instantaneous velocities. The degree of temporal averaging is determined by the length of the data acquisition window. For non-gated sequences, the latter is defined by the total imaging time. While this is sufficient for the quantitative characterization of constant flow found in much of the venous system, pulsatile arterial flow requires measurements at multiple points along the cardiac cycle. This can be achieved by combining the phase contrast technique with various forms of prospective and retrospective gating.

Cine-PC imaging combines phase-modulation with gradient echo cine-imaging. Similar to conventional cine, cine-PC employs a short repetition time and gradient-refocused echoes. Pulse repetition is independent of the electrocardiogram (ECG) signal, which is monitored and used to increment the spatial phase encoding at the beginning of each cardiac cycle retrospectively. For a single section and a single flow-encoding direction, two sequences with alternating first moments are interleaved during each cardiac cycle, yielding a two-dimensional velocity map in a vascular cross section. The temporal resolution is defined by twice the length of the repetition time.

The number of cine-PC frames which can be obtained within a cardiac cycle is inversely proportional to the length of the repetition time and the subject's heart rate. The data acquired in any one cardiac cycle can, however, be interpolated to the desired number actual of "n" frames (usually 16) regardless of the actual number of acquired phases. The total cine-PC scan time is determined by the product of desired phase encoding steps (128-256) and the length of the cardiac cycle.

To permit breathheld data acquisitions, the PC technique has recently been implemented in segmented k-space acquisitions [10, 11] as well as in ultrafast echo-planar data acquisition strategies [12]. With these techniques, between 6 and 20 quantitative data points can be obtained throughout a cardiac cycle within a comfortable breathhold.

Flow Averaging Effects

Both temporal and spatial data averaging may adversely impact PC measurement accuracy. The number of data points necessary to properly characterize a flow profile is dependent on the degree of pulsatility. Flow volume measurements without sufficient temporal resolution may contain error. These errors are unpredictable and may over- or underestimate true flow. Temporal resolution should therefore always be maximized, providing at least 16 to 20 phases for flow quantification in highly pulsatile vessels such as the aorta or superior mesenteric artery. To maximize temporal resolution, flow quantification should be limited to through-plane flow, encoded in a single direction in a single imaging location.

Spatial averaging effects are somewhat less intuitive. Intravoxel partial voluming occurs along the periphery of a vessel within voxels containing both static and flowing spins. Due to flow enhancement, the signal intensity of moving spins exceeds the signal intensity of static spins. For moving spins, the total signal intensity fraction is thus far greater than the pixel volume fraction. This results in an overestimation of true flow. The degree of error is directly proportional to the number of such peripherally located voxels relative to the total number of voxels containing flowing spins. Hence the effect increases proportionally with increases of vessel angulation, slice thickness or voxel size [1].

Another form of spatial averaging occurs in vessels subject to motion perpendicular to their flow direction [10]. This applies particularly to the quantitative analysis of intra-abdominal vessels like the portal vein and renal arteries. Motion causes blurring of the target vessel resulting in overestimation of the apparent vessel size. Around the vessel's periphery, a number of voxels contain flowing and static spins for varying degrees of time. This too causes overestimation of the flow rate, the extent of which is dependent on the degree of motion relative to the vessel size [10].

Optimal Quantitative Analysis

In order to maximize the accuracy of quantitative PC flow mapping analysis, a number of ground rules apply:

a) *Repetition time (TR)*: The shortest possible repetition time should be chosen (20-40 ms) to assure maximal temporal resolution.

b) *Echo time (TE)*: The shortest possible echo time should be chosen to minimize dephasing artifacts (5-10 ms).

c) *Flip angle*: A flip angle of 30°-45° renders good intravascular signal. Whilst preserving sufficient signal in the stationary tissue, it does not exacerbate intravoxel partial volume effects. A smaller flip angle should be chosen for ultrafast turbo gradient PC sequences.

d) *Imaging plane*: To maximize measurement accuracy and precision, vessels should be imaged perpendicular to their course. To assure an optimal PC imaging plane perpendicular to the vessel of interest, double oblique localizing strategies are imperative.

e) *Sectional thickness*: To limit partial voluming, the sectional thickness should be chosen as thin as possible, while maintaining adequate SNR. A thickness of 3-6 mm is recommended.

f) *In-plane resolution*: Field of view and matrix should be chosen to assure a minimum of 12-16 pixels within the lumen of the vessel of interest.

g) *Temporal resolution*: Temporal resolution should be maximized by only mapping through-plane flow and encoding in a single direction.

h) *Velocity encoding value (VENC)*: VENC should be chosen to exceed the maximum expected flow velocity by 25%.

i) *Frequency-encoding direction*: The frequency-encoding direction should be chosen to avoid signal contamination by pulsatility artifacts in the vessel of interest.

j) *Saturation bands*: Phase artifacts from surrounding pulsatile structures may be reduced by the placement of spatial presaturation bands. These bands should be placed carefully to avoid inadvertent saturation of inflowing spins in the vessel of interest.

k) *Data acquisition strategy*: While conventional data acquisition is sufficient for the quantitative analysis of most vessels, fast and ultrafast acquisition strategies should be chosen to quantitate flow in vessels subject to respiratory motion. To assure sufficient accuracy, these data must be acquired within a comfortable breathhold.

l) *Flow data analysis*: To reduce noise, the measurement region of interest (ROI) should be defined carefully to only include the vessel volume. These definitions should be performed separately for each frame on the magnitude images, using a threshold approach based on the maximal intravascular signal intensity. While the correct threshold value depends on a variety of factors including vessel size, velocity profile and signal intensity of the surrounding tissues, it ranges between 30% and 50% of the maximal intraluminal signal intensity for most vascular structures.

References

1. Pelc NJ, Herfkens RJ, Shimakawa A, Enzmann DR (1991) Phase contrast cine magnetic resonance imaging. Magn Reson Q 7: 229-254
2. Wehrli FW, Shimakawa A, Guliberg GT, MacFall JR (1986) Time-of-Flight MR Flow Imaging: Selective Saturation Recovery with Gradient Refocusing. Radiology 160: 781-785
3. Edelman RR, Mattle HP, Kleefield J, Silver MS (1989) Quantification of Blood Flow with Dynamic MR Imaging and Presaturation Bolus Tracking. Radiology 171: 551-556
4. Edelman RR, Zhao B, Liu C, Wentz KU, Mattle HP, Finn JP, McArdie C (1989) MR angiography and dynamic flow evaluation of the portal venous system. AJR 153: 755-760
5. Caro CG, Pediey TJ, Schroter RC, Seed WA (1978) The mechanics of the circulation. Oxford University Press, New York
6. Haacke EM, Smith AS, Lin W, Lewin JS, Finelli DA, Duerk JL (1991) Velocity Quantification In Magnetic Resonance Imaging. Topics in Magn Reson Imaging 3: 34-49
7. Pelc NJ, Bernstein M, Shimakawa A, Glover G (1991) Encoding Strategies for Three-Direction Phase Contrast MR Imaging of Flow. J Magn Reson Imaging: 405-413
8. Hausmann R, Lewin J, Laub G (1991) Phase Contrast MR Angiography with Reduced Acquisition Time: New Concepts in Sequence Design. J Magn Reson Imaging: 415-422
9. Evans AJ, Iwai F, Grist TA, et al. (1993) Magnetic resonance imaging of blood flow with a phase subtraction technique: 'in vitro' and 'in vivo' validation. Invest Radiol 28: 109-115
10. Debatin JF, Ting RH, Wegmuller H, Sommer FG, Fredrickson JO, Brosnan TJ, Bowman BS, Myers BD, Herfkens RJ, Pelc NJ (1994) Renal Artery Blood Flow: Quantitation with Phase-Contrast MR Imaging with and without Breath Holding. Radiology 190: 371-378
11. Fredrickson JO, Pelc NJ (1994) Time-resolved MR Imaging by Automatic Data Segmentation. J Magn Reson Imaging 4: 189-196
12. Debatin JF, Leung DA, Wildermuth S, Botnar R, Felblinger J, McKinnon GC (1996) Flow Quantitation with Echo Planar Phase Contrast Velocity Mapping: In Vitro and in Vivo Evaluation. J Magn Reson Imaging (in press)

Functional MRI: The Environment and Technology for Clinical Application

K.R. Thulborn[1,2], B. McCurtain[2], J. Voyvodic[1], S. Chang[1], J. Gillen[1], J.A. Sweeney[2]

MR Research Center, Departments of [1]Radiology and [2]Psychiatry, University of Pittsburgh Medical Center, Pittsburgh, PA 15213, USA

Introduction

As the applications of functional magnetic resonance imaging (fMRI) in clinical radiology become more evident, several broad requirements must be recognized. First, whereas diagnostic MRI uses visual inspection of a few dozen images in which the lesion contrast-to-noise ratio is usually high (>15%), fMRI studies use hundreds of images to detect signal changes (1-5%) well below the visual detection threshold. Second, clinically useful information must be available rapidly for efficient case management, thus requiring the enormous data load of fMRI to be reduced to interpretable form in near real time. Third, the fMRI protocol must be performed quickly and routinely by a MR technologist and nurse. Unlike structural MRI examinations in which the patient is asked merely to hold still, greater patient cooperation is required for cognitive tasks in that the paradigm requires active participation. Preparation of the subject is essential, conveniently performed away from the scanner with a scanner simulator that replicates the fMRI protocol. Such prescan preparation removes novelty effects, is inexpensive compared to scanner time and provides a measure of task performance that can be used to tailor the paradigm to the capabilities of the individual subjects. Such prescan preparation has been very useful for pediatric subjects who, in our experience, take considerable coaching for full cooperation. Acquisition of the fMRI data requires equipment that allows stimulus presentation and response monitoring without loss of scanner performance. Documentation of the timing of coincident images, stimuli and responses must be done accurately and automatically. As all fMRI data are processed off-line, automated documentation avoids delayed and inaccurate communication between technologist and data analyst and allows semi-automated processing.

The procedure and equipment used for performing fMRI studies with neuropsychological paradigms that require responses to visual stimuli during image acquisition are described and demonstrated with examples of applications in cognitive function.

Environment and Technology

1. Instrumentation and Quality Assurance

All fMRI studies were performed on a 1.5 T Signa whole body scanner (General Electric Medical Systems, Milwaukee, WI) retrofitted with echo planar imaging capabilities (Advanced NMR Systems, Inc., Wilmington, MA) and operating under Version 5.4.2 software. The superconducting magnet was passively shielded with a closely coupled shield that reduced the fringe field in the scan room. This has the advantage of allowing otherwise MR incompatible equipment in the scan room without the need for additional magnetic shielding. The magnet homogeneity was less than 2 Hz over a 22 cm diameter spherical phantom and less than 30 Hz over a human brain. The commercial head radiofrequency (RF) coil was used with head immobilization by a close-fitting pillow around the head supported by the RF coil. As most fMRI studies at this site are performed using echo planar imaging, the equipment has been customized to allow continuous acquisition of 0.5 Gbyte of image data into RAM with a total hard disk storage of 6 Gbyte. Most studies of the order of 60 min produce about 0.5 Gbyte of images that are transferred off-line for further processing as described below. Because of the rigorous performance requirements of fMRI, instrumentation quality assurance is an important daily routine. Two measures, performed daily on a standard phantom with the head RF coil are: (1) overall signal intensity stability of the system measured over 30 min using standard gradient echo, echo planar imaging (better than 1%) and (2) signal-to-noise (SNR) measurement (> 300). The absolute values are site-specific and somewhat arbitrary, but the variation in these parameters provides a valuable measure of system stability.

2. Simulator and Subject Preparation

Prior to fMRI imaging studies, subjects are trained in a simulator. The simulator was built in-house using the fiberglass patient tube used in the genuine scanner, thereby providing the same subject access (55 cm). Subject positioning is by a manually operated table mounted on ball bearings. Sounds taped during the fMRI protocol on the scanner are replicated with a high fidelity audio tape system matched in noise level to the actual scanner. Visual stimuli, where necessary, can be presented with identical equipment as described below for the scanner. As paradigms often require estimates of response times to tailor presentation timing parameters to individual subject performance, the simulator provides an inexpensive way to obtain such information prior to scanning. This allows better planning of the image acquisition strategies. The training session for most subjects is between 15 and 30 min and is directed by a trained nurse.

3. fMRI Control System

The fMRI control system, shown schematically in Fig. 1, is a Macintosh 660AV computer with a MacADIOS board (GWI, Somerville MA) containing the master

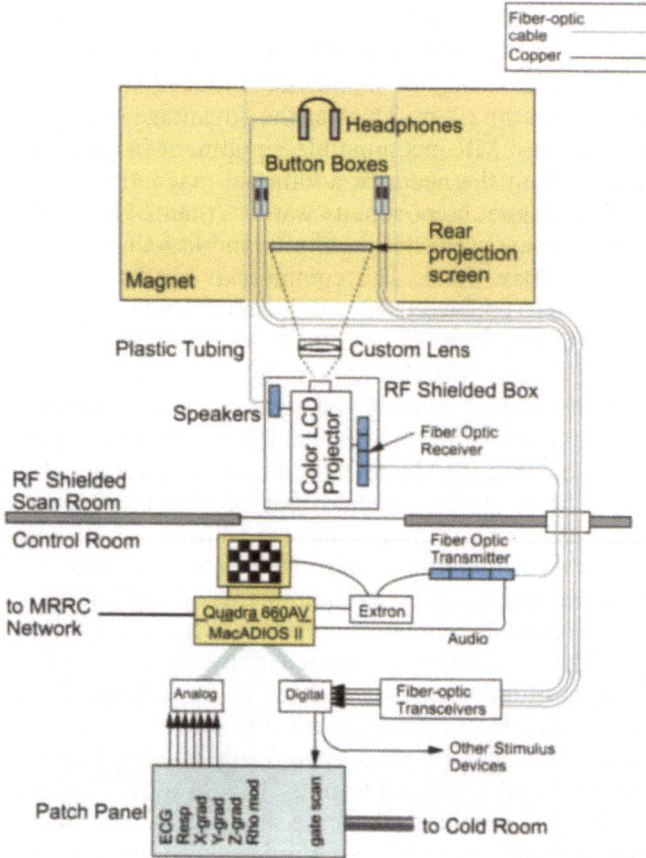

Fig. 1. *Schematic diagram of the fMRI control system.* The entire timing record of the fMRI study, including stimulus presentation, image acquisition, response time and type, and physiological parameters, is documented automatically for analysis with the images. All data transmitted into and out of the scan room are via fiber-optics thereby avoiding any degradation of SNR of the images

clock and the analog and digital inputs and outputs. The audiovisual stimuli are generated on the Macintosh 660AV. The presentation of the audiovisual stimuli is triggered in fixed temporal relationship to the image acquisition. The visual stimuli are transmitted into the shielded (acoustically, magnetically, RF) scanner room via fiber-optics to a modified LCD video projector with manufacturer's focusing lens removed and Fresnel lens replaced. This equipment is installed in an RF shielded case (MRA, Inc., Washington, PA). Light is projected through a lens (Buhl Optics, Pittsburgh, PA, 50 in. focal length) clamped to the handles of the patient table of the scanner, ensuring reproducible projection down the bore of the magnet. The vertical back-projection screen (Stewart Filmscreen Corp, Torrance, CA) is suspended by Velcro inside the bore of the magnet. Fine adjustment of the focusing of the high-resolution, 8 × 12 in. image is done by the supine subject by adjusting the screen as viewed through an angled mirror. The light intensity at the eyes of the subject is 240 lux. This configuration with the images projected into the bore allows an eye deviation of 25° across the field of view. This feature is essential for paradigms investigating eye movement control.

Sound is transmitted from the projector pneumatically (3/16" I.D. tubing) to modified ear muffs (29 dB) positioned over the subjects ears (MRA, Inc., Washington, PA) and located within the RF coil-head support assembly.

Manual responses are recorded using a finger switch which acts as a shutter in a fiber-optic circuit (MRA, Inc., Washington, PA). Electronic circuitry, located outside the scan room, transmits light into and detects light from the fiber-optic circuit. Disruption of the light path generates a TTL output pulse recorded on the digital input of the Mac ADIOS board. Four switches are available and can be operated in one or both hands as single or double units to encode different responses appropriate for a particular paradigm.

The computer produces a unique paradigm file that records the timing of scanner triggers (image timing), audiovisual transmission (stimulus timing), manual response (response timing and type) and physiological parameters of heart and respiratory rates (via fiber-optic peripheral oximetry and respiratory bellows, respectively). The timing remains accurate (≤ 0.1 ms) over acquisitions as long as 1200 images per slice (30 min). No degradation of SNR is seen in images when the fMRI control system is operational.

4. Data Management

As compared to routine clinical MRI examinations that produce about 30 MBytes of image data, fMRI produces an order of magnitude more data. It is not feasible to analyze such data on the scanner, and even the transfer of such large data sets over a 10 Mbps Ethernet local area network (LAN) to an off-line workstation is time consuming. Rapid transfer rates are achievable using a 100 rates Mbps copper distributed data interface (CDDI) based LAN. Not only is a higher transfer rate available but more importantly, the rate is maintained when the LAN is heavily loaded with other traffic. We have adapted our scanner to include the CDDI interface to allow transfer of data to a central multiprocessor computer (Silicon Graphics Challenge L, 4 CPU). The network management and archiving software has been developed in-house as has been the analysis software.

5. Data Analysis

The appropriate statistical methods for evaluating fMRI data have yet to be defined. Many variations are being used by different laboratories. The most conservative approach is the use of a simple t-test in which the voxel by voxel difference in mean signal intensity of images acquired under two paradigm conditions are tested for significance based on the signal variation in each condition. All data in this report will use this approach. It is obvious that such a test fails to use all the information available in the design of a repetitive paradigm and that other methods, such as a spectral analysis or correlation analysis, may yield a more powerful analysis. A more detailed discussion of such statistical methods goes beyond the scope of this report.

The purpose of the analysis is to detect regions of significant signal change between paradigm conditions and to localize the activation anatomically. As the functional images are acquired at high temporal but limited spatial resolution, registration of functional data over high resolution structural images is useful. Typically, functional images are acquired with gradient echo, echo planar images (acquisition matrix = 128×64; 3×3 mm in-plane resolution; 5 mm image thickness). To avoid registration errors of different geometrical distortions that may occur between echo planar and conventional spin-warp images, high-resolution structural images are acquired with spin echo, echo planar imaging (acquisition matrix = 256×128; 1.5×1.5 mm in-plane resolution; 3 mm image thickness, same plane as functional data). These images are acquired as four stacks, each stack offset by 1.5 mm, which are recombined to give a nominal isotropic resolution of 1.5 mm. Such data is treated as a three-dimensional data set that can then be viewed interactively in three orthogonal planes. Co-registration with the regions of activation allows rapid localization relative to the surface features of the brain. Co-registered data can also be displayed in planar format so that all slices can be viewed simultaneously.

6. Data Acquisition and Paradigm Development

Because the signal changes are small for fMRI, gradient echo images are the most sensitive for detecting the un-

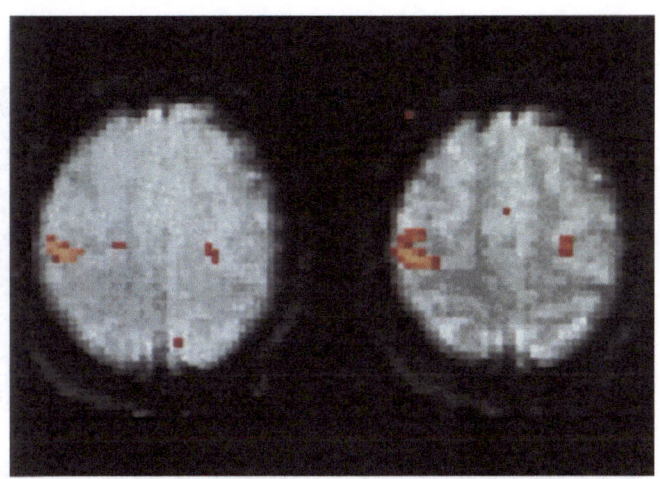

Fig. 2. *Activation maps on a representative image slice for VGS paradigm using identical acquisition scheme except for TR and the number of slices. Left acquisition performed over 7 slices at* TR = 1.5 s, *performed with the same number of images/slice as in 14 slice acquisition and Right acquisition performed over 14 slices at* TR = 3 s. *The activation maps use the same t-statistic threshold*

derlying magnetic susceptibility effects. The echo time (TE) is matched to T2* (50 ms at 1.5 T) to optimize this detection sensitivity. Although echo planar imaging allows rapid imaging, T1 saturation effects within and between slices impose a limit as to how often an image of a particular slice can be acquired without loss of SNR. Hence echo planar imaging allows images to be acquired over a large volume of the brain. The duty cycle of the scanner determines the repetition time (TR) for the coverage required. Typically, the cerebral hemispheres can be covered with 14 slices of 5 mm thickness with 1 mm gap using a TR of 3 s. If more intense signal averaging is desired with less coverage, 7 slices can be obtained every 1.5 s. The comparison between these two approaches is demonstrated in Fig. 2 for a visually-guided saccade (VGS) paradigm described below. The volume of activation in the frontal eye fields bilaterally, determined at the same t-statistic threshold for the same number of images per slice, is clearly larger for the longer TR which allowed coverage of the entire cerebral hemispheres. Hence, whole brain imaging is not only desirable for examining broadly distributed neuronal pathways but also for obtaining optimal SNR.

A balance must be reached in that signal averaging improves statistical reliability but extended imaging increases the problem of subject motion. Also task performance for cognitive paradigms can change during extended imaging as attention levels change. Experience suggests that paradigms around 10 min are suitable for highly motivated subjects but may be excessive for many patients with cognitive dysfunction. This clinical concern remains an area for further investigation. Head motion must be less than voxel dimensions and generally is below 0.5 mm.

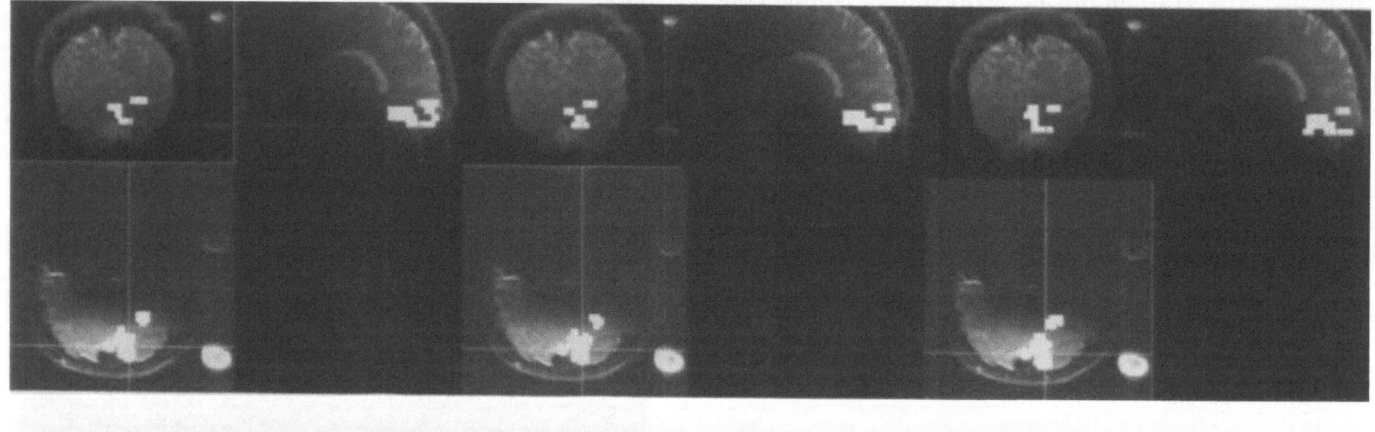

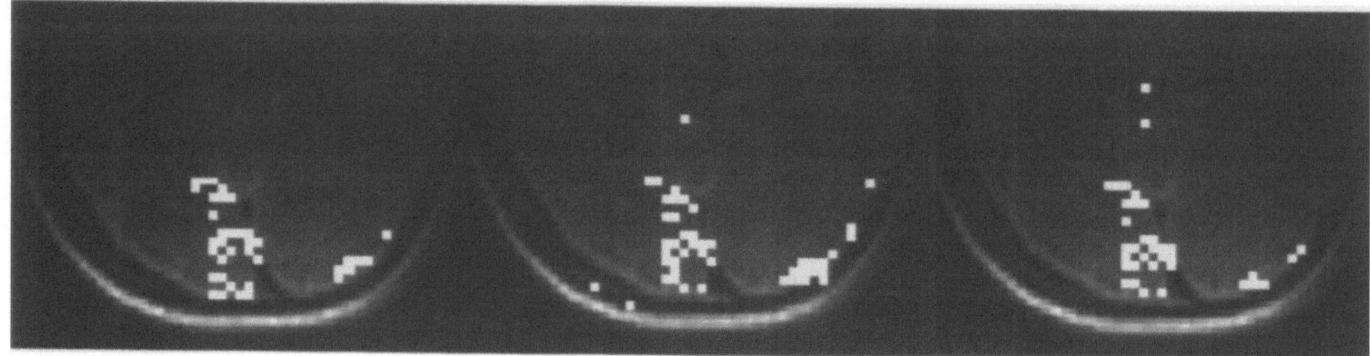

Fig. 3. *Activation maps for photic stimulation on a single individual.* Images are presented as three orthogonal views (*top*) and at higher magnification in a selected axial plane (*bottom*) for three different trials . The small round high signal outside the brain on the axial images is a reference sample. Imaging was performed using gradient echo, echo planar imaging (occipital RF surface coil, TE = 50 ms, TR = 1000 ms, 5 mm thickness, 1 mm gap, 128 × 64 acquisition matrix, 4 axial slices, 630 images/slice acquired over 10.5 min)

Another aspect of fMRI is the test-retest reliability of the method. This is demonstrated in Fig. 3 using a photic stimulation paradigm. The visual paradigm was an alternating hemifield, flashing checkerboard stimulus (8 Hz) in which central fixation without checkerboard (50 s) was subtracted from central fixation with flashing hemifield checkerboard (left or right, 30 s) over 5 cycles of alternation. This was done three times with 10 min rest between trials. These trials used the same experimental setup without moving the subject thereby reducing variability due to subject position. This was repeated in three separate sessions. Such data incorporated both instrumental and biological changes across sessions. With adequate quality assurance, the activation maps are robust as shown in Fig. 3. The distribution of voxels is highly reproducible on a voxel by voxel basis when care is taken to sample the target regions in exactly the same way by appropriate choice of head positioning and imaging plane. Changes in signal intensity as used to detect activation also appear to be reproducible.

7. Paradigm Development

For clinical applications, mapping of brain function in the vicinity of known lesions may prove fruitful for surgical planning and radiation planning. In psychiatric dis-

ease, a specific anatomic lesion is often not present. Although it may be possible to develop specific paradigms that probe each region of the brain, another approach is to use a paradigm that activates a widely distributed neuronal pathway. This would be a global probe to look for disruption of that pathway, possibly localizing a region of dysfunction. A paradigm that can be used for each of these approaches is the eye movement control pathway, being a widely distributed pathway well documented in non-human primates.

The eye movement control paradigm has several variations. The visually-guided saccade (VGS) paradigm is a broadly distributed probe. VGS consists of a comparison between images during a period of central visual fixation (condition 1) and images acquired during a period of saccadic eye movement to follow a target appearing in an unpredictable way at random locations along the horizontal meridian (condition 2). The two conditions, each of 30 s duration, are alternated for 6 cycles. An example of the activation maps that are derived from such a study is shown in Fig. 4. As a more specific probe of dorsolateral prefrontal cortex, believed to be involved in spatial working memory, a memory-guided saccade (MGS) paradigm can be used. MGS consists of a comparison between images obtained during a period of VGS (condition 1) and images acquired during a period

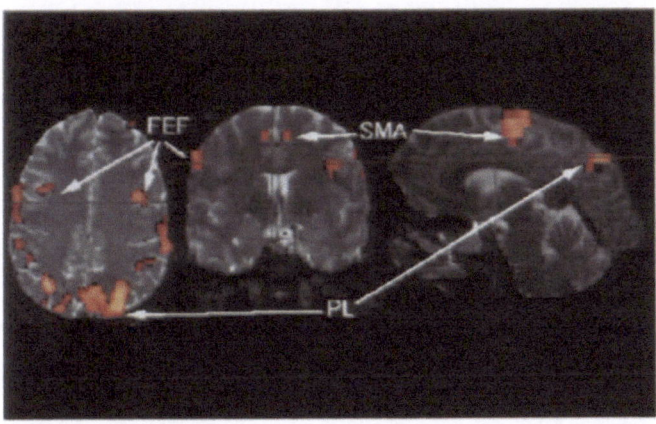

Fig. 4. *Activation maps for visually guided saccades (VGS) in a volunteer, presented in axial, coronal and sagittal planes, respectively.* The low spatial resolution activation voxels are painted over the high resolution structural echo planar images as described in Data Analysis. Regions of activation shown are in the frontal eye fields (FEF), supplementary motor area (SMA), and parietal lobes (PL)

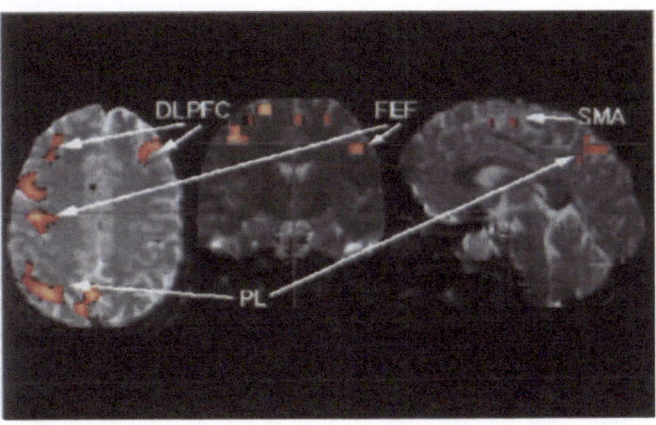

Fig. 5. *Activation maps for memory guided saccades (MGS) in a volunteer, presented in axial, coronal and sagittal planes, respectively.* The low spatial resolution activation voxels are painted over the high resolution structural echo planar images as described in Data Analysis. In addition to the regions of activation in Fig. 4, dorsolateral prefrontal cortex (DLPFC) is activated and appears to be involved in spatial working memory

in which central fixation is maintained while a light flashes briefly (100 ms) at a random peripheral location that the subject is instructed to remember. When the central fixation point disappears at a specified time after the peripheral flash, the subject looks towards the remembered location of the flash (condition 2). The result of such a MGS study is shown in Fig. 5. The task can be repeated at different delay times to increase the difficulty of the task. The degree of difficulty of such eye movement tasks can be tailored to subject performance. Considerable behavioral information is already available from neuropsychological testing in patient studies of a wide range of dysfunctional states, making it an appropriate starting point for fMRI.

Conclusions

Both the hardware and software components of the technology which allows a fMRI protocol to be performed

routinely by a MR technologist have been described. As subject cooperation beyond that expected in a routine MRI examination is required, the simulator allows the nurse to prepare the subject in a timely fashion for the fMRI study. The fMRI control system ensures that a complete summary of the study is automatically prepared for subsequent data analysis. The accurate timing available allows stimulus-gated imaging to be performed. Judicious choice of paradigms and imaging conditions allows widely distributed regions of the brain to be assessed in little time. Within this environment, we are able to produce activation maps within minutes of acquisition. These considerations provide the basis for routine implementation of fMRI studies for clinical service.

Acknowledgments

The authors acknowledge support from General Electric Medical Systems and Advanced NMR Systems, Inc.

NEUROFUNCTIONAL MRI:
TECHNIQUES

Diffusion, Perfusion and Functional MRI

D. Le Bihan

Service Hospitalier Frédéric Joliot, Département de Recherche Médicale, Commissariat à l'Energie Atomique,
4, Place du Général Leclerc, 91401 Orsay cedex, France

Introduction

Recent developments in the use of magnetic resonance (MR) imaging to measure and image molecular diffusion and blood microcirculation (perfusion) hold significant promise in the evaluation of anatomic and functional disorders of the brain. Although diffusion and perfusion are often conceptually mixed, they actually refer to different phenomena. Molecular diffusion is the result of the thermal, so-called Brownian, spontaneous random translational motion that involves all molecules. Perfusion, in contrast, relates to blood delivery to the tissues.

Noninvasive imaging of perfusion is recognized to have widespread applications in tissue characterization, treatment monitoring, and function studies. Perfusion imaging is currently performed with non-MR imaging methods such as contrast agent-enhanced computed tomography (which depicts blood distribution in tissues but is also sensitive to nonspecific blood-brain barrier disruption), conventional angiography and positron emission tomography (PET) with radioisotopes. All these methods provide accurate blood flow measurements. Yet one would like to employ an inexpensive, safe, reliable, and accurate technique that provides perfusion images with high spatial and temporal resolution. MR imaging might be such a technique, and important research efforts are dedicated to this field.

Diffusion imaging, in contrast, is a completely new field. For the first time, it has been possible to noninvasively measure and depict molecular diffusion coefficients in vivo with MR imaging. Studying molecular displacements over distances comparable to cell dimensions may provide information about the geometry and spatial organization of the tissue compartments and about water exchange between these compartments in normal or disease states. Although the information provided by diffusion measurements needs further assessment, several reports have shown that diffusion MR imaging could quickly become a powerful tool for both diagnostic and therapeutic imaging. The early diagnosis and treatment of stroke, the assessment of white matter diseases, and the monitoring of tissue temperature changes during hyperthermia or laser surgery are medical research areas likely to benefit.

Magnetic resonance imaging (MRI) has been for the last ten years the method of choice to visualize brain *structural anatomy* in vivo and in a completely noninvasive manner. MRI is now also becoming an important technique for the visualization of *brain function*. MRI may be one of the best tools available to study mental and cognitive processes underlying the function of the human brain. Ultimately such studies may help to prevent or stop brain disorders and aging.

Diffusion MR Imaging

The principles of diffusion MR imaging have been outlined elsewhere [1]. Diffusion imaging of water is based on the natural sensitivity of MR signals to motion. In presence of a magnetic field gradient, protons carried by moving water molecules undergo a phase shift of their transverse magnetization. Because diffusion is characterized by the random nature of the molecular displacements, these phase shifts are widely dispersed, interfere with each other and finally attenuate the MR signal amplitude. This attenuation depends directly on the amplitude of the molecular displacements (related to the diffusion coefficient) and on the intensity and duration of the magnetic field gradient.

Diffusion effects are small and usually invisible on conventional images. In practice, diffusion-weighted images are obtained by incorporating strong magnetic field gradient pulses into an imaging pulse sequence. The degree of diffusion weighting is set by the gradient pulse strength and duration (integrated into the so called gradient factor, b) as the degree of T2-weighting in a spin-echo sequence is set by the echo time, TE. In a diffusion-weighted image, structures with fast (high) diffusion are dark because they are subject to greater signal attenuation, whereas structures with slow (low) diffusion are bright. Calculated (quantitative) diffusion images may also be generated from a series of diffusion-weighted images. In these images, diffusion alone is responsible for the contrast, not T1 nor T2. Usually, contrast is such that structures with a fast diffusion are bright, whereas those with a slow diffusion are dark. Calculated diffusion images require important post-processing and generally have a noisier appearance than diffusion-weighted images, which may, therefore, be preferred for clinical use. Only calculated images, however, provide the quantitative information necessary to validate new results and are independent of T1 or T2 contamination. Moreover, because other kinds of intravoxel incoherent motion (IVIM) such as capillary perfusion may produce effects similar to those of true diffusion, it has been suggested that the term *apparent diffusion coefficient* (ADC) be used to quantitatively describe the results of diffusion imaging experiments in vivo.

The clinical use of diffusion MR imaging has been limited by its high sensitivity to motion artifacts and by hardware limitations on conventional MR scanners. Recently, there have been technical improvements such as shielded gradient coils which reduce eddy currents generated by the switching of the diffusion-sensitizing gradient pulses, and small dedicated low-inductance coils which allow large gradient amplitudes to be switched rapidly. These coils also enable implementation of echo planar imaging (EPI). This single-shot technique directly benefits diffusion imaging because it greatly reduces the possibiliy of motion artifacts and increases the accuracy of the measured diffusion coefficient by allowing many differently sensitized diffusion images to be obtained within short time intervals. This technique is thus compatible with a clinical protocol.

Diffusion Imaging in Normal Brain

The diffusion coefficient of water in the normal brain does not vary much among subjects if measurements are made with great care [2]. However, when compared to that of pure water, the diffusion coefficient of water in tissues is 2 to 10 times less. This difference is understandable given that water molecules are obliged to move tortuously around obstructions presented by fibers, intracellular organelles, or macromolecules. In addition, there is a continual exchange between free water molecules and water molecules which associate with more slowly moving macromolecules. Diffusion in thus more likely to be hindered by random obstacles than be strictly restricted by the closed spaces of tissue microcompartments.

Diffusion of water in cerebrospinal fluid (CSF) is similar to that of pure water at the same temperature (2.95×10^{-3} mm^2/s at 37.5°C). Sometimes ADC may be surprisingly larger (3×10^{-3} to 6×10^{-3} mm^2/s), which seems physically nonsensical for diffusion but is perfectly understandable considering that the CSF flows incoherently in some locations. The distribution of CSF velocities

in a voxel, for instance in the foramina of Monro or in the fourth ventricle, will produce a signal attenuation (flow-void effect) similar to that of diffusion but larger. This finding has been used to map and evaluate CSF flow, especially when CSF pathways are obstructed by tumors or mass effect (e.g., obstructive hydrocephalus).

In gray matter, diffusion is isotropic and roughly 2.5 times lower than in pure water at the same temperature. In white matter, diffusion is extremely variable. The value of the diffusion coefficient depends directly on the relative orientation of the fibers and the magnetic field gradients. This phenomenon is known as anisotropic diffusion. Diffusion coefficients appear to be significantly decreased when the myelin fiber tracts are perpendicular to the direction of the magnetic field gradient used to measure molecular displacements. Color coded maps of the myelin fiber orientation can be generated on the basis of diffusion anisotropy.

A simple way to explain this anisotropy is to consider that water molecules are enclosed in the axonal spaces and that water diffusion outside the axons is prevented by the myelin sheath. When diffusion measurements are made parallel to the direction of the fibers, diffusion is not restricted, resulting in higher measured diffusion coefficients. The situation is more complex, however, because it has been shown that the myelin sheath is somewhat permeable to water. Such diffusion studies could thus provide estimates of the permeability of myelin to water. The measurement of anisotropic diffusion in white matter offers exciting potential applications. Mapping myelin fiber orientation may be useful in understanding white matter diseases such as multiple sclerosis, Wallerian degeneration or delayed white matter myelination in neonates. The coupling between the degree of diffusion anisotropy and the degree of white matter myelination during central nervous system maturation makes it likely that diffusion ansiotropy in white matter is related to the myelin sheath.

Diffusion Imaging in Brain Ischemia

1. Subacute and Chronic Ischemia

In subacute ischemia, when conventional MR images appear abnormal (showing an increase in T2), the diffusion coefficient in white matter increases about two- or threefold above its normal value. This increase is probably due to the presence of vasogenic edema, in which bulk water motion in the extracellular space is an important phenomenon. Earlier work showed that edema could be easily recognized on diffusion images. Typically, vasogenic edema is visible as a large homogeneous area with an increased diffusion coefficient. In some instances of chronic ischemia, abnormalities in brain parenchyma (low diffusion) have been seen on diffusion images, although conventional T1- or T2-weighted images appeared normal [3]. Diffusion may also help detect encephalomalacic cysts, which have diffusion coefficients similar to that of pure water.

2. Acute Ischemia

The most promising application of diffusion imaging in stroke has been suggested by the finding that it can detect brain ischemia at an early stage. Recently, MR diffusion imaging in a cat brain model showed that the diffusion coefficient of water after an ischemic injury decreased significantly within minutes, a time when all other imaging techniques, including conventional MR, did not show any change [3]. The decrease in diffusion developed progressively within the first hour. The mechanism of this decrease in water mobility is still unclear. It is unlikely that it is related to nondiffusion phenomena, such as a decrease in bulk tissue pulsatility caused by microcirculatory arrest. It is also difficult to explain on the basis of a decrease in temperature. A 30% decrease in the diffusion coefficient would imply a temperature decrease of about 10°C, which is unrealistic. This decrease in diffusion more likely reflects a modification of the water balance or transport between tissue compartments, such as intra- and extracellular spaces. It is known that ischemia is responsible for the massive entry of ions and accompanying water into the intracellular space, accompanied by an increase in osmolarity. The cell swelling that results is responsible for an increased tortuosity in the extracellular space. A modern, but still debated, theory of cytotoxic edema is that calcium channels open because of the excitation of N-methyl-D-aspartate receptors by the release and accumulation of neurotoxic dicarboxylic amino acids, such as glutamate, in the extracellular spaces. Cytologic changes in terms of microvacuolation are visible as early as 20 min after complete ischemia. This process results in the cellular release of potassium ions and the massive entry of sodium ions which quickly overtake the capacity of transmembrane ion pumps. An interesting finding in favor of this mechanism is that calcium channel blockers prevent or lessen the decrease in diffusion. Furthermore, artificially induced cytotoxic edema in animals also produces a decrease in the diffusion coefficient. Diffusion imaging could also reflect the intracellular active transport mechanisms that cease operating when energy metabolites are no longer available.

Diffusion imaging thus offers the unique opportunity to address, noninvasively and in a clinical setting, fundamental issues about the response of brain tissue to different stages of ischemia; this may not be possible with other techniques, including conventional MR and MR spectroscopy [4]. Detection of stroke at an early stage when tissue damage is still reversible may justify more aggressive and controversial reperfusion or other therapies designed to protect CNS tissues. It will be of extreme interest to find out if diffusion can be used as a reliable marker of the extent and potential reversibility of tissue damage.

Perfusion MR Imaging

Several proposed techniques to measure perfusion follow basic nuclear medicine principles and use radioactive diffusible tracers. By introducing a tracer into the circulation and monitoring its concentration in a tissue over time, one can determine the rate of delivery of the tracer and, hence, blood flow to this tissue. In MR imaging tracers no longer need to be radioactive. MR tracers comprise molecules containing nonproton MR-sensitive nuclei such as ^{19}F, ^{2}H in the form of deuterium oxide, and ^{17}O used as oxygen gas or as $H_2^{17}O$. None of these techniques has been used clinically because of safety concerns or because of low signal-to-noise ratios. A potentially great improvement is expected from the use of hyperpolarized gases, such as xenon or helium. The use of intrinsic tracers has also been suggested, and an extensive review has been published.

The most clinically relevant method to date is based on magnetic susceptibility-enhanced imaging, using a paramagnetic agent such as gadopentetate dimeglumine (Gd-DTPA) injected as an intravenous bolus. When the bolus reaches the brain capillaries it induces a difference in magnetic susceptibility between the blood compartment and the brain tissue, where the contrast agent does not penetrate because of the blood-brain barrier. This susceptibility difference is responsible for internal magnetic field gradients between capillaries and tissues. Diffusion of water through these internal gradients produces a signal attenuation. Diffusion of bulk water in the tissue is not a concern because only the water molecules in the vicinity of the capillaries are involved. Furthermore, the presence of the effect outside the capillaries results in an amplification, so that this method has a high sensitivity. Ultrafast imaging techniques such as EPI or a turbo-fast low-angle shot sequence can monitor the first passage of contrast agent through the brain tissue; this period lasts a few seconds. Quantifying blood flow remains difficult partly because the relationship between the signal drop and the tissue concentration of Gd-DTPA is known only empirically and may be tissue dependent. Calculating actual blood flow also requires knowledge of the time course of the contrast agent's arterial concentration (input function); this concentration is still difficult to determine, especially with a high temporal resolution. Another consideration is the permeability of the blood-brain barrier and the leakage of Gd-DTPA into the tissue, especially in brain tumors. This leakage decreases the concentration gradient through the capillary wall and leads to underestimates of blood volume and perfusion. Nevertheless, promising clinical results have been reported, after restrictive assumptions were made, in terms of relative blood volume and blood-brain barrier permeability maps.

Brain function studies have been carried out, until recently, using techniques which record brain electrical activity (electroencephalography or EEG), or which measure magnetic fields produced by neurons (magnetoencephalography or MEG). In addition, brain function can be measured using tomographic methods such as single photon emission tomography (SPECT) and positron emission tomography (PET) which employ radioactive nuclides. The 'electrical' techniques have excellent time resolution (typically 1 ms), but lack spatial resolution if electrodes are placed on the scalp. Imaging methods based on radioactive tracers are slow, are limited in spatial resolution, and result in subject irradiation, precluding repetitive studies. MRI already appears as a complementary approach with broad advantages. MRI does not use ionizing radiation and is completely noninvasive. Spatial resolution is high (typically better than 1 mm) and images may be obtained in any orientation at any level over the whole brain. Temporal resolution may be in the subsecond range with new ultra-fast acquisition schemes. MRI installations do not require extensive chemistry laboratories and are becoming available to most neurological patients.

MRI, as well as neuroimaging techniques such as SPECT and PET, is sensitive to changes in metabolism (glucose and oxygen utilization) and hemodynamics (perfusion). The monitoring of brain activity with these techniques is possible because of the tight coupling between neuronal activity and regional blood flow (hemodynamics).

The first successful attempt to investigate brain activity with MRI was made by the group of Belliveau et al. [5] using a perfusion method based on a bolus injection of the paramagnetic contrast agent gadolinium-DTPA. The transit of this bolus through the brain microvasculature resulted in a transient signal decrease due to a magnetic susceptibility difference between capillaries containing the agent and the surrounding tissues. From the signal time course, the relative blood volume in each voxel of the image was approximated. The contrast agent had to be injected twice: the first time when the subject was resting; the second time when performing a task. Because blood volume increases in activated cortical areas, a comparison of the two relative blood volume maps reveals which areas of the brain have been activated. This method has been succesfully used to show activation of the human primary visual cortex during visual stimulation by external flashing light. A clear drawback of this technique is that one has to inject contrast agent for each task, so that repetitive studies on a single subject are precluded. Furthermore, calculation of blood volume maps requires somewhat extensive modeling.

The most common approach for studying brain activation so far has been using Blood Oxygen Level Dependent (BOLD) contrast [6-8]. This technique, which is sensitive to both changes in metabolism and hemodynamics induced by brain activation, requires no external contrast agent and is relatively easy to implement. Deoxyhemoglobin is paramagnetic due to the presence of four unpaired electrons (oxyhemoglobin is diamagnetic). Deoxyhemoglobin in red cells behaves as a natural, endogenous paramagnetic contrast agent present in the blood stream at high concentration and modulated by variations in oxygen supply (blood flow) and oxygen utilization (tissue metabolism). During brain activation, tissue oxygen consumption increases only slightly, while blood volume and blood flow increase by up to 50%. One thus expects a sharp increase in oxygen supply to the tissue and a decrease in deoxyhemoglobin content which lead to an increased signal intensity.

One should keep in mind that this hemodynamic response is delayed with respect to the neuronal response, so that deoxyhemoglobin contrast only indirectly reflects neuronal activity. Although quantification of blood flow or oxygen consumption remains out of reach at this stage, this technique is very sensitive and allows mapping of activated areas of the brain in real time.

Monitoring deoxyhemoglobin contrast for brain activation studies has been performed at 1.5 T [6-8] and on experimental systems at high field (4 T) [9, 10]. Echo planar imaging [6, 8, 10], as well as conventional fast gradient echo sequences [9-11], has been used. As deoxyhemoglobin is permanently present in the blood stream, studies may be performed by acquiring images continuously using ultra-fast imaging schemes while subjects are performing tasks. A typical paradigm is to alternate periods of rest and stimulation. Signal intensity in cortical areas activated by the stimulus thus presents easily recognizable step pattern. The relative amplitude of the signal change remains low (typically 3% to 7% at 1.5 T and up to 25% at 4 T) [10] and stable hardware, as well as good patient head immobilization, is required to visualize the effect. Surface coils may be used to increase the signal-to-noise ratio. As changes in MR signal intensity related to changes in blood flow during brain activation are small, measurements depend on algorithms that allow one to distinguish the patterns of MR signal intensity during the mental task from the resting or control pattern, with statistical significance.

Applications of Functional MRI

The unmatched combined spatial and temporal resolution of functional MRI (fMRI) and the possibility to conduct totally noninvasive studies on an individual basis, without the need for intersubject averaging should reveal new aspects of the working brain which were hidden until now. Initial MRI studies have demonstrated activation in the primary cortices (visual, sensorimotor and auditory). More refined studies have shown that MR signal changes in these cortices were correlated with the rate of stimulation (or task performance), suggesting that MR signal changes are actually related to some underlying neuronal activity. Of greater interest to neuroscientists is the demonstration that fMRI detects activation during higher-order cognitive processes such as language tasks (word generation or listening), motor learning and motor ideation, or visual mental imagery [12]. Besides exploration of the normal brain, there are at least four potential clinical applications of fMRI: presurgical mapping, imaging of epileptic foci, monitoring recovery after stroke or head trauma, and following treatments using neuropharmacological agents. Presurgical mapping of the brain may identify tissue to be removed or spared during surgery, as for brain tumors [13]. For epilepsy, fMRI could also be used for presurgical mapping, for instance in intractable complex partial seizures if language is to be spared during lobectomy. Currently, hemispheric language dominance is determined from invasive and risky tests such as the Wada test, based on intracarotid amobarbital injection, and electrical cortical recording through electrodes positioned intraoperatively. It is becoming clear that fMRI language studies have the potential to replace such invasive tests [14]. On the other hand, fMRI could also be used to visualize epileptic foci with or even without associated clinical seizure. The use of fMRI for monitoring functional recovery after stroke or head trauma appears especially important for patients with hemiplegia or aphasia. Studies may be repeated at will on individuals during the recovery period without concerns about irradiation. Regarding neuropharmacological agents, PET still remains the gold standard in terms of receptor binding imaging. MRI does not have the necessary sensitivity to directly detect such small amount of molecules. However, fMRI could be used to visualize regions of the brain where receptors have been activated or inhibited through effects on blood flow and blood oxygenation, as we recently suggested in the monkey brain using neurochemical activation by arecoline [15]. Also, the modulation by such drugs of the brain response to specific stimuli or cognitive tasks could be evaluated.

Brain activation can be detected non-invasively with unmatched spatial/temporal resolution using deoxyhemoglobin contrast MRI. There are, of course, some limitations. First, as with conventional MRI, patients with pacemakers and magnetic implants must be excluded. Patient cooperation is also particularly necessary: not only is their direct participation required for the activation tasks, but also they are required to maintain absolute immobility during scanning to avoid misregistration artifacts. Another important issue relates to the accuracy of the localization of the activated regions. It has been argued that since brain activation is sometimes seen in large vessels (arteries through inflow effects or veins containing deoxygenated blood), the actual site of activation could be distant from that visualized.

It remains that MRI brain activation studies have tremendous potential to answer important questions re-

garding the functional organization of the brain. Recent studies show that MRI, in addition to being an exquisite anatomical study tool, is a powerful functional tool for clinicians to understand, detect and manage functional disorders of the brain.

References

1. Le Bihan D (1991) Molecular diffusion nuclear magnetic resonance imaging. Magn Reson Q, 7:1-30
2. Le Bihan D, Turner R, Douek P, Patronas NJ (1992) Diffusion MR Imaging: Clinical Applications. AJR, 159:591-599
3. Moseley ME, Kucharczyk J, Mintorovitch J, Cohen Y, Kurhanewicz J, Derugin N, Asgari H, Norman D (1990) Diffusion-weighted MR imaging of acute stroke: correlation with T2-weighted and magnetic susceptibility-enhanced MR imaging in cats. AJNR, 11:423-429
4. Warach S, Chien D, Li W, Ronthal M, Edelman RR (1992) Fast magnetic resonance diffusion-weighted imaging of acute human stroke. Neurology, 42:1717-1723
5. Belliveau JW, Kennedy DN, McKinstry RC, Burchbinder BR, Weisskoff RM, Cohen MS, Vevea JM, Brady, Rosen BR, Buchbinder BR (1991) Functional mapping of the human visual cortex by magnetic resonance imaging. Science, 254:716-719
6. Kwong KK, Belliveau JW, Chesler DA (1992) Dynamic magnetic resonance imaging of human brain activity during primary sensory stimulation. Proc Natl Acad Sci, USA, 89:5675-5679
7. Edelman RR, Siewert B, Darby DG, Thangaraj V, Nobre AC, Mesulam MM, Warach S (1994) Qualitative Mapping of Cerebral Blood Flow and Functional Localization with Echo-planar MR Imaging and signal Targeting with Alternating Radio Frequency. Radiology, 192:513-520
8. Bandettini PA, Wong EC, Hinks RS, Tikofski RS, Hyde JS (1992) Time Course EPI of Human brain Function during Task Activation. Magn Reson Med, 25:390-397
9. Ogawa S, Tank DW, Menon RS, Ellerman JM, Kim SG, Merkle H, Ugurbil K (1992) Intrinsic signal changes accompanying sensory stimulation brain mapping with magnetic resonance imaging. Proc Natl Acad Sci, USA, 89:5951-5955
10. Turner R, Jezzard P, Wen H (1993) Functional mapping on the human visual cortex at 4 tesla and 1.5 tesla using deoxygenation contrast EPI. Magn Reson Med, 29:277-279
11. Frahm J, Bruhn H, Merboldt KD, Hanicke W (1992) Dynamic MR imaging of human brain oxygenation during rest and photic stimulation. J Magn Reson Imaging, 5:501-506
12. Le Bihan D, Turner R, Zeffiro A, Cuenod CA, Jezzard P, Bonnerot (1993) Activation of human primary visual cortex during visual recall: A magnetic resonance imaging study. Proc Natl Acad Sci USA, 90:11802-11805
13. Jack CR, Thompson RM, Butts RK, Sharbrough FW, Kelly PJ, Hanson DP, Riederer SJ, Ehman RL, Hangiandreou NJ, Cascino GD (1994) Sensory motor cortex: correlation of presurgical mapping with functional imaging and invasive cortical mapping. Radiology, 190:85-92
14. Hertz-Pannier L, Gaillard WD, Motts, Cuenod CA, Bookheimer S, Weinstein S, Conry J, Theodore WH, Le Bihan D (1994) Preoperative assessment of language localization by fMRI in children with complex partial seizures: A preliminary study. Book of abstracts, Metting of the SMR, p 236
15. Cuenod CA, Chang MCJ, Arai T, Pannier L, Posse S, Despres D, Frank JA, Rapoport S, Le Bihan D (1993) Local brain response to cholinergic receptor stimulation detected by MRI. Book of abstracts, Meeting of the SMRM, p 1387

Tumor Viability Assessed by Cerebral Blood Volume Measurements

P. Turski[1], B. Mock[2], E. Baker[2], S. Terae[3], M. Bahn[4]

[1] Department of Radiology E3/311, and [2] Department of Medical Physics, University of Wisconsin Medical School, Madison, WI, USA,
[3] Hokkaido University School of Medicine, Sapporo, Japan [4] Mallinckrodt Institute of Radiology, St. Louis, MO, USA

Introduction

A common clinical problem in neuroradiology is the differentiation of recurrent malignant glioma from radiation necrosis. Frequently, patients present one to two years after surgery and radiation therapy with large intracranial lesions. The lesions enhance with intravenous contrast material and have associated vasogenic edema. It is virtually impossible to distinguish recurrent tumor from radiation necrosis based solely on the imaging characteristics. Previous studies using positron emission tomography (PET) and fluorodeoxyglucose (FDG) have been successful in differentiating these entities based on variations in metabolic activity [1-3].

Subsequent PET studies using oxygen-15 revealed that there was a relative uncoupling of oxygen consumption and blood flow in malignant gliomas. The regional fractional extraction of oxygen was decreased, but a major portion of the tumors had sufficient blood supply to meet oxygen metabolic demand. A reduction in blood flow was observed in regions of vasogenic edema [4].

Recent investigations using the susceptibility properties of a series of lanthanide chelates have opened a new avenue of investigation regarding tumor blood flow and tumor viability. Investigations performed by Rosen et al. [5] revealed that the concentration of a contrast agent (in the setting of rapid passage through the microcirculatory bed) can be used to calculate cerebral blood volume. Subsequent investigations by Rosen et al. [6] outlined the techniques for determining regional cerebral blood volume (rCBV). These results were based on the application of tracer kinetics to the concentration time data obtained from bolus injections of lanthanide chelates followed by rapid T2-weighted echo planar magnetic resonance (MR) imaging. The ability to generate regional cerebral blood volume maps has been used to determine tumor vascularity [7] and glioma tumor grade [8]. In these investigations, relative cerebral blood volume maps were able to stratify high-grade gliomas from lower-grade gliomas.

The maximum cerebral blood volume was associated with increasing mitotic activity and vascularity, but did not correlate with cellular atypia, endothelial proliferation or cellularity.

In this investigation, relative cerebral blood volume, maps were obtained using dysprosium DTPA (Sprodiamide) and gadodiamide (OmniScan). The rCBV maps were compared to deoxyglucose PET scans to determine the feasibility of using rCBV mapping for differentiating viable tumor from radiation necrosis.

Methods

Under an approved protocol from the University of Wisconsin Human Subjects committee, 19 patients were selected from the neuro-oncology clinic who presented with computed tomography (CT) and MR scans suggestive of recurrent malignant glioma or radiation necrosis. The patients underwent a series of diagnostic examinations including clinical history and physical examination, clinical laboratory studies, MR imaging without and with contrast, and susceptibility dynamic imaging using dysprosium DTPA. Following the dysprosium scans, additional rCBV maps were obtained in 10 of the patients using gadodiamide.

Cerebral blood volume maps were generated from a series of echo planar data sets obtained during the first pass of the contrast agent through the capillary bed. The acquisition consisted of echo planar T2-weighted images obtained using echo time (TE) = 100 ms, repetition time (TR) = 1500 ms, 7 mm slice thickness, 128×128 matrix and 40 cm field of view [9, 10].

The pixel signal intensity data were then converted to tissue concentration curves using a signal modeling conversion to delta R2. The subsequent tissue concentration curves were subjected to a nonlinear least squares fit (4 parameter) of the tissue concentration curve to a gamma variant function. The analytic result was integrated or calculated using a trapezoid integration to estimate regional cerebral blood volume for each pixel. The composite pixel mosaic was then represented as a cerebral blood image or map [11].

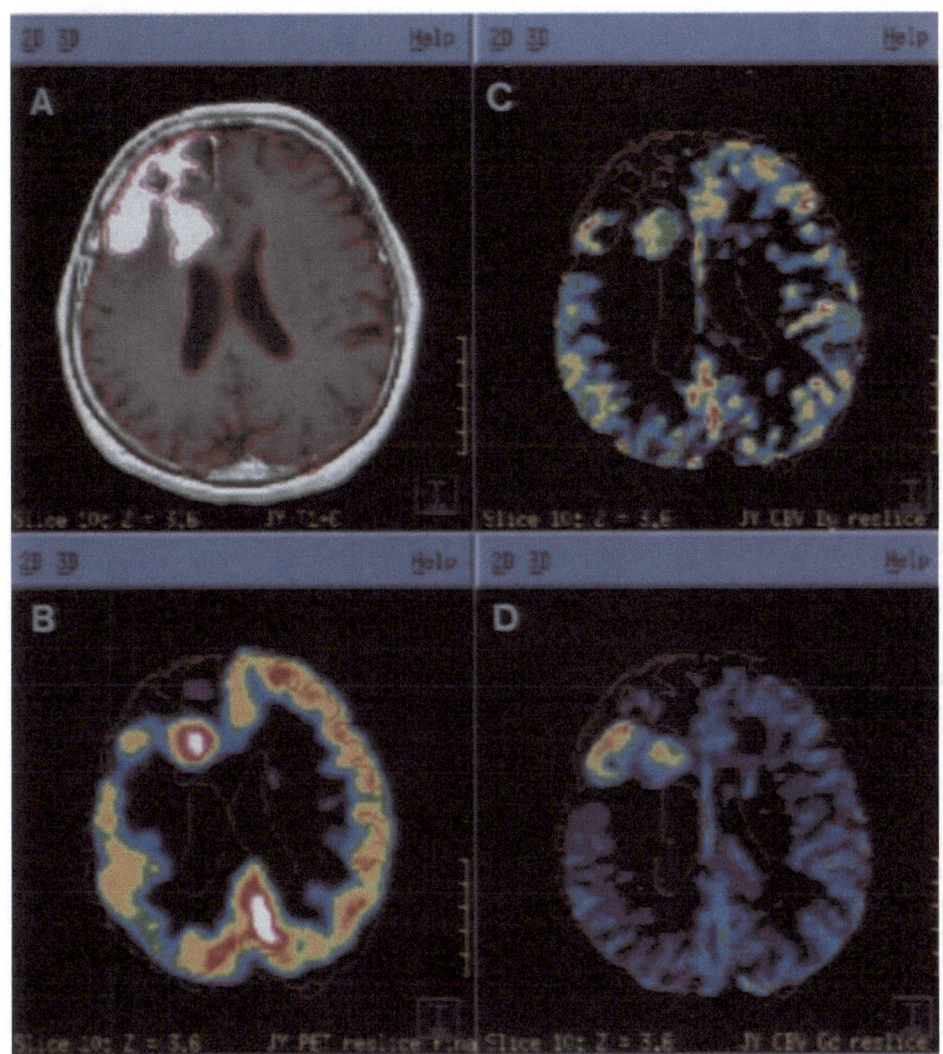

Fig. 1a-d. Recurrent grade IV astrocytoma. **a** The T1-weighted image reveals areas of contrast enhancement adjacent to the right frontal horn and along the surface of the right frontal lobe. The regions of contrast enhancement as well as the surface of the brain have been outlined in red and superimposed on the subsequent images. **b** The fluorodeoxyglucose PET scan indicates that the enhancing region adjacent to the right frontal horn represents viable tumor. The region along the anterior surface of the right frontal lobe, however, has no glycolytic activity and indicates an area of necrosis. **c** The rCBV map generated following a bolus injection of dysprosium DTPA reveals increased cerebral blood volume in the region of the recurrent tumor. There is reduced blood volume in the region of necrosis. **d** The rCBV map generated from a bolus injection of gadodiamide reveals similar results with increased blood volume adjacent to the right frontal horn. There is also reduced blood volume in the superficial aspect of the anterior right frontal lobe. Subsequent biopsy of the lesion adjacent to the right frontal horn revealed recurrent grade IV astrocytoma.

Within one week of the MR examinations, the patients also underwent deoxyglucose PET scanning. The images were then coregistered and regions of contrast enhancement were traced on the cerebral blood volume maps as well as on the fluorodeoxyglucose PET scans. Histology material from the primary surgical procedure was available for all 19 patients. Relative cerebral blood volume maps were also obtained at Sprodiamide concentrations of 0.05, 0.10 and 0.20 mmol/kg of body weight [11-13]. For the gadolinium studies an initial 0.1 mmol/kg was administered to compensate for permeability effects in the tumor. This was followed by a 0.2 mmol/kg bolus of gadodiamide. The subsequent image sets were correlated with the fluorodeoxyglucose PET scans. In six patients additional biopsy material was obtained from specific regions of interest.

Results

The regions of contrast enhancement on the T1-weighted images were scored as viable tumor or necrosis based on the deoxyglucose PET scan. Regions were considered to be viable tumor if the fluorodeoxyglucose PET scan revealed glycolytic activity equal to or greater than that of the cerebral cortex. The cerebral blood volume maps were considered positive for viable tumor if the cerebral blood volume was equivalent to or greater than that of normal cerebral cortex. Both the dysprosium cerebral blood volume maps and the gadolinium cerebral blood volume maps were correlated with the FDG studies.

Four exams were disqualified by patient motion, hardware/software malfunction or inadequate contrast bolus. Of the remaining 15 patients, 13 were found to have viable neoplasms. Of these, 11 were correctly identified as having viable tumor by relative cerebral blood volume mapping. In two instances, rim-like viable tumor was not clearly defined on the cerebral blood volume maps and was incorrectly interpreted as adjacent normal cortical tissue. In an additional two patients, the cerebral blood volume maps and the fluorodeoxyglucose PET scans suggested that the predominance of the enhancing process was radiation necrosis. Subsequent biopsy confirmed the diagnosis of radiation necrosis. None of the patients experienced any severe adverse reactions to the bolus injection of either Sprodiamide or gadodiamide. One patient complained of headache and one patient experienced a transient episode of dizziness with a slight decrease in blood pressure.

Discussion

In this preliminary investigation it was possible to distinguish regions of tumor necrosis and large areas of radiation necrosis from viable tumor using fluorodeoxyglucose PET scanning and regional cerebral blood volume maps. Coregistration of the image data sets improved the analysis of the images. Although only 10 patients underwent cerebral blood volume mapping using gadodiamide, it appears that this agent has promise for cerebral blood volume mapping and warrants further investigation.

Relative cerebral blood volume maps correlated well with fluorodeoxyglucose PET scans for the detection of viable tumor and regions of tumor necrosis as well as larger areas of radiation necrosis. Adequate cerebral blood volume maps required that a bolus of 0.1 mmol of dysprosium or 0.2 mmol of gadodiamide per kilogram of body weight is used to obtain adequate bolus characteristics. A minor limitation is that the echo planar acquisition was more sensitive to susceptibility artifacts from metallic sutures and air-tissue interfaces. Nonetheless, cerebral blood volume maps appear to be a useful tool for the evaluation of patients with recurrent malignant gliomas.

References

1. DiChiro G, Oldfield E, Wright DC, DeMichele D, Katz DA, Patronas NJ, Doppman JL, Larson SM, Ito M, Kufta CV (1988) Cerebral Necrosis After Radiotherapy and/or Intraarterial Chemotherapy for Brain Tumors: PET and Neuropathologic Studies. Am J Roentgenol 150: 189-197
2. DiChiro G, DeLa Paz RL, Brooks RA, et al (1982) Glucose utilization of cerebral gliomas measured by ^{18}F-fluorodeoxyglucose and PET. Neurology 32: 1323-1329
3. Mazziotta JC (1991) The Continuing Challenge of Primary Brain Tumor Management: The Contribution of Positron Emission Tomography. Ann Neurology 29: 345-346
4. Ito M, Lammertsma AA, Wise RJS, Bernardi S, Frackowiak RSJ, Heather JD, McKenzie CG, Thomas DGT, Jones T (1995) Measurement of Regional Cerebral Blood Flow and Oxygen Utilisation in Patients with Cerebral Tumours Using ^{15}0 and Positron Emission Tomography: Analytical Techniques and Preliminary Results Proocedings of the Society of Magnetic Resonance in Medicine, p. 394
5. Rosen BR, Belliveau JW, Vevea JM, Brady TJ (1990) Perfusion Imaging with NMR Contrast Agents. Magn Reson Med 14: 249-265
6. Rosen BR, Belliveau JW, Buchbinder BR, McKinstry RC, Porkka LM, Kennedy DN, Neuder MS, Fisel CR, Aronen HJ, Kwong KK, Weisskoff RM, Cohen MS, Brady TJ (1991) Contrast Agents and Cerebral Hemodynamics. Magn Reson Med 19: 285-292
7. Maeda M, Itoh S, Kimura H, Iwasaki T, Hayashi N, Yamamoto K, Ishii Y, Kubota T (in press) Tumor Vascularity in the Brain: Evaluation with Dynamic Susceptibility-Contrast MR Imaging. Magn Reson Med
8. Aronen HJ, Gazit IE, Louis DN, Buchbinder BR, Pardo FS, Weisskoff RM, Harsh GR, Cosgrove GR, Halpern EF, Hochberg FH, Rosen BR (1994) Cerebral Blood Volume Maps of Gliomas: Comparison with Tumor Grade and Histologic Findings. Radiology 191: 41-51
9. Rosen BR, Aronen HJ, Kwong KK, Belliveau JW, Hamberg LM, Fordham J (1993) Advances in Clinical Neuroimaging: Functional MR Imaging Techniques. RadioGraphics 13: 889-896
10. Rempp KA, Brix G, Wenz F, Becker CR, Gückel F, Lorenz WJ (1993) Quantification of Regional Cerebral Blood Flow and Volume with Dynamic Susceptibility Contrast-enhanced MR Imaging. Radiology 193: 637-641
11. Roberts TPL, Kucharczyk J, Cox I, Moseley ME, Prayer L, Dillon W, Bleyl K, Harnish P (1994) Sprodiamide-Injection-Enhanced Magnetic Resonance Imaging of Cerebral Perfusion. Invest Radiol 29: S24-S26
12. Tzika AA, Massoth RJ, Ball, Jr WS, Majumdar S, Dunn RS, Kirks DR (1993) Cerebral Perfusion in Children: Detection with Dynamic Contrast-enhanced T2*-weighted MR Images. Radiology 187: 449-458
13. Bahn MM (1995) A Single-Step Method for Estimation of Local Cerebral Blood Volume from Susceptibility Contrast MRI Images. Magn Reson Med 33: 309-317

Cerebral Perfusion Imaging with Gadolinium Chelates and Iron Oxides in Humans

P. Reimer, G. Schuierer, A. Tigges, C. Fischer, P.E. Peters

Institute of Clinical Radiology, Westfalian Wilhelms-University Muenster, Germany

Introduction

Susceptibility-induced signal loss following the bolus injection of paramagnetic contrast agents coupled with dynamic magnetic resonance imaging (MRI) has enabled the generation of cerebral blood volume (CBV) maps which reflect cerebral perfusion [1-4]. Both gadolinium- and dysprosium-based paramagnetic contrast agents and endogenous substances have been used for CBV and functional MRI (fMRI) studies [1-6]. More recently, superparamagnetic iron oxides (SPIO) with a stronger susceptibility effect than paramagnetic chelates have been applied in humans as well [7, 8]. We describe clinical results with the current approved dose of gadolinium chelates (0.1 mmol/kg body weight), present results with a neutral gadolinium chelate at higher doses (0.1-0.5 mmol/kg bodyweight), and take a look into the future with the first clinical results of a novel bolus-injectable SPIO contrast agent (Resovist, SH U 555A, Schering AG, Berlin) to induce susceptibility contrast in the brain [9].

Methods

MRI studies were performed on a 1.0 T system (Magnetom Impact, Siemens AG) equipped with 15 mT/m gradients (Software A 2.1 Numaris) and a 1.5 T system (Magnetom SP 4000, Siemens AG) equipped with 10 mT/m gradients (Software A 2.7 Numaris). Patients were examined with a circular polarized head coil and individual shimming. Following a T1-weighted sagittal scout, single slice axial T2*-weighted FLASH images were acquired with a repetition time of 32 ms, an echo time of 22 ms, a 10° flip angle, 1 acquisition, and a pixel bandwidth of 130 Hz/pixel. Within 87 s, 40 images were acquired at a 128×64 matrix (slice thickness 5 mm at a field-of-view of 230 mm yielding voxel dimensions of $5 \times 1.8 \times 1.8$ mm) and post-processed to generate cerebral blood volume (CBV) maps by numerical integration of the relative concentration ($\Delta R2$) for the first-pass bolus through each voxel based on kinetic principles for nondiffusible traces [10, 11].

Results

1. Cerebral Perfusion Imaging with the Standard Dose

Four different chelates (gadopentetate dimeglumine, Magnevist, Schering; gadodiamide, Omniscan, Nycomed; gadoteridol, Prohance, Bracco; and gadolinium-DOTA, Dotarem, Guerbet) have been clinically approved in different countries. All contrast agents have been approved for cerebral imaging at a dose of 0.1 mmol/kg body weight with patients ≥ 18 years and may be administered by means of bolus injections in Europe. Magnevist was approved for two separate bolus injections of 0.1 mmol/kg body weight at the time of the study.

A total of 52 patients were studied with Magnevist with 2 manual injections (0.1 mmol gadopentetate dimeglumine /kg body weight per bolus) in each patient (104 perfusion studies); this protocol is clinically approved in the FRG. Patients without cerebral pathology (n = 7) were used to obtain normal values for signal changes following manual injections of the contrast agent. The mean percent signal drop in cerebral white matter was 6.9 ± 3.1% and 10.2 ± 2.9% in cerebral gray matter with no difference in the transit time (9.2 ± 3.4 s). Patients with carotid occlusive disease (n = 10) did not show a significant hemispheric difference with a mean signal drop in cerebral white matter of 5.3 ± 2.2% (normal hemisphere) vs. 5.3 ± 1.5% (diseased hemisphere) and in cerebral gray matter of 11.0 ± 4.3% vs. 11.2 ± 3.9% with no difference in the transit time (6.5 ± 2.7 s vs. 7.0 ± 1.0 s). Enhancing brain tumors (n = 14) demonstrated significant signal changes within the tumor of 15.5 ± 5.0% compared to gray matter with 9.2 ± 2.1%. Patients (n = 11) with brain infarcts showed significantly lower signal changes (3.3 ± 1.1%) within old infarcted areas compared to gray matter (7.9 ± 1.8%) or white matter (5.6 ± 1.3%). Similar values were obtained in 10 patients with small vessel disease; a mean signal drop of 3.7 ± 1.5% in cerebral white matter was measured for these patients which we used for the diagnostic work-up of this disease entity.

P. Reimer, G. Schuierer, A. Tigges, C. Fischer, P.E. Peters

Table 1. Maximum signal drop and transit time in normal hemispheres following bolus injection of Gadovist at different doses

Dose	Thalamus (%)	Nucl. lent. (%)	Cortex (%)	Transit time (s)
0.1 mmol	7.5 ± 5.5	7.8 ± 5.2	21.4 ± 13.6	6.5 ± 1.5
0.2 mmol	9.8 ± 5.9	9.7 ± 6.7	27.3 ± 18.3	7.1 ± 1.3
0.3 mmol	16.1 ± 12.2	16.3 ± 8.5	34.6 ± 15.0	8.9 ± 3.6
0.4 mmol	23.3 ± 6.3	21.1 ± 7.9	52.6 ± 19.7	10.3 ± 3.9
0.5 mmol	14.6 ± 3.5	14.6 ± 3.5	19.0 ± 11.1	13.8 ± 2.5

Nucl. lent, lentiform nucleus.

2. High-dose Cerebral Perfusion Imaging

The potential value of a neutral or so called non-ionic gadolinium chelate (gadobutrol, Gadovist, Schering AG) was evaluated within a dose-finding study. Gadovist was administered by i.v. bolus injection at five different doses: 0.1 mmol, 0.2 mmol, 0.3 mmol, 0.4 mmol, and 0.5 mmol/kg body weight. Bolus injections were performed with a commercially available MR-compatible injector (Ulrich AG) at a flow rate of 5 ml/s with an automatic saline flush through the i.v. line (20 ml). A total of 40 patients with either hemispheric infarcts or significant (> 70%) internal carotid stenosis and normal contralateral hemispheres were scanned. The mean signal drop and the transit time were estimated in a subgroup of patients using the routine mean-curve program. Further analysis with dedicated software will be required for final analysis.

The current approved dose for gadolinium chelates of 0.1 mmol/kg body weight showed significantly lower mean signal drops in cerebral gray and white matter as compared to all other doses (Fig. 1 and Table 1). Signal changes increased from 0.2 mmol/kg body weight up to 0.4 mmol/kg body weight (Fig. 2). The highest dose of

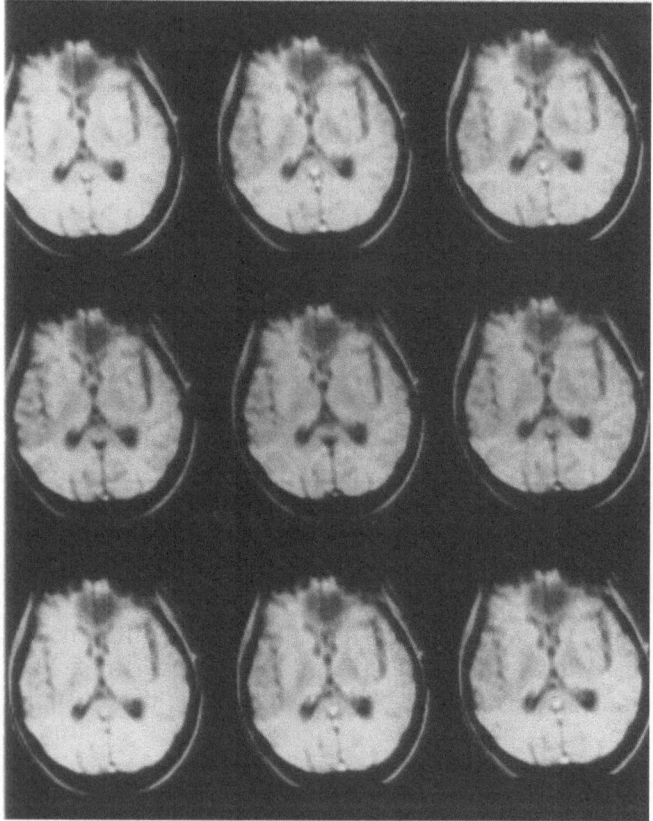

Fig. 1. *Cerebral perfusion imaging with 0.1 mmol/kg Gadovist.* Sequential images before (*upper left*), during peak signal loss and 60 s (*lower right*) following bolus i.v. administration of Gadovist at a dose of 0.1 mmol/kg body weight demonstrate weak signal changes in cerebral gray and white matter

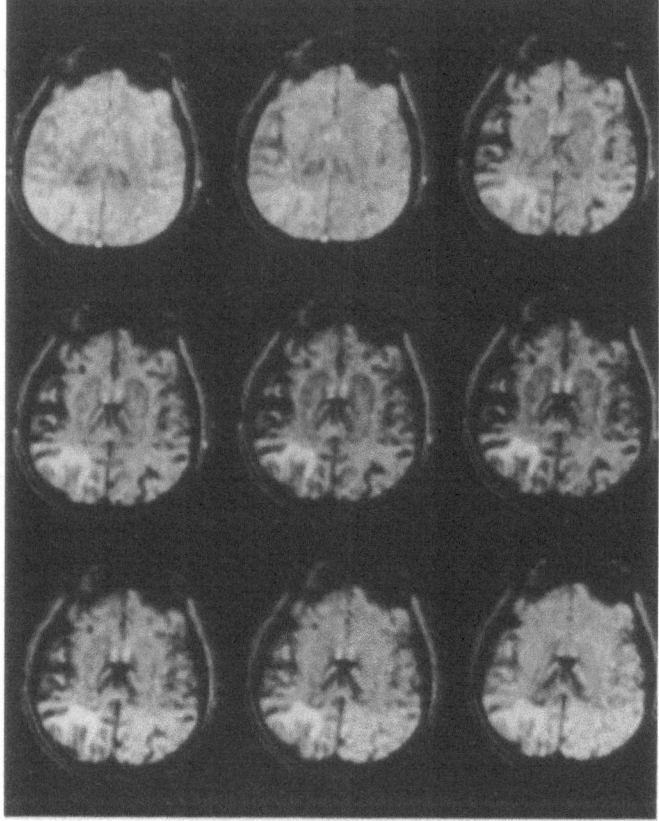

Fig. 2. *Cerebral perfusion imaging with 0.3 mmol/kg Gadovist.* Sequential images before (*upper left*), during peak signal loss and 60 s (*lower right*) following bolus i.v. administration of Gadovist at a dose of 0.3 mmol/kg body weight demonstrate strong signal changes in cerebral gray and white matter with a significant increase compared to 0.1 mmol/kg body weight

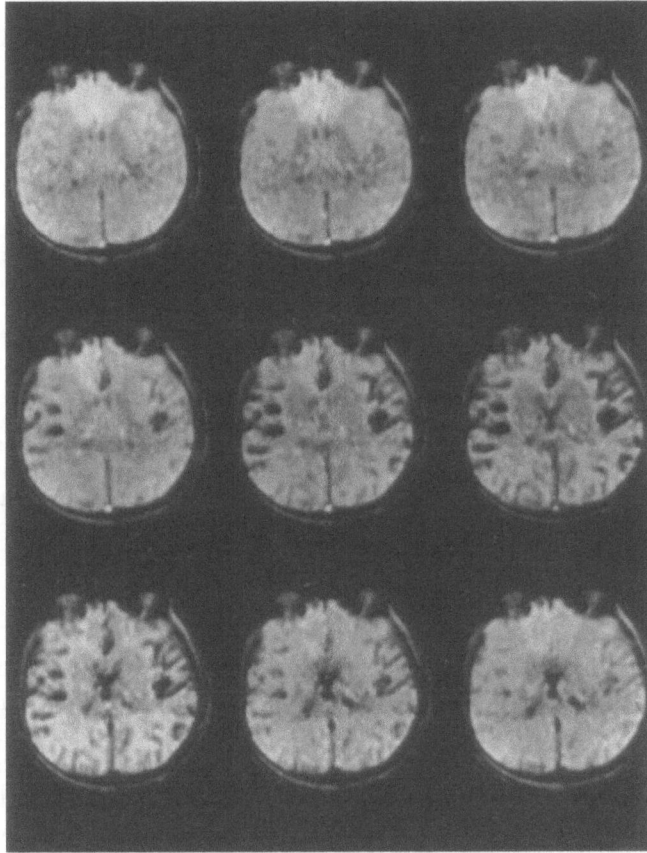

Fig. 3. *Cerebral perfusion imaging with 0.5 mmol/kg Gadovist.* Sequential images before (*upper left*), during peak signal loss and 60 s (*lower right*) following bolus i.v. administration of Gadovist at a dose of 0.5 mmol/kg body weight demonstrate strong signal changes in cerebral gray and white matter without a further increase compared to 0.3 mmol/kg body weight

0.5 mmol/kg body weight showed decreasing signal changes (Fig. 3). Both doses of 0.3 mmol and 0.4 mmol/kg body weight provided strongest signal changes. The transit time increased with the dose, because the injection volume increased and was ejected over more cardiac cycles. This may explain why the highest dose showed weaker signal effects than did either dose of 0.3 mmol or 0.4 mmol/kg body weight.

3. SPIO for Cerebral Perfusion Imaging

Resovist (SH U 555 A, Schering AG, Berlin) comprises superparamagnetic iron oxide microparticles (magnetite – Fe_3O_4/maghemite – gFe_2O_3), coated with a carboxydextran shell. These microparticles exhibit a hydrodynamic diameter of 61.1 nm as measured by photon correlation spectroscopy and an iron oxide core of 4.2 nm as measured by electron microscopy. The carboxydextran coating (27-35 mg/ml with an iron to carboxydextran ratio of 1:1 (w/w)) provides aqueous solubility of the microparticles and prevents aggregation [12]. Resovist was administered in a feasibility study in 3 patients

as a bolus intravenously (i.v.) through an indwelling cubital catheter (18 gauge) with adequate extension tubing to permit injections outside the bore of the magnet. The extension tubing was loaded with the contrast agent via a 5 µm filter and flushed with 20 ml saline at a rate of 4 ml/s for bolus injections. The injection volume for a 75 kg patient for the lowest dose of 4 µmol Fe/kg body weight was 0.6 ml, for 8 µmol Fe/kg body weight it was 1.2 ml, and for a dose of 16 µmol Fe/kg body weight it was 2.4 ml.

Dynamic studies with Resovist decreased gray matter and white matter signal intensity in a dose-dependent fashion during the first pass of the contrast agent without a saturation effect: 4 µmol Fe/kg body weight-gray matter 13% and white matter 7%; 8 µmol Fe/kg body weight – gray matter 28% and white matter 16% (Fig. 4); and 16 µmol Fe/kg body weight – gray matter 44% and white matter 20%. A decrease in normalized signal intensity of approximately 5% remained for the duration of the acquisitions after i.v. administration of 16 µmol Fe/kg body weight. Following i.v. administration of gadopentetate dimeglumine in the control group, decreases of 11.3 ± 2.3% in gray matter signal and 5.3 ± 0.8% in white matter signal were measured. These signal changes are comparable to the dose of 4 µmol Fe/kg body weight. CBV maps showed improved visibility of cerebral anatomy with increasing dose of Resovist.

Discussion

The utility of cerebral perfusion imaging with the clinically approved dose of 0.1 mmol gadolinium/kg body weight and standard hardware/software is limited because of limited signal changes and therefore insufficient perfusion maps. Signal changes are directly related to the concentration of contrast agents, their magnetic moment, the bolus quality, the patient's cardiovascular situation, and imaging technique. The use of dedicated power injectors with flow rates > 3 ml/s is likely to improve bolus quality. The bolus geometry may furthermore be improved by using more concentrated gadolinium chelates which significantly reduces the injection volume. Clinical results with commercially available equipment demonstrate decreased cerebral blood volume in brain infarcts and small vessel disease. However, the time resolution and signal changes do not allow the discrimination of differences in hemispheric perfusion of patients with carotid occlusive disease.

Another problem of the standard dose in combination with manual injections and conventional hardware is the reproducibility of adequate signal changes required to generate sufficient perfusion maps. Schuierer et al. [13] analyzed a total of 126 perfusion studies with Omniscan in 21 patients (hemispheric brain infarction and brain tumors). All patients received three manual injections of 0.1 mmol/kg gadodiamide in two sessions,

P. Reimer, G. Schuierer, A. Tigges, C. Fischer, P.E. Peters

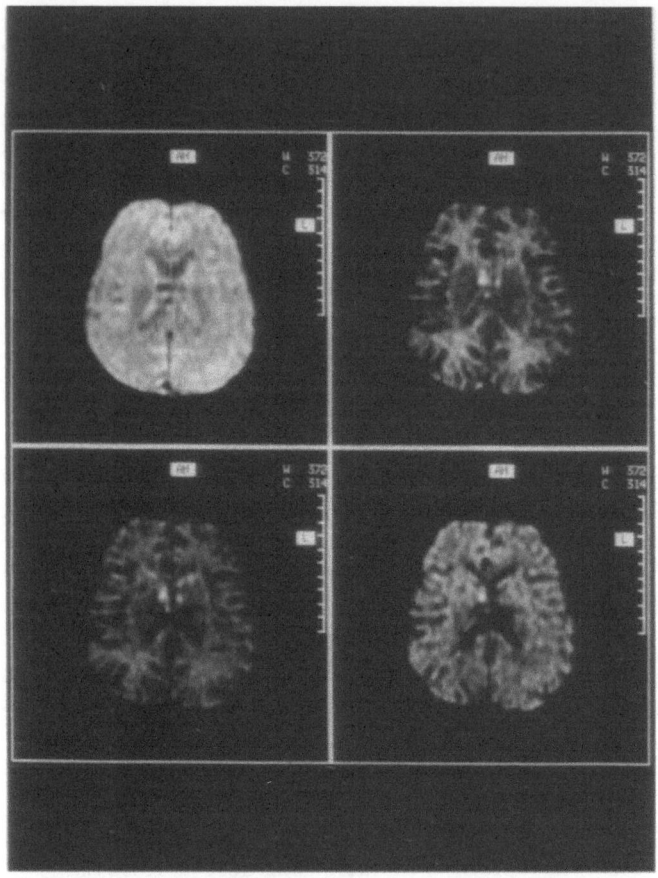

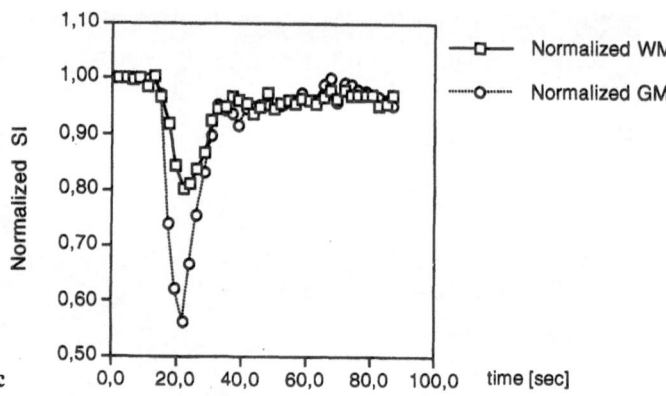

Fig. 4a-c. *16 μmol Fe/Kg body weight.* **a** Sequential images before (*upper left*), during peak signal loss (*upper right* and *lower left*) and after 60 s (*lower right*). **b** CBV map. **c** Normalized signal intensity curve following bolus i.v. administration of Resovist at a dose of 16 μmol Fe/kg body weight. WH, white matter; GM, gray matter; SI, signal intensity

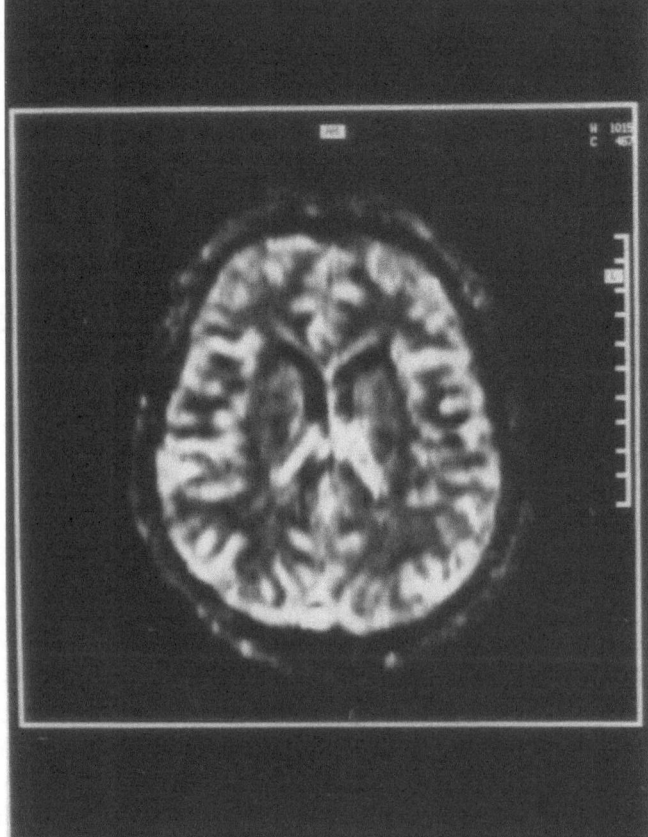

with the second as a follow-up session between 1 week and 3 months following the first session which accounts for 6 injections in each patient. The mean signal drop in cerebral white matter was 4.8 ± 1.4% and in cerebral gray matter it was 8.8 ± 3.0%. Technical or motion artifacts were present in 9.5% (11 injections), 14.3% of studies (16 injections) showed no clear signal drop, 11 studies could not be analyzed due to the individual brain anatomy, and 22 studies (17.4%) revealed an insufficient white matter/gray matter ratio (< 2.0 ± 0.7). Thus, only 50% of the perfusion studies (63/126) were technically sufficient. Considering the follow-up sessions, results were even worse. Only 33% of follow-up sessions showed sufficient signal changes following all three injections [13].

The benefit of higher gadolinium concentrations is clearly demonstrated when comparing Gadovist at different doses with an escalation up to 0.5 mmol/kg body weight. It appears that the optimal dose for the hardware/software used is in the range of 0.3-0.4 mmol/kg body weight, because signal changes are decreased at higher doses. Since an increasing volume limits the effects of higher doses because the bolus is ejected over more cardiac cycles, even more concentrated contrast agents (> 1 mol/l) would be necessary. However, a dose of 0.3-0.4 mmol/kg body weight is probably a good compromise. The study also indicates the benefit of power injectors, because signal changes with 0.1 mmol/kg bodyweight were weaker with manual injections than with machine-driven injections (percent signal decrease in gray matter: Magnevist – 10.2 ± 2.9 vs. Gadovist – 21.4 ± 13.6).

Our preliminary results with Resovist show that dynamic imaging with SPIO using susceptibility contrast is feasible in humans and allows a stronger reduction in gray and white matter signal intensity (28% and 44% respectively with 16 μmol Fe/kg body weight) compared to paramagnetic chelates such as gadopentetate dimeglumine using the same imaging technique. Gadopentetate dimeglumine at a dose of 0.1 mmol/kg body weight leads to a signal decrease comparable to the lowest dose of 4 µmol Fe/kg body weight [14]. The small volume (< 4 ml) of Resovist required for injection because of its high concentration and the dose reduction are advantageous, and none of our patients perceived any discomfort or pain during the injection [15]. Iron oxides have been evaluated for dynamic MR imaging of the brain [8, 16, 17]. Immediately after intravenous administration, brain signal intensity decreased but more than 90% of the original signal intensity was recovered within 5 blood half-times [7, 8, 16]. Resovist enables rapid injection without cardiovascular side effects, appears to be suited for dynamic MR imaging, and may play a role in contrast-enhanced fMRI [18, 19].

References

1. Frahm J, Haase A, Matthaei D (1986) Rapid NMR imaging of dynamic processes using the FLASH technique. Magn Reson Med 3: 321-327
2. Fisel CR, Ackerman JL, Buxton RB, et al (1991) MR contrast due to microscopically heterogeous magnetic susceptibility: Numerical simulations and applications to cerebral physiology. Magn Reson Med 17: 336-347
3. Villringer A, Rosen BR, Belliveau JW, et al (1988) Dynamic imaging with lanthanide chelates in normal brain: Contrast due to magnetic susceptibility effects. Magn Reson Med 6: 164-174
4. Rosen BR, Belliveau JW, Aronen HJ, et al (1991) Susceptibility contrast imaging of cerebral blood volume: Human experience. Magn Reson Med 22: 293-299
5. Aronen HJ, Gazit IE, Louis DN, et al (1994) Cerebral blood volume maps of gliomas: Comparison with tumor grade and histologic findings. Radiology 191: 41-51
6. Belliveau JW, Kennedy DN, McKinstry RC, et al (1991) Functional mapping of the human visual cortex using magnetic resonance imaging. Science 254: 716-719
7. Bulte JWM, De Jonge MWA, Kamman RL, et al (1992) Dextran-magnetite particles: Contrast-enhanced MRI of blood-brain barrier disruption in a rat model. Magn Reson Med 23: 215-223
8. Kent TA, Quast MJ, Kaplan BJ, Lifsey RS, Eisenberg HM (1990) Assessment of a superparamagnetic iron oxide (AMI-25) as a brain contrast agent. Magn Reson Med 13: 434-443
9. Reimer P, Schuierer G, Balzer T, Peters PE (1995) Application of a superparamagnetic iron oxide (Resovist) for MR imaging of human cerebral blood volume. Magn Reson Med (in press)
10. Axel L (1980) Cerebral blood flow determination by rapid-sequence computed tomography: a theoretical analysis. Radiology 137: 679-686
11. Rosen BR, Belliveau JW, Chien D (1989) Perfusion imaging by nuclear magnetic resonance. Magn Reson Q 5: 263-281
12. Hamm B, Staks T, Taupitz M (1994) A new superparamagnetic iron oxide contrast agent for magnetic resonance imaging. Invest Radiology 29: S87-S89
13. Schuierer G, Tigges A, Reimer P, Daldrup H, Peters PE (1995) The repeatability of MR-perfusion studies: a clinical study. Twelth Annual Meeting and Exhibition of the Society of Magnetic Resonance and European Society for Magnetic Resonance in Medicine and Biology, Nice, p. 84
14. Edelman RR, Mattle HP, Atkinson DJ, et al (1990) Cerebral blood flow: Assessment with dynamic contrast-enhanced T2*-weighted MR imaging at 1.5 T. Radiology 176: 211
15. Reimer P, Rummeny EJ, Daldrup HE, et al (1995) Clinical results with Resovist: A phase 2 clinical trial. Radiology 195: 489-496
16. Majumdar S, Zoghbi S, Gore JC (1988) Regional differences in rat brain displayed by fast MRI with superparamagnetic contrast agents. Magn Reson Med 6: 611-615
17. White DL, Aicher KP, Tzika AA, Kucharzyk J, Engelstad BL, Moseley ME (1992) Iron-dextran as a magnetic susceptibility contrast agent: Flow-related contrast effects in the T2-weighted spin-echo MRI of normal rat and cat brain. Magn Reson Med 24: 14-28
18. Prichard JW, Rosen BR (1994) Functional Study of the Brain by NMR. Cereb Blood Flow Metab 14: 365-372
19. Frahm J, Merboldt KD, Hänicke W (1993) Functional MRI of human brain activation at high spatial resolution. Magn Reson Med 29: 139-144

High Resolution Studies of Oxygen, Carbogen and Carbon Dioxide in the Brain - with Supporting Findings from Peripheral Muscle

I.R. Young, J.V. Hajnal, A. Oatridge, J.A. Wilson, G.M. Bydder

Robert Steiner Magnetic Resonance Unit, Hammersmith Hospital, London W12 0NN, UK

Introduction

This article reviews a number of experiments in which volunteers inhaled air, oxygen, carbon dioxide (5%) in air, and carbogen (5% carbon dioxide, 95% oxygen). Most of the experiments described used the registration methods described elsewhere in this Syllabus (*MRI Using True 3D Sequences and Full Positional Registration*, JV Hajnal et al.) and the reader is referred there for descriptions of the methodology. Following the investigations of the effects of the inhaled gases on the brain and its surrounds, we discuss briefly experiments on volunteer calf muscle, in which we produced extreme depletion in tissue oxygenation, (going far beyond anything that could normally be tolerated in the brain), in order to try to understand the development of signals such as those attributed to the BOLD (blood oxygenation level dependent) effect [1, 2].

Experiments in which subjects have been given 100% oxygen to breath have been performed by a number of workers [3, 4]. These have shown effects which have seemed to confirm the BOLD model with increasing signals in the cerebral cortex when oxygen was supplied. Studies with carbon dioxide have also shown the expected changes with a substantial increase in tissue perfusion [5]. We describe here experiments which raise questions about the role of changes in cerebrospinal fluid (CSF) signals in mimicking the effects seen. Finally, we describe experiments in peripheral muscle tissue which suggest that changes in T2* are much less than those to be found in another magnetic resonance (MR) parameter (the chemical shift of the water peak).

Methods

All the experiments discussed here were performed at 1.0 T using a Picker Vista HPQ machine. Except where otherwise stated, volume data sets were acquired for registration. These had spatial resolutions of $1.6 \times 1.6 \times 1.6$ mm^3 (A acquisition) or $3.2 \times 3.2 \times 3.2 \times$ mm^3 (B ac-

quisition). Both echo time used the same T1-weighted three-dimensional (3D) sequence with a repetition time (TR) of 21 ms, an echo time (TE) of 6 ms, and a flip angle of 35°. The former acquisition (A) took 12 min; the latter (B) 1 min 30 s.

Other sequences (such as FLAIR) were used in studies of oxygen and carbogen uptake but the results are not reported here for lack of space. Similarly, angiographic studies in which volunteers breathed oxygen in comparison with those performed while they breathed air are also not described. However, all results were consistent with those presented in this paper.

Specific studies are then as follows:

1. Volunteers breathed air during data acquisition A. They then breathed 100% oxygen during a further acquisition A, with a subsequent reversion to air, and further A acquisition. The cycle was repeated with A acquisitions during the breathing of air, then carbogen, followed by air.
2. In another study the same form of protocol was used, but with 5% carbon dioxide in air (referred to hereafter as "carbon dioxide") used as well as carbogen.
3. In another experiment of the same general structure as the previous two, volunteers breathed air, followed by oxygen. They were then given 100 μmol of gado pentetate dimeglumine (Gd-DTPA)/kg body weight, while continuing to breath oxygen, followed by air. At each stage, an A acquisition was completed.
4. Time course experiments were performed using the B acquisition. In these, the volunteers initially breathed air to establish a baseline; thereafter they were given oxygen for a period of 12-15 min, followed by a reversion to air. During the cycle, about 12-14 volume acquisitions were obtained at approximately 1 min 50 s intervals.

Results are also reported of experiments in which the level of oxygen in blood and tissue was dramatically reduced. Since this cannot acceptably be achieved in the brain of a human volunteer, a standard ischaemia protocol was applied to the leg. This consisted of the application to one thigh of a pneumatic cuff pressurised to 300 mm Hg for 25-30 min. The subject rested for 1 1/2 hours

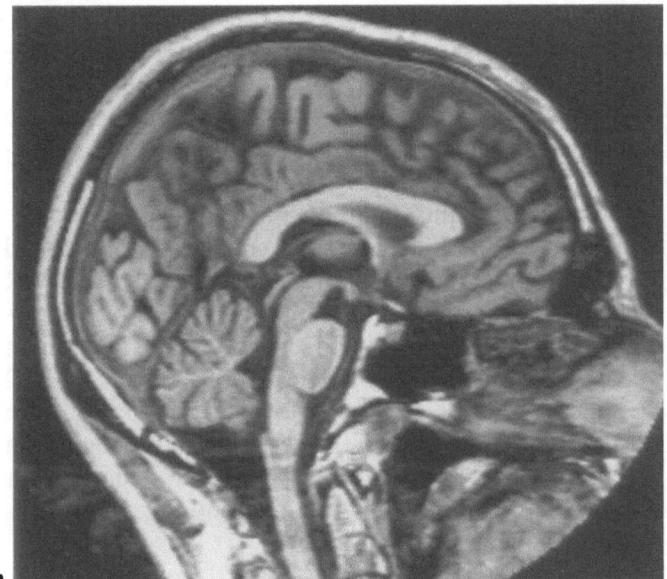

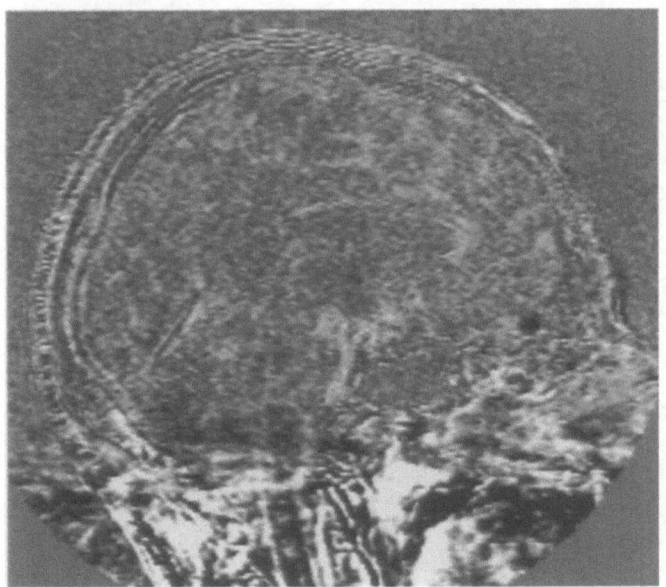

Fig. 1a-c. *Difference images.* From co-registered 3D volume sets (acquisition A) from the first experiment discussed. **a** Anatomical slice, **b** Oxygen-air, **c** Carbogen-air

prior to the start of the challenge. This was followed by MR imaging (MRI) and near infrared spectroscopy (NIR) for 30 min prior to, during and for 30 min after the period of application of the cuff. The NIR measurements (Hamamatsu 500) were performed on a separate occasion and provided a direct measure of changes in concentrations of the oxy- and deoxy-forms of haemoglobin and myoglobin. It did not differentiate between the two oxygen carrying molecules, though the oxygen binding characteristics of the two mean that most of the haemoglobin is in its deoxy- form before there is a significant formation of deoxymyoglobin [6].

The MRI study employed a long TR, short TE spin echo (TR/TE 2000/20 ms) to assess proton density changes, and a dual echo field echo sequence (TR 225, TE 9, 60 ms; flip angle 65°) to measure changes in T2* and phase changes associated with susceptibility varia-

tions. Images of 3 transverse sections of 10 mm thickness were acquired using an enveloping coil that accommodated both the cuffed leg and the other leg, which acted as a control.

Results

Only sample results from this range of experiments can be displayed here for reasons of space. All the images are either directly the result of three-dimensional registration or are derived from such data. Results from experiment 1 are shown in Fig. 1, showing the anatomical sagittal slice (Fig. 1a) from which the other results were derived: the differences between oxygen and air breathing on the one hand (Fig. 1b), and carbogen and air on the other (Fig. 1c). Figure 2 shows a similar difference

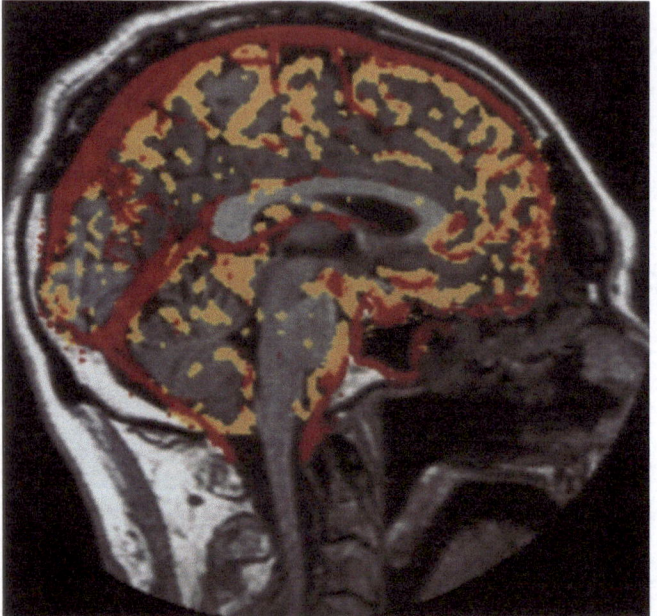

Fig. 2. *Difference image*. As in Fig. 1, but between air with 5% CO_2 added and air.

image from the second experiment in which the volunteer breathed carbon dioxide and air. Figure 3 is a composite coloured image obtained from experiment 3. This shows one image from the initial three-dimensional set. Overlaid on it in yellow are regions showing changes in the difference set between oxygen and air, while the red areas correspond to those showing differences between the volunteer breathing air, having received Gd-DTPA,

and breathing air prior to the contrast agent being injected.

Figure 4 plots the time courses measured from experiment 4 observed for a number of regions of the brain and for CSF. Note that the locations displaying a time course which changes significantly lie in the extracerebral region. For the rest, including the cortex, white matter and sagittal sinus, there was no significant change.

In Fig. 5a, the time course of changes of deoxy- and oxy-components in the tissue as observed by the NIR system (measured in µmol/l) are shown. Figure 5b shows phase differences observed from the long TE gradient recalled echo sequence, showing average results from 12 regions of interest distributed over the 3 slices for the cuffed leg, as well as average results from 11 regions in the unrestricted leg. Figure 5c shows the T2* pattern for the two legs from the same regions, and Fig. 5d displays the proton density variations.

Oxygen time course

(9008)

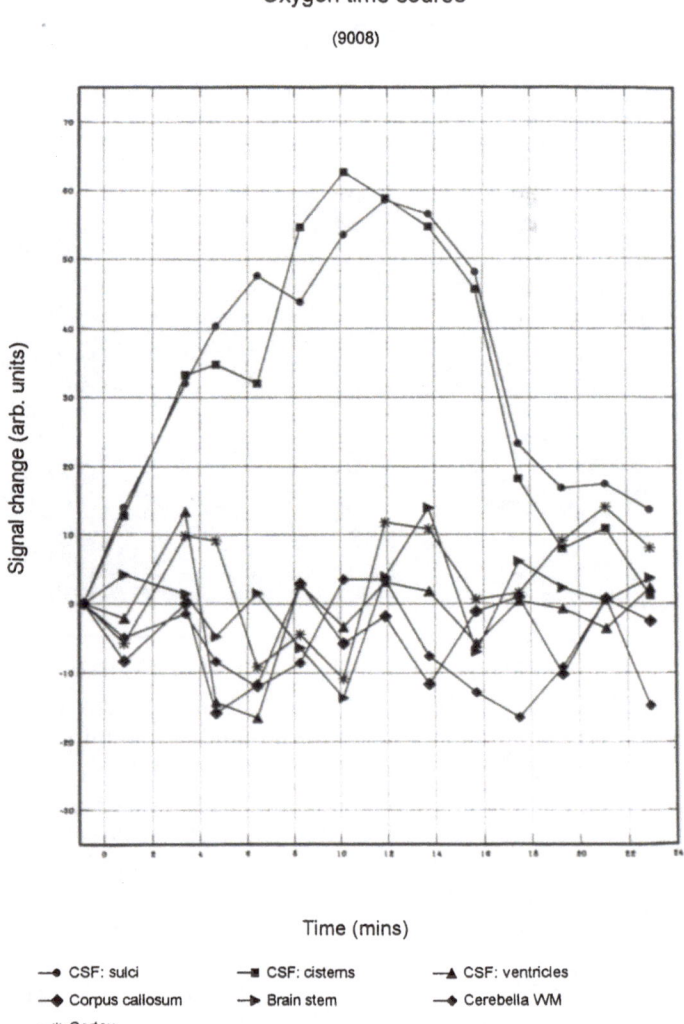

Time (mins)

→● CSF: sulci   →■ CSF: cisterns   →▲ CSF: ventricles
→◆ Corpus callosum   →► Brain stem   →● Cerebella WM
→✳ Cortex

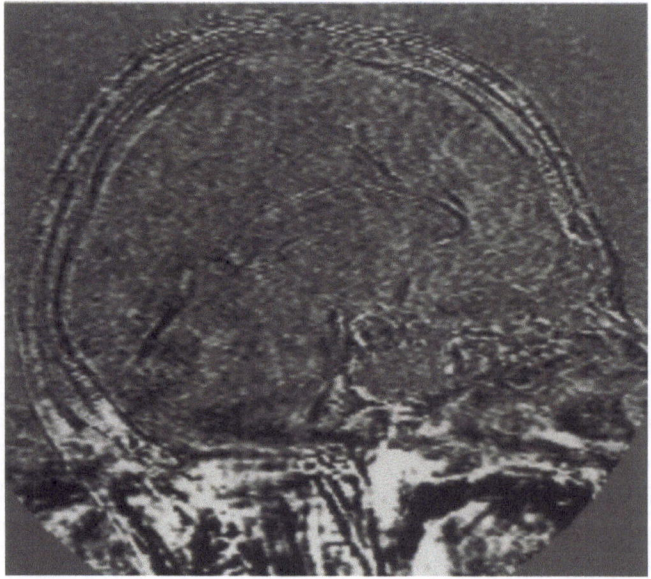

Fig. 3. *Overlaid image*. A baseline image (from one of the air data sets) was overlaid with data derived from difference images between oxygen and air data sets (yellow) and between pre- and post-Gd-DTPA injection (with the volunteer breathing air) (red). (Data acquisitions were type A)

Fig. 4. *Plots of the time course of oxygen uptake response from the brain of a volunteer derived from registered type B acquisitions.* The plot shows data from a number of locations in the head – but only significant changes in signals from CSF surrounding the brain and in the sulci

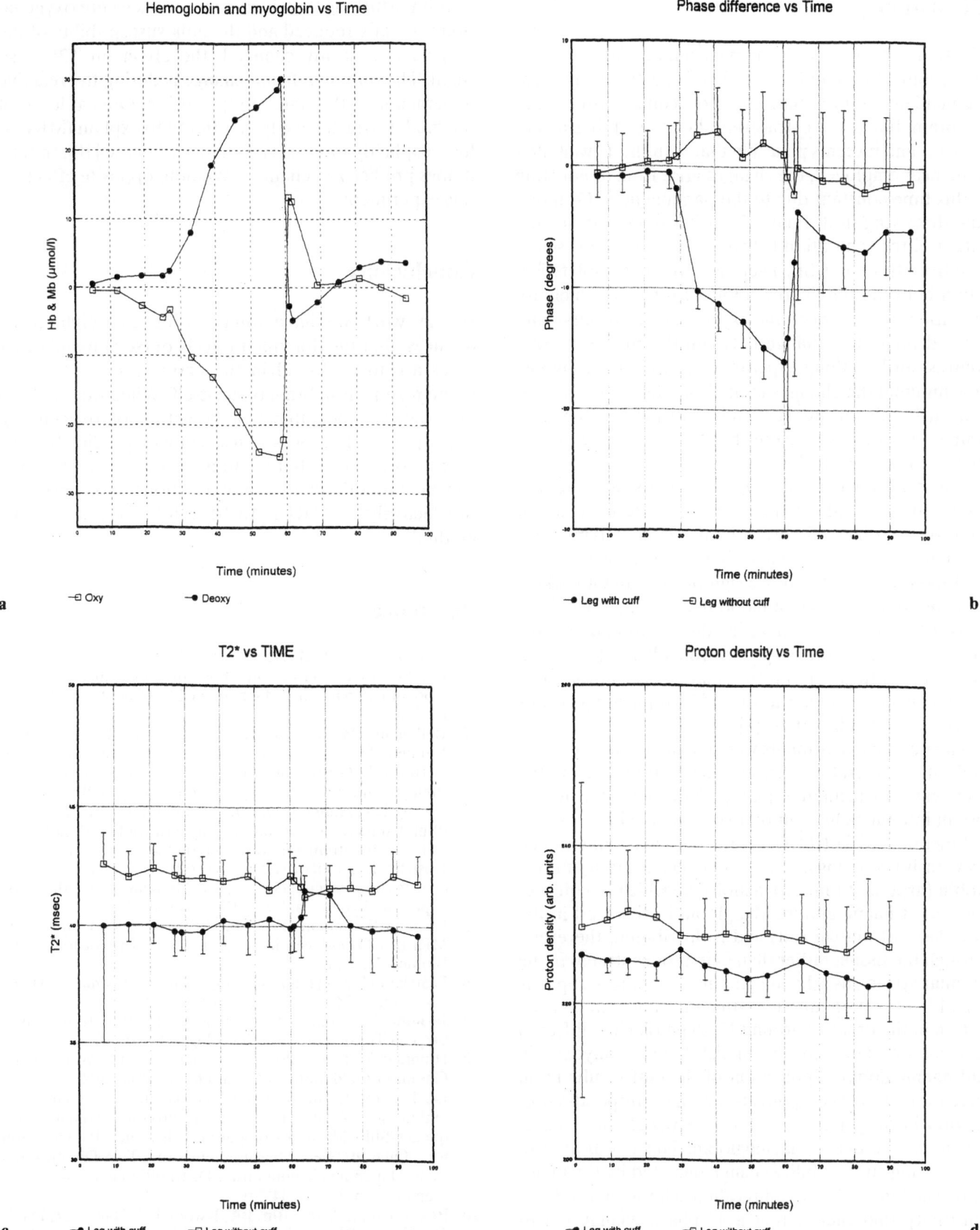

Fig. 5a-d. *Data derived from the cuffed leg experiment described in the text.* Signals from both the restricted and unrestricted legs are shown in **b**, **c** and **d**. **a** Near infrared data – unlocalised, and showing the changes in tissue oxy- and deoxy- components, **b** Phase changes observed using NMR during the cuff experiment. The kink in the characteristic of its initially rapid decline is the subject of ongoing investigations, **c** T2* changes during the cuff experiment, **d** Proton density changes during the cuff experiment

Discussion

The first conclusion to be drawn from the data, which is well demonstrated in Figs. 1b, 3 and 4, is that changes in the head due to breathing 100% oxygen are not seen in the brain, but in the extracerebral CSF. CSF has a very long T1, and it seems plausible that with the T1weighted sequences employed, the changes arise from a reduction in this time constant due to the paramagnetic O_2 molecule dissolving in it. Figure 3 further demonstrates the extent of the separation between effects in the vasculature from those in CSF. There is virtually complete isolation between the yellow coloured regions (which are the differences between the oxygen and air results), and the red ones (the change between the pre- and post-contrast air breathing experiments). It is surprising just how minimal the changes in the brain tissue are, as evidenced by all the images, and confirmed in the time course data of Fig. 4. Note that there is no significant change in ventricular CSF.

The experiment with CO_2, the results of which are shown in Fig. 2, also appears to show the presence of additional oxygen dissolved in the CSF. Giving CO_2 (5%) in air is not expected to change the oxygenation of the blood reaching the tissue significantly, but it is likely to increase the volume of blood reaching it. Since there is no change in activation during the experiment, the tissue's requirement for oxygen is probably little changed. Though the effect is relatively small, it is clear that oxygen has been dissolved in the CSF (replicating results observed in man by others [7]).

The muscle experiments were conducted originally to calibrate temperature measurements in vivo using the chemical shift technique [8, 9,]. They yielded a further insight into the behaviour of tissue signals with relevance to functional MRI (fMRI). Some muscle (as mentioned previously) contains a significant concentration of myoglobin (around 0.1 mmol), a molecule which is a quarter the size of haemoglobin. Myoglobin is dissolved in the cytoplasm of muscle cells and is distributed, therefore, through the tissue, rather than being concentrated in the vascular system, as is haemoglobin. Blood makes up perhaps 1% of resting muscle, with a haemoglobin concentration in the tissue of around 15-25 µmol. Near infrared spectroscopy does not distinguish between myoglobin and haemoglobin. Application of the cuff results in an increase in deoxy-components, and a corresponding reduction in oxygenated ones. Deoxymyoglobin is paramagnetic, like deoxyphaemoglobin. This is reflected in the growing susceptibility change detected by the phase shift. The long TE gradient recalled echo sequence has a sensitivity that means that a 1° phase change corresponds to a susceptibility difference of about 1 part in 10^9. The changes and values observed, both with NIR and NMR are consistent with this calibration.

It is perturbing that, in circumstances where oxygenation is greatly reduced and the bulk susceptibility of the tissue has radically changed, the effect on T2* is so small. The only significant change is during the reactive hyperaemia at the time of reperfusion. One, at least, of the models which have been offered to explain fMRI effects explicitly forecasts no change of phase [10], though it does predict T2* changes. We note opposite effects in this experiment.

Conclusions

In this work we have found, using T1-weighted sequences, that the dominant effects of oxygen and other gases are to be found in the extracerebral CSF. We found no effects in brain tissue itself. When we sought to investigate some effects of depletion of oxygen, we found phase differences, consistent with predictable susceptibility changes, but we found no effect on T2*. We conclude that there are many questions to be answered satisfactorily if fMRI is to be validated as a reliable method.

References

1. Ogawa S, Lee T-M, Nayak AS, Glynn P (1990) Oxygenation-Sensitive Contrast in Magnetic Resonance Image of Rodent Brain at High Magnetic Fields. Magn Reson Med 14 68-781
2. Belliveau JW, Rosen BR, Kantor HL, Rzedzian RR, Kennedy DN, McKinstry RC, Vevea JM, Cohen MS, Pykett L, Brady TJ (1990) Functional Cerebral Imaging by Susceptibility Contrast NMR. Magn Reson Med 14: 538-546
3. Kwong KK, Hanke L Devahue K et al. (1995) EPI imaging of global increase of brain MR signal with breath hold preceded by breathing O_2. Magn Reson Med 33: 448-452
4. Rostrup LS, Larson HBW, Toft PB et al (1995) Signal changes on gradient echo images of human brain induced by hypo- and hyperexia, NMR Biomed 8: 41-47
5. Rostrup E, Larson BW, Toft PB et al (1994) Functional MRI of CO_2 induced increase in cerebral perfusion. NMR Biomed 7: 29-34
6. Biörck G (1956) Hematin Compounds in Mammalian Heart and Skeletal Muscle, Am Heart J 52: 624-539
7. Jarnum S, Lorenzen I, Skinhoje E (1964) External Fluid Oxygen Tension in Man. Neurology 64: 703-707
8. Hindman JC (1966) Proton Resonance Shift of Water in the Gas and Liquid States. J Chem Phys 4: 4852-4592
9. De Poorter J, De Wagter C, De Deene Y, Thomsen C, Stahlberg F, Achten E (1994) The Proton-Resonance-Frequency-Shift Method Compared with Molecular Diffusion for Quantitative Measurement of Two-Dimensional Time-Dependent Temperature Distribution in a Phantom. J Magn Reson B 103: 234-241
10. Boxerman JL, Bandettini PA, Kwong KK, Baker JR, Davis TL, Rosen BR, Weisskoff RM (1995) The Intravascular Contribution to fMRI Signal Change: Monte Carlo Modeling and Diffusion-Weighted Studies in Vivo. Magn Reson Med 34: 4-10

fMRI Using True 3D Sequences and Full Positional Registration

J.V. Hajnal, A. Oatridge, N. Saeed, G.M. Bydder, I.R. Young

Robert Steiner Magnetic Resonance Unit, Hammersmith Hospital, London W12 OHS, UK

Introduction

Numerous studies of brain activation using magnetic resonance imaging (MRI) [1-5] have demonstrated spatially localised signal changes that correlate with the temporal format of the study protocol being used. In most cases the studies consist of repeated acquisition of single or multiple two-dimensional slices of a chosen region of the brain. The time course of signals from each individual voxel is then analysed to extract components that correlate with the time course of the applied stimulus [6, 7]. This procedure has high sensitivity, but is vulnerable to the presence of correlated signal changes that arise from sources other than brain activation. In a previous paper [8] we showed that head motion which correlated with the motor or visual stimuli being applied was present in all subjects that were investigated. These displacements changed the anatomical content of image voxels and resulted in signal changes that simulated activation of the brain.

Several groups have attempted to reduce head motion during functional MRI (fMRI) using foam padding, head moulds, polystyrene beads in evacuated bags and dental fixation. However, even with these methods, residual displacements of 1-2 mm are common (e.g. [5]). This creates difficulties because displacements of much less than 0.5 mm may produce spurious activation signals [8].

Recognition of Displacement Induced Signal Changes

At first sight it appears trivial to recognise image displacements by inspection. This may be true for large inplane effects, but it is much more difficult when the displacements are small and/or they are in the through-plane direction. Figure 1 illustrates the effect of 1 mm shifts on the signals in a transverse slice of a high resolution T1-weighted three-dimensional (3D) data set acquired at 1.0 T on a Picker HPQ system. The signal differences for a left-right (Fig. 1b) or an antero-posterior (Fig. 1c) shift are clearly related to the anatomy seen in Fig. 1a. However a head-foot (through-plane) shift produces a quite

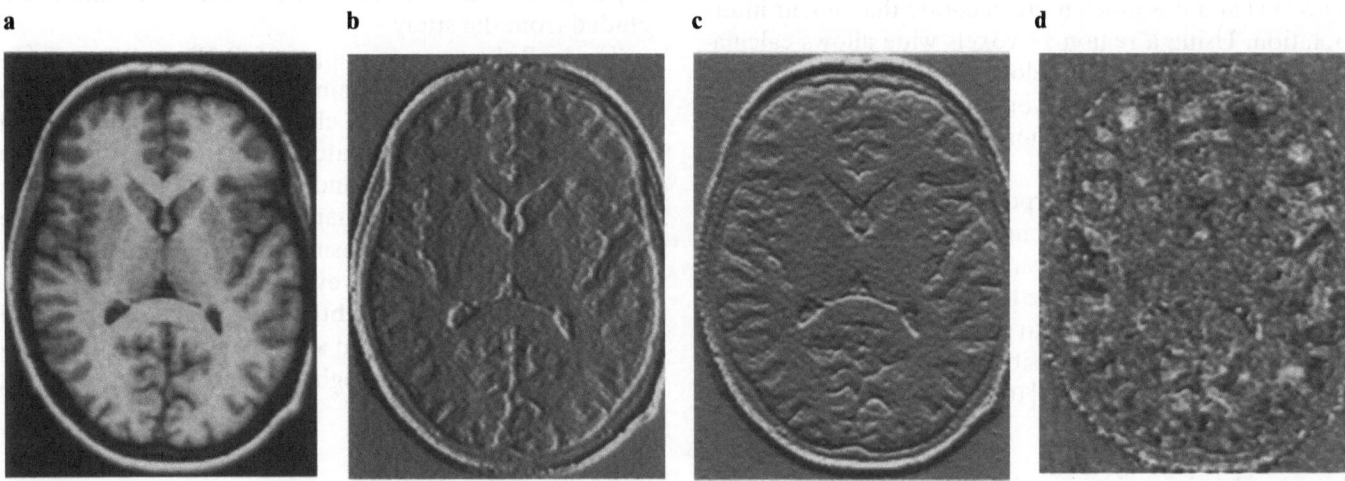

Fig. 1a-d. *Effects of a 1 mm shift.* **a** Transverse image from a 3D T1-weighted (TR 21 ms, TE 6 ms) data set with $1 \times 1 \times 1$ mm^3 voxels. Difference signals produced by a 1 mm shift in the **b** left-right, **c** antero-posterior and **d** head-foot (through-plane) directions. The inplane shifts (**b, c**) produce curvilinear intensity patterns that are clearly related to the anatomy within the slice. The through-plane shift (**d**) produced a quite different appearance with patches of changed signal that are difficult to relate to the image in **a**

different appearance (Fig. 1d) which is very difficult to predict from the in-plane structure. Whereas in-plane shifts tend to produce curvilinear signal changes, through-plane shifts often produce diffuse, patchy regions of signal change. fMRI studies are highly vulnerable to unrecognised through-plane motion effects, and these can readily lead to stimulus correlated signals [8, 9]. In single slice fMRI experiments no information is obtained from adjacent tissues and so it is not possible to correct for stimulus correlated motion effects in the through-slice direction even if one is aware of the problem.

This situation can be remedied by acquiring data covering a 3D region of the brain. The simplest way of achieving this is by using multislice techniques. However, before proceeding with this approach it is prudent to verify that full positional correction can be achieved with this type of data without introducing unacceptable errors.

Image Interpolation

To correct for small changes in position, image shifts of fractions of a voxel are required. This can be achieved using image interpolation, in which updated voxel intensity values are calculated from the original image voxels that are closest to each voxel of interest in the shifted image. The simplest and fastest interpolation algorithm is linear interpolation in which only nearest neighbour voxels are considered; the assumption is made that these contribute intensities in direct proportion to their proximity to the voxel of interest. However this approach is not very suitable for fMRI because it introduces intensity errors which may be much larger than the activation effects being sought [10].

A much more appropriate interpolation algorithm is available for fMRI data, namely "sinc interpolation" [10]. This algorithm matches the interpolation function precisely to the in-plane point spread function of the images [11] and it is much more accurate than linear interpolation. Using a region 14 voxels wide allows calculational errors to be kept below 1% [10]. However, sinc interpolation is much slower than linear interpolation because it includes many more voxels in the calculation of new intensity values.

Unfortunately sinc interpolation is not useful in the through-plane direction of multislice data, because the slice profile is not generally a sinc function. For this reason we do not use multislice techniques. Instead we employ true 3D sequences, with phase encoding in two spatial directions. These acquisitions can be faithfully shifted using sinc interpolation [10].

Image Registration

The capability to shift an image without introducing unacceptable intensity errors is only part of the requirement for fMRI. Some means is also required for determining the positional correction that is needed. There are many approaches to this problem (see for example [12-14]), but we use a least squares method [10]. The two images to be matched are compared voxel by voxel and the sum of squares of the voxel intensity differences is calculated and divided by the number of voxels. This number, which we refer to as χ^2, is a global measure of image differences. A computer program then automatically reduces the value of χ^2 by simple rigid body rotation and translation of one 3D image set relative to the other. The shifts required to minimise χ^2 result in an optimal positional match between the image sets. The information so obtained can then be used in conjunction with sinc interpolation to reposition one image set so that its signal content is exactly what it would have been had it been obtained in the position to which it has been shifted. Quantitative comparisons can then be made between the voxel intensities in the matched image sets to determine if physiological signal changes have occurred.

Tissue Model

The previous section employed a rigid body model for the tissues being imaged. Such a model is clearly inappropriate for soft tissues outside the cranial cavity since these are readily deformed by the slight changes in head position within the head support system of the scanner. In addition, the brain itself may change shape under the influence of gravity if the head is tilted by more than a few degrees [15]. However, this latter effect has not proved to be a major problem for our fMRI studies so far.

To avoid obtaining an incorrect positional match as a result of extraneous tissue changes we limit the calculation of χ^2 to brain tissue only. This is achieved by image segmentation [10,15]. Once the required rotations and translations have been determined, the full images are repositioned and compared. In this way no data is excluded from the study.

Figure 2 shows an example of full 3D registration applied to 3D data sets obtained by repeat scanning of a normal volunteer with a change of position between scans. Approximately matched anatomical slices are shown in Figs. 2a and 2b, and a simple subtraction image is shown in Fig. 2c. The change in position between the scans produced large intensity changes that make Fig. 2c difficult to interpret. However, if the data sets are first registered and then a subtraction image is produced (Fig. 2d), it is clear that no significant changes have occurred in the brain although there are extracranial soft tissue changes.

3D fMRI

We have applied this methodology to a simple motor stimulation study that is similar to the work of Lai et al.

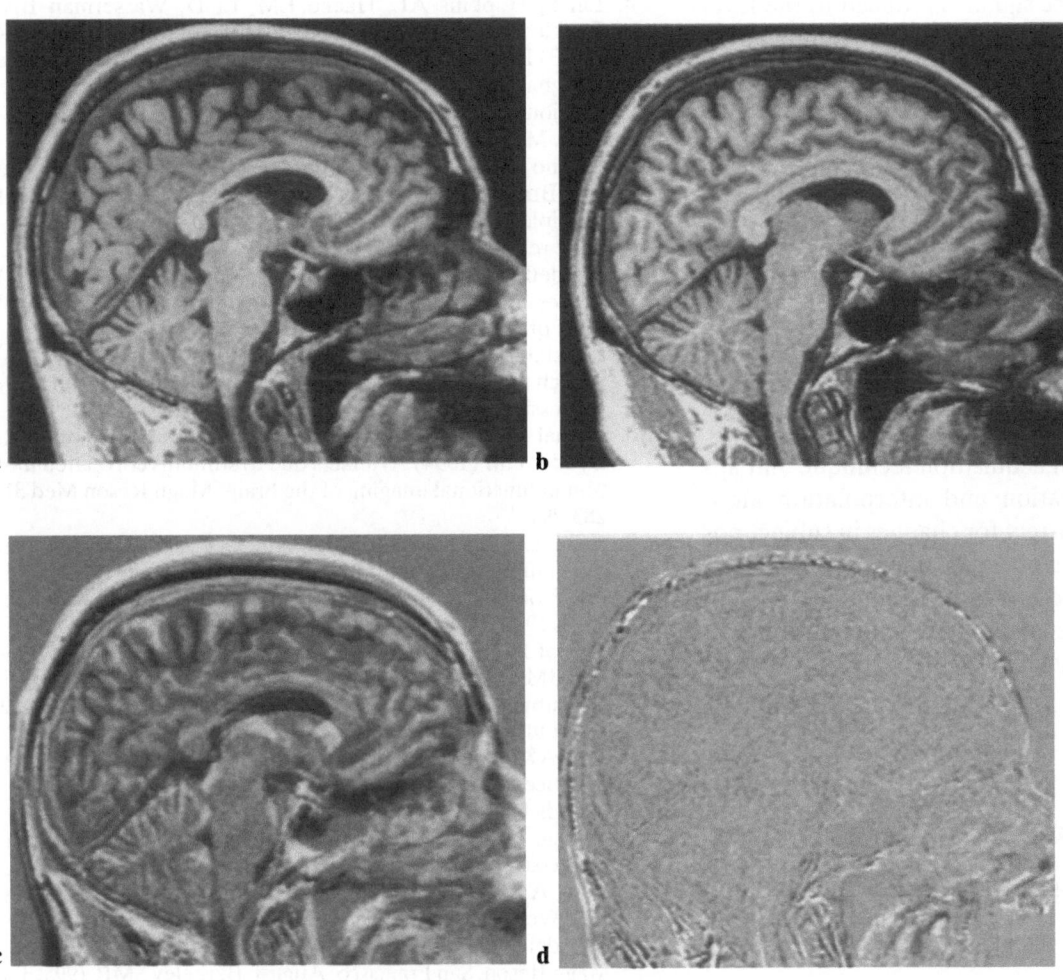

Fig. 2a-d. *Registration of true 3D images.* A subject was imaged twice with the same T1-weighted 3D sequence (TR 21 ms, TE 6 ms, 1.6 mm isotropic resolution). **a, b** Approximately matched slices from the two acquisitions, **c** a simple subtraction of **a** from **b**, and **d** a subtraction image obtained after image alignment using an automatic registration algorithm and sinc interpolation. Differences within the brain are reduced to approximately the noise level in **d**, but residual signals are seen from superficial soft tissue

[4]. Three-dimensional angio-sequences were acquired in which subjects exercised first with one hand for the duration of a complete scan and then with the other hand for the next scan and so on for six repetitions. The images were then all registered to one another and difference images and t-test maps were computed to look for significant changes.

Figure 3 shows an example of one slice extracted from the 40 partitions that made up a volume set. The anatomy is seen in Fig. 3a, with prominent draining veins on each side of the brain. The mean difference image, right hand activation minus left hand activation (Fig. 3b), shows a signal change in the left draining vessel. This is as might be expected. However after image

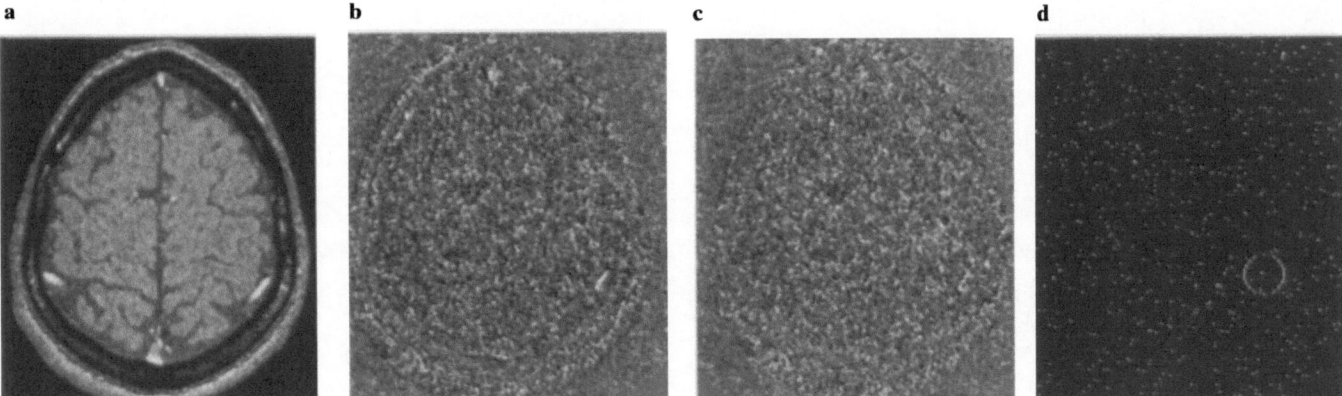

Fig. 3a-d. *A motor stimulation study and full positional registration.* (TR 40, TE 8, 20° flip angle, 192 × 180 × 40 matrix, 21 cm field of view (FOV) with 40 × 1 mm partition) **a** A representative anatomical slice shows two prominent draining vessels at the left and right of the brain. **b** A simple comparison between images acquired with right hand activation and left hand activation shows a signal increase in the left draining vessel. **c** After image registration the difference signal is reduced to approximately the noise level and **d** is not found to be statistically significant at the 5% level. The speckled appearance in **d** results from isolated random voxels that exceed the threshold of significance by chance

registration this difference signal is reduced to the level of the background noise (Fig. 3c) and is not significant at the 5% level (Fig. 3d). The speckled appearance in Fig. 3d arises from isolated random voxels that exceed the threshold for significant signal difference by chance.

Use of surface coils to locally improve signal-to-noise ratio also did not result in the detection of significant signals. In repeat examinations on five subjects with both enveloping and surface coils no significant signals that could be attributed to brain activation were detected.

Conclusion

With care in the choice of acquisition technique and appropriate use of registration and interpolation algorithms, it is possible to correct for changes in subject position without introducing unacceptable errors. However when this was achieved in a motor stimulation study, no significant activation signals could be identified in 10 examinations of five subjects.

References

1. Kwong KK, Belliveau JW, Chesler DA, Goldberg IA, Weisskoff RA, Poncelet BP, Kennedy DN, Hoppel BE, Cohen MS, Turner R, Cheng H-M, Brady TJ, Rosen BR (1992) Dynamic magnetic resonance imaging of human brain activity during primary sensory stimulation. Proc Natl Acad Sci USA 89: 5675-5679
2. Ogawa S, Tank DW, Menon R, Ellerman JM, Kim S-G, Merkle HH, Ugurbil K (1992) Intrinsic signal changes accompanying sensory stimulation: functional brain mapping with magnetic resonance imaging. Proc Natl Acad Sci USA 89: 5951-5955
3. Bandettini PA, Wong EC, Hinks RS, Tikofsky RS, Hyde JS (1992) Time course EPI of human brain function during task activation. Magn Reson Med 25: 390-397
4. Lai S, Hopkins AL, Haake EM, Li D, Wasserman BA, Buckley P, Friedman L, Meltzer H, Hedera P, Friedland R (1993) Identification of vascular structures as a major source of signal contrast in high resolution 2D and 3D functional activation imaging of the motor cortex at 1.5 T: preliminary results. Magn Reson Med 30: 387-392
5. Sereno MI, Dale AM, Reppas JB, Kwong KK, Belliveau JW, Brady TJ, Rosen BR, Tootell RBH (1995) Borders of multiple visual areas in humans revealed by functional magnetic resonance imaging. Science 268: 889-893
6. Bandettini PA, Jesmanowicz EC, Wong EC, Hyde JS (1993) Processing strategies for time-course data sets in functional MRI of the human brain. Magn Reson Med 30: 161-173
7. Constable RT, Skudlarski P, Gore JC (1995) An ROC approach for evaluating functional brain MR imaging and post-processing protocols. Magn Reson Med 34: 57-64
8. Hajnal JV, Myers R, Oatridge A, Schwieso JE, Young R, Bydder GM (1994) Artefacts due to stimulus correlated motion in functional imaging of the brain. Magn Reson Med 31: 283-291
9. Hill DLG, Simmons A, Studholme C, et al (1995) Removal of stimulus correlated motion from echo planar fMRI studies. Proc Soc Magn Reson (SMR) Third Annual Meeting, Nice, 19-25 August. Berkeley SMR: 840
10. Hajnal JV, Saeed N, Oatridge A, Soar EJ, Young IR, Bydder GM (1995) A registration and interpretation procedure for subvoxel matching of serially acquired MR images. J Comput Assist Tomogr 19: 289-296
11. Jain AK (1989) Fundamentals of digital image processing. Prentice Hall, Englewood Cliffs
12. Woods RP, Cherry SR, Mazziota JC (1992) Rapid automated algorithm for aligning and reslicing PET images. J Comput Assist Tomogr 16: 620-633
13. Jiang A, Kennedy D, Woods R, Baker J, Tootell R, Kwong KK, Weisskoff R, Belliveau J, Brady T, Rosen B (1994) Motion detection and correction in functional MRI. Proc Soc Magn Reson, San Francisco, August. Berkeley SMR 1995: 351
14. Risinger R, Hertz-Pannier L, Schmidt M, Maisog JM, Cuenod CA, Le Bihan D (1995) Evaluation of image registration in functional brain MRI. Proc Soc Magn Reson, San Francisco, August. Berkeley SMR: 649
15. Hajnal JV, Saeed N, Oatridge A, Williams EJ, Young IR, Bydder GM (1995) Detection of subtle brain changes using subvoxel registration and subtraction of serial MRI. J Comput Assist Tomogr 19: 677-691

Functional Magnetic Resonance Imaging Using Photic and Motor Stimulation: Comparison of Results Obtained at 1.0 T and 1.5 T

R. Wirestam[1], M. Bolling[1], O. Rudling[2], S. Brockstedt[1], P. Åkeson[3], S. Holtås[3], F. Ståhlberg[1, 3]

[1] Department of Radiation Physics, Lund University Hospital, [2] Department of Diagnostic Radiology, Helsingborg Hospital,
[3] Department of Diagnostic Radiology, Lund University Hospital, Sweden

Introduction

Since the demonstration of blood oxygenation level dependent (BOLD) contrast in magnetic resonance (MR) imaging at 7 and 8.4 T by Ogawa et al. in 1990 [1], the concept of functional magnetic resonance imaging (fMRI) has developed rapidly. Techniques of different complexity have been employed, ranging from conventional gradient echo imaging to advanced echo planar imaging, and a variety of applications have been suggested [2-4]. However, an accurate interpretation of observed BOLD effects in MR images is not always trivial, since the contrast mechanism reflects the combination of several parameters, for example, alterations in blood flow, blood volume, blood oxygenation and oxygen consumption. Furthermore, the possibility to correctly localize an activated region is hampered by the fact that larger vessels or draining veins can generate signal at a distance from the site of true tissue activation, and this large vessel signal contribution is not readily distinguishable from the signal arising from the capillary system within the tissue. In gradient echo imaging, the signal from the capillary system of the activated region is dominated by the T2*-sensitivity, while the signal from large vessels is likely to be a combination of susceptibility effects and inflow effects [3]. Theoretical modelling has suggested that the relative signal enhancement during stimulation ($\Delta S/S_0$) is the sum of a contribution from small vessels, showing a quadratic dependence on field strength, and a large vessel component with a linear dependence on field strength [5]. Consequently, experiments at different field strengths could provide further information on the origin of the fMRI contrast in gradient echo imaging. The aim of this study was to experimentally demonstrate activation of human visual and motor cortex at 1.0 T as well as at 1.5 T, and to investigate different aspects of the field strength dependence in fMRI using identical pulse sequences and identical volunteers at both field strengths.

Methods

The MR imaging units used in this study were a Siemens Magnetom Impact 1.0 T and a Siemens Magnetom Vision 1.5 T. Informed consent was obtained from all volunteers, after full explanation of the experimental procedure. Anatomical imaging and experimental procedures were similar to what was used in a previously presented investigation at 1.5 T [6]. Sagittal imaging for localization was performed using spin echo pulse sequences (echo time (TE) = 15 ms, repetition time (TR) = 300 or 650 ms). For registration of morphology in the slice selected for fMRI, a spin echo pulse sequence (TE = 15 ms, TR = 650 ms) was used. Statistical analysis was performed using stand-alone C programs, executed on a SUN Sparc 10 computer.

1. Activation of Visual Cortex

For the fMRI experiments, a gradient echo pulse sequence with TE = 60 ms, TR = 85 ms and a flip angle of 30° was used. The field of view was 300 × 300 mm², the slice thickness was 4 mm and the matrix size 128 × 128 or 190 × 256, giving a minimum voxel volume of 7.4 mm³. The slice was parallel to the long axis of the visual cortex. The acquisition bandwidth was 78 Hz/pixel, and in the readout and slice-selecting directions a three-lobe gradient structure was used to reduce motion artifacts from pulsatile CSF and intracranial vessel blood flow. Eight healthy volunteers (5 males and 3 females, 24-49 years old) were investigated at 1.0 T as well as at 1.5 T, in supine position and with their heads carefully immobilized. For stimulation, constant white/yellow light was used, reflected by a mirror. Both eyes were stimulated simultaneously, and all stimulations were performed during a time interval of 110 s, followed by an equally long period of rest (5 images were acquired during each period). Totally, three activation periods and three rest periods were employed during each investigation. All images obtained during stimulation and all images obtained during rest were averaged and the two resulting averaged images were subtracted to give a difference map. In order to identify pixels showing a statistically significant activation during stimulation, two statistical evaluation procedures were performed pixelwise on signal data from all volunteers: t-test and correlation. In the correlation procedure, measured signal was correlated to a function reflecting the stimulation pattern, i.e. a function given the value 0 during rest and the value 1 during stimulation. Within a large region-of-interest (ROI) including the visual cortex, the numbers of pixels considered to show significant activation during stimulation at 1.0 T and at 1.5 T were compared (t-test $p < 0.10$ or correlation coefficient $cc > 0.4$). Furthermore, for an equal number of significant pixels at both field strengths (i.e. the pixels showing the highest significance levels at 1.0 T and at 1.5 T, respectively), all signal values obtained during rest ($n = 15$ for each pixel) and all signal values obtained during stimulation ($n = 15$ for each pixel) were averaged, and the functional contrast-to-noise ratio $\Delta S/N$ was calculated. N denotes system and thermal noise and it was approximated by the signal standard deviation within a ROI outside the brain in one of the gradient echo images used for fMRI. The functional contrast-to-noise values from all volunteers, obtained at 1.0 T and at 1.5 T, respectively, were averaged, and the ratio of $\Delta S/N$ at 1.5 T to $\Delta S/N$ at 1.0 T was determined for the large ROI including the visual cortex. In order to gain information on the field strength dependence of physiological noise, the procedure was repeated for a large ROI in a non-activated region within the brain.

2. Activation of Motor Cortex

A gradient echo pulse sequence with TE = 56 ms, TR = 90 ms and a flip angle of 30° was used. The field of view was 300 × 300 mm², the slice thickness was 4 mm and the matrix size was 190 × 256. The slice was parallel to the orbitomeatal line, and positioned at the level of the motor cortex. A three-lobe gradient design for reduction of motion artifacts was used in the readout and slice-selecting directions, and the acquisition bandwidth was 19 Hz/pixel. Four healthy volunteers (3 males and 1

Table 1. Summary of results obtained for a large ROI including the visual cortex.

	1.0T		1.5T	
	T test	Correlation	T test	Correlation
No. of significant pixels	456 ± 311	248 ± 161	922 ± 544	598 ± 406
$\Delta S/N$	2.12 ± 0.79	2.04 ± 0.60	3.10 ± 0.90	3.06 ± 0.91

Given as mean ± 1 SD (n = 8). The numbers of significant pixels were obtained from the statistical analysis (p < 0.10 and cc > 0.4, respectively). The functional contrast-to-noise ratios $\Delta S/N$ were obtained using an equal number of significant pixels at both field strengths.

female, 24-31 years old) were investigated at 1.0 T and 1.5 T. During stimulation, the volunteer was asked to repeatedly touch the fingers (denoted 1-4) of his right hand with the thumb of the same hand. The thumb was touching the four fingers according to the following paradigm: "1-2-1-3-1-4-1-2-1-3-1-4-...". The stimulus was applied during a time interval of 115 s, and followed by an equally long period of rest. Similar to photic stimulation, each investigation consisted totally of three activation periods and three rest periods. The statistical evaluation and the calculation of functional contrast-to-noise effects at the two different field-strengths were also similar to the procedure described above for photic stimulation, although in this case significance levels of p < 0.05 and cc > 0.5 were used in the comparison of the number of significant pixels at the two field strengths.

Results

1. Visual Cortex

A summary of the results is given in Table 1. For the large ROI including the visual cortex, the ratios of sig-

a   b   c

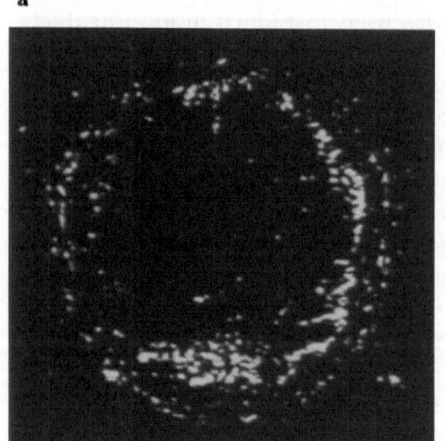 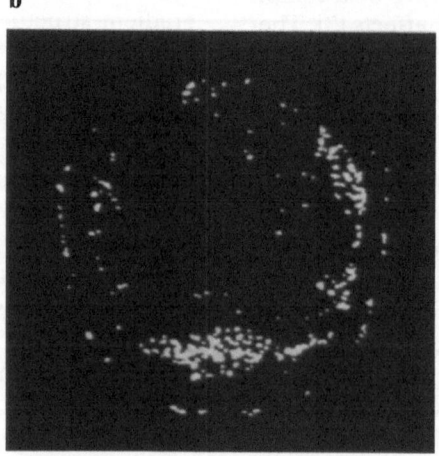 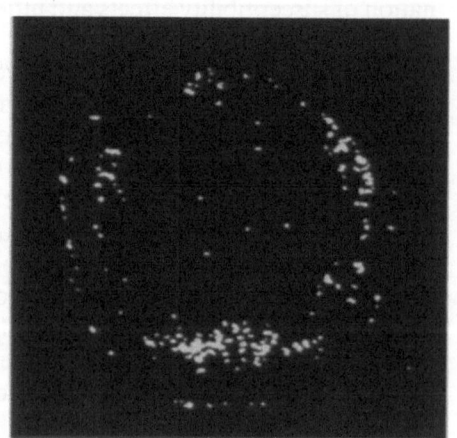

Fig. 1a-c. *Activation of visual cortex in a healthy volunteer at 1.5 T using a photic stimulation described in the text.* **a** Difference map obtained by averaging all images obtained during stimulation and all images obtained during rest, and subtracting the two averaged images; **b** Pixels displayed white were considered to show significant activation according to a t-test evaluation (p < 0.10); **c** Pixels displayed white were considered to show significant activation according to a correlation analysis (cc > 0.40)

Table 2. Summary of results obtained for a large ROI including the motor cortex.

	1.0 T		1.5 T	
	T test	Correlation	T test	Correlation
No. of significant pixels	66 ± 37	28 ± 18	186 ± 32	112 ± 37
$\Delta S/N$	1.77 ± 0.12	2.19 ± 0.31	4.04 ± 0.86	5.21 ± 1.09

Given as mean $\pm$ 1 SD (n = 4). The numbers of significant pixels were obtained from the statistical analysis ($p < 0.05$ and $cc > 0.5$, respectively). The functional contrast-to-noise ratios $\Delta S/N$ were obtained using an equal number of significant pixels at both field strengths.

nificant number of pixels at 1.5 T to significant number of pixels at 1.0 T were 2.03 (t-test) and 2.41 (correlation), and the ratios of $\Delta S/N$ at 1.0 T to $\Delta S/N$ at 1.5 T were 1.46 (t-test) and 1.49 (correlation). For comparison, $\Delta S/S_0$ was also calculated, and the 1.5-to-1.0 T ratio was approximately 1.9. For the large ROI in a non-activated region, the ratios of significant number of pixels at 1.5 T to significant number of pixels at 1.0 T were 1.50 (t-test) and 1.36 (correlation). The difference map from one volunteer is given in Fig. 1a, and corresponding maps showing pixels with a significant activation during stimulation are given in Fig. 1b (t-test, $p < 0.10$) and Fig. 1c ($cc > 0.4$).

2. Motor Cortex

A summary of the results is given in Table 2. For the large ROI including the motor cortex, the 1.5-to-1.0 T ratios regarding number of significant pixels were 2.80 (t-test) and 3.99 (correlation), and the 1.5-to-1.0 T ratios of $\Delta S/N$ values were 2.29 (t-test) and 2.38 (correlation). For comparison, $\Delta S/S_0$ was calculated, and the 1.5-to-1.0

T ratio was approximately 0.9. For the large ROI in a non-activated region, the ratios of significant number of pixels at 1.5 T to significant number of pixels at 1.0 T were 1.01 (t-test) and 1.35 (correlation). Motor-cortex activation at 1.0 T and 1.5 T, in one volunteer, is illustrated in Fig. 2.

Discussion

The results on field strength dependence presented in this report can be compared with previous studies [7-10]. As expected, BOLD contrast appeared more clearly at 1.5 T. For example, the number of pixels showing a significant activation was approximately a factor of 2 to 4 higher at 1.5 T than at 1.0 T. Regarding the number of significant pixels, a slight increase with field strength was indicated also in the non-activated region, and this observation might be related to a rather obvious field strength dependence seen for physiological noise [3, 11]. Although an unexpectedly low ratio of $\Delta S/S_0$ at 1.5 T to $\Delta S/S_0$ at 1.0 T was observed in the motor-cortex activation study, an obvious field strength dependence was seen in $\Delta S/N$. In the functional contrast-to-noise parameter, N is representing only system and thermal noise. Assuming that S_0/N of the systems used increased approximately linearly with field strength and that $1/T2^*$ of the tissue itself showed somewhere between a zero and first order dependence on field strength [11], it is not unreasonable for the functional contrast-to-noise ratio $\Delta S/N$ to show somewhere between a linear and a third order dependence on field strength, depending on the relative contributions from large and small vessels. For visual cortex, the ratio $(\Delta S/N)_{1.5T}/(\Delta S/N)_{1.0T} \approx 1.5$, obtained in the present study, is very close to $(1.5/1.0)^1$, while for motor cortex the obtained ratio $(\Delta S/N)_{1.5T}/(\Delta S/N)_{1.0T} \approx 2.3$ is close to $(1.5/1.0)^2 = 2.25$.

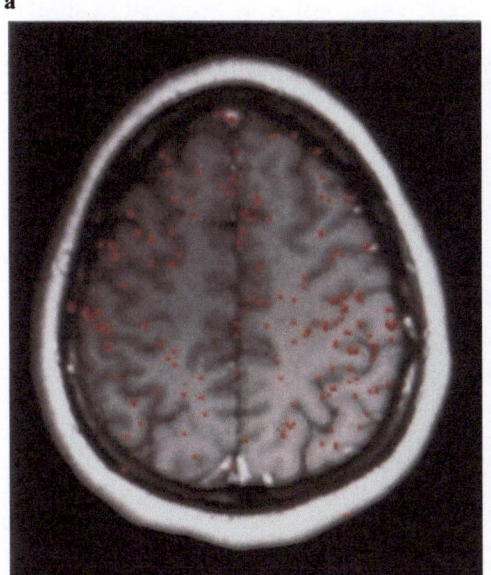
a

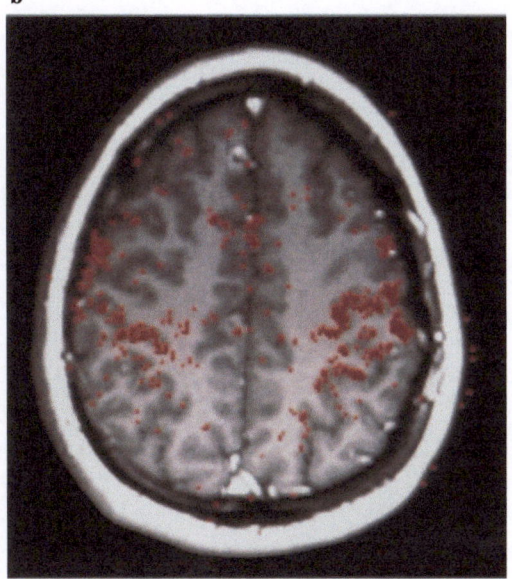
b

Fig. 2. a Functional MR imaging of activated motor cortex in a healthy volunteer at 1.0 T using a paradigm described in the text. Pixels displayed red showed a correlation coefficient $cc > 0.45$ in a correlation analysis used for identification of significantly activated voxels; **b** Corresponding results in the same volunteer at 1.5 T ($cc > 0.45$). Observed activation not only of left motor cortex, but also of right motor cortex and supplementary motor cortex is probably related to the complexity of the finger-movement paradigm used [12]

Obviously, the presented material is small, the noise is not fully characterized and the effects of altered relaxation times with field strength were neglected, but the results might nevertheless indicate that, in our experiments, the BOLD contrast observed in visual cortex was more influenced by large vessels than what was the case in the motor-cortex activation study. Finally, it is concluded that functional MRI can be performed at 1.0 T with reasonable results, although with a lower accuracy than at higher field strengths.

References

1. Ogawa S, Lee T-M, Nayak AS, Glynn P (1990) Oxygenation-sensitive contrast in magnetic resonance image of rodent brain at high magnetic fields. Magn Reson Med 14: 68
2. Frahm J, Merboldt K-D, Hänicke W (1993) Functional MRI of human brain activation at high spatial resolution. Magn Reson Med 29: 139
3. Kwong KK (1995) Functional magnetic resonance imaging with echo planar imaging. Magn Resonance Q 11: 1
4. Le Bihan D (ed) (1995) Diffusion and perfusion magnetic resonance imaging. Applications to functional MRI. Raven, New York
5. Ogawa S, Menon RS, Tank DW, Kim S-G, Merkle H, Ellermann JM, Ugurbil K (1993) Functional brain mapping by blood oxygenation level-dependent contrast magnetic resonance imaging. Biophys J 64: 803
6. Henriksen O, Larsson HBW, Ring P, Rostrup E, Stensgaard A, Stubgaard M, Ståhlberg F, Søndergaard L, Thomsen C, Toft P (1993) Functional MR imaging at 1.5 T. Initial results using photic and motoric stimulation. Acta Radiol 34: 101
7. Turner R, Jezzard P, Wen H, Kwong KK, Le Bihan D, Zeffiro T, Balaban RS (1993) Functional mapping of the human visual cortex at 4 and 1.5 tesla using deoxygenation contrast EPI. Magn Reson Med 29: 277
8. McKenzie CA, Drost DJ, Carr TJ (1994) The effect of magnetic field strength on signal change $\Delta S/S$ in functional MRI with BOLD contrast. Proc II Soc Magn Reson, p. 433
9. Bandettini PA, Wong EC, Jesmanowicz A, Prost R, Cox RW, Hinks RS, Hyde JS (1994) MRI of human brain activation at 0.5 T, 1.5 T, and 3.0 T: Comparisons of $\Delta R2^*$ and functional contrast to noise ratio. Proc II Soc Magn Reson, p. 434
10. Gati JS, Menon RS, Ugurbil K, Rutt BK (1995) Experimental determination of the BOLD field dependence in tissue and vessels. Proc III Soc Magn Reson, p. 771
11. Menon RS, Kim S-G, Hu X, Ogawa S, Ugurbil K (1995) Functional MR imaging using the BOLD approach. Field strength and sequence issues. In: Le Bihan D (ed) Diffusion and perfusion magnetic resonance imaging. Applications to functional MRI. Raven, New York, pp 327-334
12. Umeda M, Tanaka C, Ebisu T, Fukunaga M, Aoki I, Higuchi T, Naruse S (1995) Comparison of supplementary motor area activation between simple and complex motor task. Proc III Soc Magn Reson, p. 1326

Functional Activity Mapping of the Perirolandic Cortex During Motor Performance and Motor Imagery

C.A. Porro[1], V. Cettolo[2], M.P. Francescato[1], M.E. Diamond[1], P. Baraldi[3], C. Zuiani[2], M. Bazzocchi[2]

[1] Dipartimento Scienze Tecnologie Biomediche, Università di Udine, Via Gervasutta 48, I-33100 Udine, [2] Cattedra di Radiologia, Università di Udine, Policlinico Universitario, Piazza S. Maria della Misericordia, I-33100 Udine - [3] Dipartimento di Scienze Biomediche, Università di Modena, Via Campi 287, I-41100 Modena, Italy

Introduction

The development of noninvasive magnetic resonance imaging (MRI) techniques sensitive to the local changes of blood flow, volume, and oxygenation which accompany neuronal activation has provided the scientific community with a new and powerful tool for investigating the spatio-temporal dynamics of human brain function [1,2]. One of the most exciting application of brain mapping techniques, such as single photon emission tomography (SPET), positron emission tomography (PET), and functional MRI (fMRI) is the study of neural correlates of mental activity, such as the internal representation of sensory events or motor acts. It is still debated to what extent brain networks activated during mental rehearsal of, for instance, a visual scene or a motor sequence (visual or motor imagery) overlap those involved in the perception of visual stimuli or the preparation and execution of motor acts, respectively [3]. With regard to the motor system, the results of previous SPET and PET studies have demonstrated the activation of higher-order motor areas (such as the supplementary motor cortex) during motor imagery, whereas no change was found in the primary sensory-motor cortex [4]. However, the relatively poor spatial resolution of the employed techniques may have prevented the detection of areas characterized by less intense activation. The present study was therefore undertaken to evaluate by high-resolution fMRI the activity pattern of the perirolandic region (including pre- and postcentral gyri) during execution and imagery of a sequential motor task.

Methods

Twelve healthy right-handed volunteers (4 males, 8 females, aged 20-39 years) were studied. All gave their informed consent for the procedure, and none had a history of neurological disease. MR imaging was performed on a Magnetom SP 4000 (Siemens, Erlangen, Germany) superconducting 1.5 T whole body MR equipment, using a standard circularly polarized head coil. Field homogeneity was adjusted by a global shimming procedure for each subject, with typical line widths of about 20 Hz. To locate the pre- and postcentral gyri, multislice T1-weighted spin echo sagittal, axial, and coronal images (repetition time (TR) = 600 ms; echo time (TE) = 15 ms) were acquired. Two adjacent oblique planes between axial and sagittal planes were then defined along the central sulcus of the left hemisphere, covering the gray matter at the convexity of the pre- and postcentral gyri and the depth of the central sulcus, respectively. The anatomy of the two selected planes was shown on T1-weighted images (field of view (FOV) = 220 mm; 256×256 matrix; slice thickness = 4 mm). For the activation studies, the selected planes were imaged using a gradient echo fast low angle shot (FLASH) sequence (TR = 91 ms, TE = 60 ms, flip angle = 40°; 128×128 matrix; same FOV and slice thickness as in the corresponding anatomic images), sensitive to T2* relaxation rates. The FLASH images were interpolated to and displayed as a 256×256 matrix. Total single scan time for one slice was 14 s. Head motion during the experiments was minimized by an adjustable headholder.

Each subject performed three different tasks sequentially: mental representation of a stationary visual scene (visual imagery-VI), mental representation of self-paced, sequential finger-to-thumb opposition movements of the right hand at a frequency of about 2 Hz (motor imagery-MI), and actual execution of the same motor sequence (motor performance-MP). Visual imagery was assumed as a reference state to control for aspecific effects related to mental imagery. A total of 36 images (12 for each test) was acquired for each plane of interest over a period of about 10 min. Functional images were aligned by a software procedure implemented by R. Cox and based on a previously described algorithm [5]. In order to evaluate the intensity and time profile of signal changes, data were normalized in every subject and for each pixel by dividing the actual value in each image by the mean signal intensity of the same pixel in the 12 images acquired during the control (visual imagery) condition. Mean val-

Precentral Gyrus

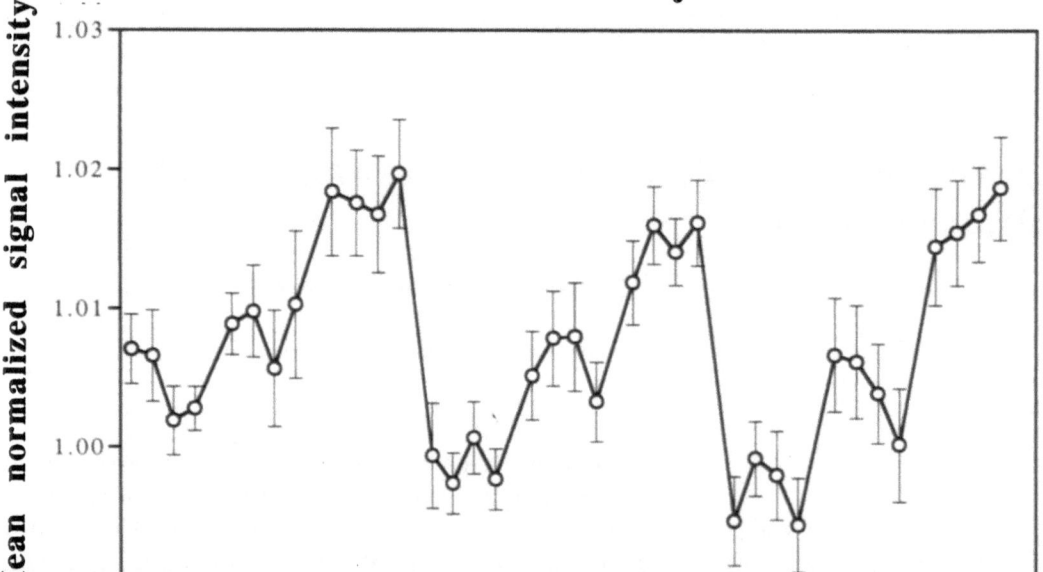

Fig. 1. *Time course of mean signal changes in the precentral gyrus (PreCG) during the execution of the three tasks.* Dynamic data sets were acquired in blocks of 4 images, each lasting 14×4 = 56 s. Subjects started the execution of the next task immediately after the end of each block; the acquisition of functional data, however, began 12 s later to avoid the hemodynamic changes occurring during the transition periods. Each point represents the mean ± S.E.M. (n = 12) of the normalized value of all pixels within the PreCG in one image

Visual imagery

Motor imagery

Motor performance

ues of signal intensity of all pixels lying within the precentral gyrus (PreCG) and postcentral gyrus (PostCG) were then calculated, and the results analyzed by repeated-measures analysis of variance (ANOVA). To locate activated foci during MI and MP, the signal time courses in each pixel were correlated with a box-car waveform [6], thus creating statistical maps based on correlation coefficients (possible range -1 to 1) comparing MI/VI and MP/VI, respectively.

Results

The results of a combined ANOVA showed that mean normalized signal intensity was higher in PreCG than in PostCG (p < .01), and that it was differently modulated in the two regions during the three tasks (Task: p < .001; Task by Region: p < .005). The mean signal time course in the precentral gyrus is shown in Fig. 1. Higher values were found both during the execution of the finger tap-

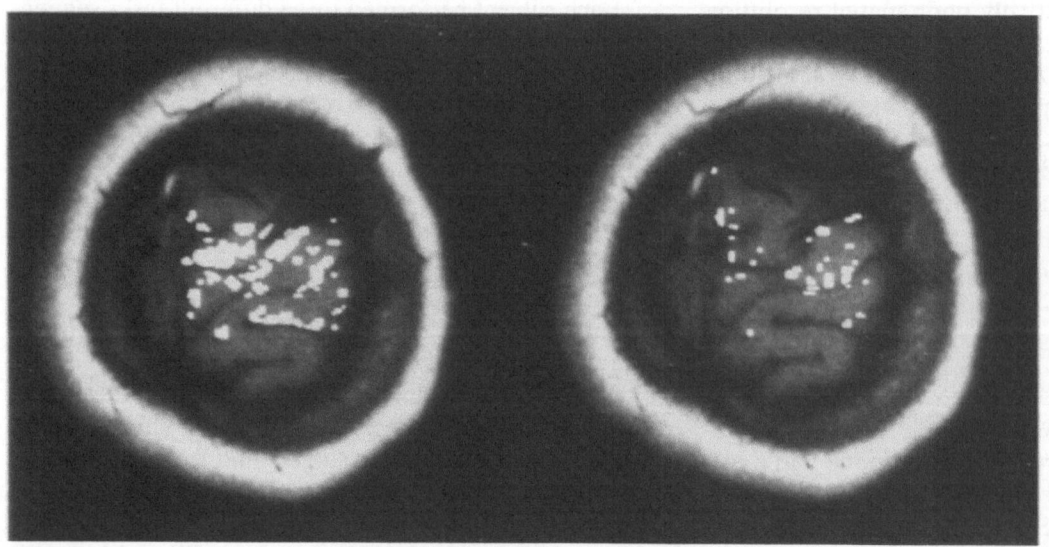

Fig. 2. *Representative statistical maps, overlaid on T1-weighted anatomic images of oblique planes along the left central sulcus, showing the location of activated points (r > .625) in the perirolandic cortex of one subject.* Maps were created from functional images acquired during a sequential finger opposition task (*left*) or mental representation of the same motor sequence (*right*). In each image, *top* is anterior, *right* is lateral. Both the precentral and postcentral gyri display widespread activation during the actual movement. More discrete foci are activated in the precentral gyrus during motor imagery

ping task (MP: p < .001) and mental representation of the same motor sequence (MI: p < .05) than during the control (VI) condition; the mean percentage increases were approximately 1.60% during MP and 0.60% during MI. In the postcentral gyrus, a significant increase over control values was detectable only during actual execution of the motor task (about 0.7%; p < .01).

Representative statistical maps are shown in Fig. 2. Activated foci (r > .625) in the PreCG were found in all subjects during motor performance and in 9/12 subjects during motor imagery, corresponding values for PostCG being 11/12 (MP) and 7/12 (MI). In the entire subject population, the number of significantly activated voxels was higher in the PreCG than in the PostCG both during actual motor performance (mean activated volume, 550 vs. 290 mm^3, p < .001) and motor imagery (70 vs. 30 mm^3, p < .05). The postero-lateral region of the PreCG, including the rostral bank of the rolandic sulcus, and the antero-medial portion, extending towards the precentral sulcus, displayed a comparable number of activated voxels during MI, whereas the posterior region appeared more activated during MP (p < .05).

Discussion

The present results confirm and extend those of previous fMRI investigations on the pattern of functional activation of the contralateral perirolandic cortex during the execution of hand movements (e.g. [7,8]). The precentral area showed a greater activation, consistent with its role in motor control, whereas the less pronounced signal changes in the postcentral gyrus, corresponding to the primary somatosensory cortex, are likely to be related primarily to processing movement-related proprioceptive and mechanoceptive information. The involvement of the postero-lateral portion of the precentral gyrus, the likely location of the primary motor cortex, during motor imagery was not detected in previous fMRI investigations using echo planar imaging [8, 9], whereas in a recent PET study [10] only 2 out of 6 subjects showed blood flow increases at this site. Cortical activation-related changes in blood flow, blood volume, and oxygenation, the likely sources of T2*-weighted fMRI signals [1], occur predominantly in the thin (a few mm) gray matter layer. As previously discussed [11], a small voxel size (as obtained in the present study) is more likely to allow detection of small areas of activation or less intense signal changes, avoiding partial volume averaging with, for instance, the white matter underlying active foci.

Additional studies are required to further establish the source and significance of the observed signal changes. However, the observed activation of the primary motor region during motor imagery supports the hypothesis that mental representation of motor acts and motor programming are both distributed processes involving largely the same central neural circuits.

Acknowledgements

We thank R. Cox, Biophysics Research Institute, Medical College of Wisconsin, USA, for providing software for image registration and analyses. Supported by funds of Consiglio Nazionale delle Ricerche and Ministero Università Ricerca Scientifica e Tecnologica, Italy, and by a grant from Siemens Italia SpA to V.C.

References

1. Kwong KK (1995) Functional magnetic resonance imaging with echo planar imaging. Magn Reson Q 11: 1
2. Le Bihan D, Karni A (1995) Applications of magnetic resonance imaging to the study of human brain function. Curr Opin in Neurobiol 5: 231
3. Jeannerod M (1994) The representing brain: neural correlates of motor intention and imagery. Behav Brain Sci 17: 187
4. Roland PE (1993) Brain activation. Wiley, New York
5. Irani M, Peleg S (1991) Improving resolution by image registration. Comput Vision Graphics Image Process 53: 213
6. Bandettini PA, Jesmanowicz A, Wong EC, Hyde JS (1993) Processing strategies for time-course data sets in functional MRI of the human brain. Magn Reson Med 30: 161
7. Kim S, Ashe J, Georgopoulos AP, Merkle H, Ellermann JM, Menon RS, Ogawa S, Ugurbil K (1993) Functional imaging of human motor cortex at high magnetic field. J Neurophysiol 69: 297
8. Rao SM, Binder JR, Bandettini BS, Hammeke TA, Yetkin FZ, Jesmanowicz A, Lisk LM, Morris GL, Mueller WM, Estkowski LD, Wong EC, Haughton VM, Hyde JS (1993) Functional magnetic resonance imaging of complex human movements. Neurology 43: 2311
9. Sanes JN, Stern CE, Baker JR, Kwong KK, Donoughe JP, Rosen BR (1993) Human frontal motor cortical areas related to motor performance and mental imagery. Soc Neurosci Abstr 18: 1208
10. Stephan KM, Fink GR, Passingham RE, Silbersweig D, Ceballos-Baumann AO, Frith CD, Frackowiak RSJ (1995) Functional anatomy of the mental representation of upper estremity movements in healthy subjects. J Neurophysiol 73: 373
11. Frahm J, Merboldt K-D, Hanicke W (1993) Functional MRI of human brain activation at high spatial resolution. Magn Reson Med 29: 139

BRAIN FUNCTIONAL ANATOMY AS ASSESSED WITH MRI: CLINICAL APPLICATIONS OF FUNCTIONAL BRAIN MRI

Basic Aspects of Magnetic Resonance Functional Neuroimaging: Physiology, Signals and Maps

J. Frahm, A. Kleinschmidt, G. Krüger, M. Requardt, K.D. Merboldt, W. Hänicke

Biomedizinische NMR Forschungs GmbH am Max-Planck-Institut für biophysikalische Chemie, Am Faßberg 11, 37077 Göttingen, Germany

Introduction

The noninvasive window on human brain "function" offered by magnetic resonance imaging (MRI) is based on the fact that functional challenge causes regional changes in perfusion and metabolism affecting blood flow, volume, and oxygenation [1]. This contribution deals with the detectability of pertinent phenomena by MRI and their use for high-resolution functional neuroimaging. In particular, it covers physiologic and physical aspects of image acquisition as well as strategies for data evaluation and paradigm design. Although a variety of techniques have been proposed to monitor changes in perfusion and metabolism, we will focus on gradient echo MRI sequences that are sensitized to changes in cerebral blood oxygenation (CBO) and thus allow mapping of neuronal activation.

Physiologic Aspects of Brain Activation

In a recent study using combined proton magnetic resonance spectroscopy and gradient echo MRI we have provided evidence for an initial prevalence of nonoxidative glycolysis in human visual cortex in response to a major increase in neural activity [2]. During such transitions blood flow and glucose uptake increase and show a physiologic "uncoupling" from largely unaffected oxygen consumption [3, 4]. In the aforementioned study we reconciled this observation with the classic understanding that perfusion and oxidative metabolism are stoichiometrically coupled [5] by demonstrating that with *sustained* visual stimulation the initially elevated MRI signal decreased toward pre-stimulus baseline. Since the interpretation of this observation as an upregulation of oxidative metabolism with a concomitantly enhanced oxygen consumption assumes that blood flow remains

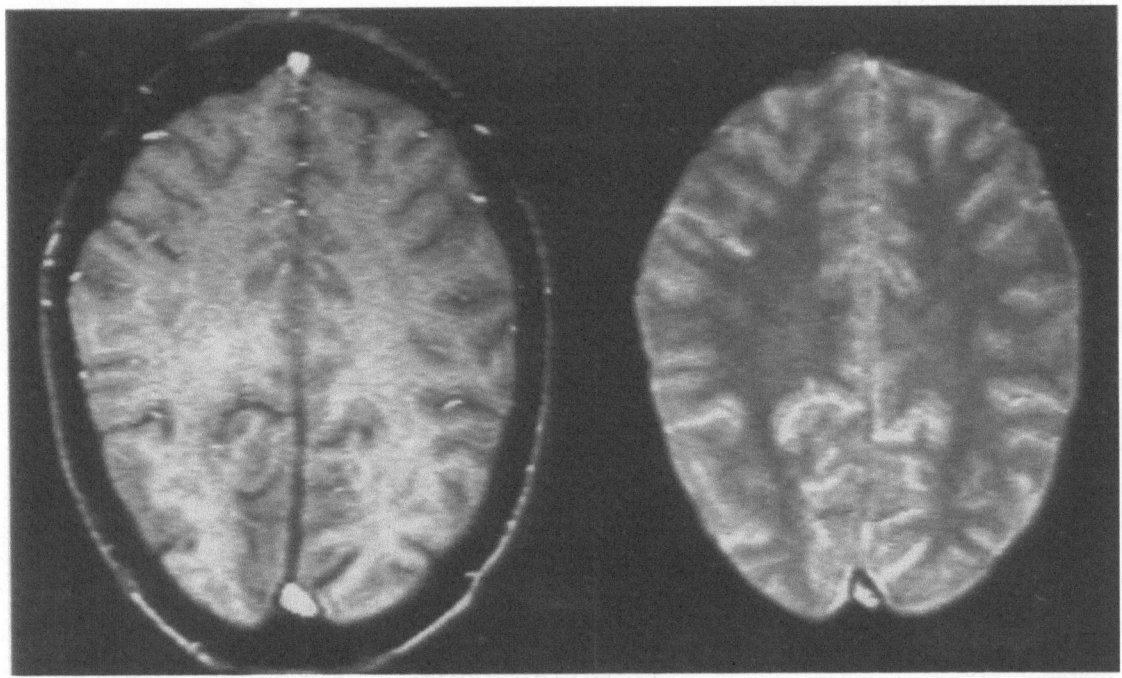

Fig. 1. *Rapid gradient echo MRI covering the calcarine cortex of a healty volunteer. Left Flow-sensitive acquisition using strong T1-weighting without T2* sensitivity (RF spoiled FLASH, TR = 62.5 ms, TE = 7.5 ms, flip angle 50°, inplane resolution 0.78 × 1.56 mm² interpolated to 0.78 × 0.78 mm², slice thickness 4 mm). Right CBO-sensitive acquisition using spin density weighting with T2* sensitivity (TE = 30 ms, flip angle 10°, other parameters as before)*

elevated throughout stimulation, additional experiments focused on changes in both regional CBO and blood flow using gradient echo MRI with respective contrasts.

All studies presented here were conducted at 2.0 T (Siemens Magnetom SP4000, Erlangen) and used a standard imaging headcoil. Visual stimulation involved a 6 min presentation of an educational video (color, no sound) using a specially designed MRI projection setup (Schäfter & Kirchhoff, Hamburg). In addition, subjects underwent a repetitive protocol comprising 6 cycles with 18 s of stimulation and 36 s of darkness each. Written informed consent was obtained in all cases. Dynamic CBO-sensitive radiofrequency-spoiled FLASH (repetition time TR = 62.5 ms, echo time TE = 30 ms, flip angle 10°) was performed using spin-density weighting with T2* sensitivity [6, 7]. Flow-sensitive recordings emphasized in-flow phenomena by means of strong T1 weighting and T2* insensitivity (TE = 7.5 ms, flip angle 50°).

Figure 1 shows corresponding T2*- and T1-weighted gradient-echo images used to dynamically monitor changes in CBO and blood flow, respectively. Figure 2 summarizes the mean responses to sustained visual stimulation from a group of 10 subjects [8]. In agreement with results obtained using a 10 Hz flickerlight [2], the CBO data reveal a rapid signal increase (hyperoxygenation) after stimulus onset and a subsequent signal decrease (relative deoxygenation) extending over 4-5 min. The end of stimulation yields a pronounced and rapid signal drop (deoxygenation) that mirrors the initial hyperoxygenation in magnitude and recovery time.

In contrast, the flow-sensitive data reveal a constant elevation of signal intensity due to inflow enhancement during sustained stimulation. Post-stimulus intensity shows no undershoot phenomenon. These findings support a model in which not only hemodynamic but also oxidative metabolic adjustments occur in response to functional challenge. Differences in their temporal evolution are responsible for both the initial hyperoxygenation and the deoxygenation at the end of stimulation. Figure 3 sketches the underlying sequence of events. The initial rise in perfusion (oxygen and glucose delivery) remains without a corresponding increase in oxygen consumption yielding a post-capillary oxygenation overshoot and CBO-sensitive MRI contrast. In the first 2-3 min, increased glucose consumption with transient lactate accumulation indicates enhanced nonoxidative glycolysis (uncoupling of perfusion and oxidative metabolism). After 4-5 min persistent elevation of blood flow and glucose consumption is progressively matched by an upregulation of oxidative metabolism that recouples oxygen consumption in a new steady-state and reduces CBO to near baseline values. Finally, terminating activation causes a rapid normalization in blood flow that yields a transient oxygenation undershoot due to the persistence and gradual attenuation of elevated oxygen consumption (transient negative uncoupling of perfusion and oxidative metabolism).

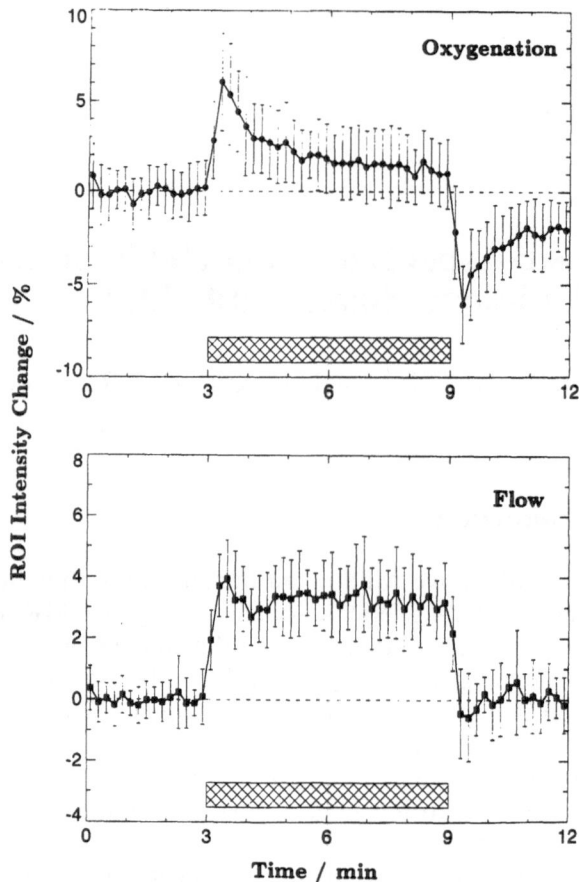

Fig. 2. *Normalized regional time courses of MRI signal intensities (12 s temporal resolution) sensitized to changes in CBO and blood flow.* 12 min protocol comprising 6 min of visual stimulation (cross-hatched bar). The values represent mean ± SD for 10 subjects in areas exhibiting stimulus-related signal alterations (primary visual cortex). (Reproduced with permission from [8])

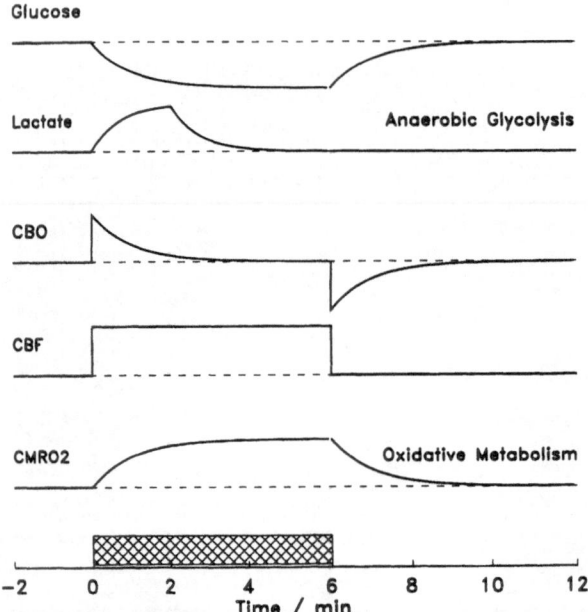

Fig. 3. *Schematic representation of the temporal evolution of hemodynamic and metabolic events associated with functional brain activation (cross-hatched bar).* For details see text (CBF = cerebral blood flow, CRM02 = cerebral metabolic rate of oxygen)

Table 1. The consequences of magnetic field inhomogeneities in a gradient echo image.

	Change in Field or Frequency Distribution	
MRI Gradient	Broadness	Mean
Frequency-encoding	Intravoxel Dephasing ($\rightarrow$ Signal Loss)	Echo Shift ($\rightarrow$ Image Distortion)
Phase-encoding	Intravoxel Dephasing ($\rightarrow$ Signal Loss)	Echo Shift ($\rightarrow$ Image Distortion)
Slice Selection	Intravoxel Dephasing ($\rightarrow$ Signal Loss)	Incomplete Refocusing ($\rightarrow$ Signal Loss)

Changes in broadness or mean of the underlying field or frequency distribution cause either signal loss or geometric distortions depending on the functionality of the MRI gradients [9].

Physical Aspects of MRI Data Acquisition

"Functional contrasts" in CBO-sensitive gradient echo MRI are due to regional and transient changes in the concentration of deoxyhemoglobin. Corresponding susceptibility effects represent alterations of the intravoxel magnetic field distributions. As indicated in Table 1, a change in magnetic field homogeneity may affect the broadness of the frequency distribution of nuclear spin moments in an image voxel and/or shift its mean value [9]. As far as frequency- and phase-encoding gradients are concerned, a change in distribution broadness causes an intravoxel signal loss, while a change in mean frequency only shifts the echo position along pertinent dimensions of the 2D data matrix ("k-space"). Depending on relative strengths this may lead to geometric distortions during image reconstruction but does not result in signal loss unless the gradient echo signal is shifted outside the acquisition window. Conversely, however, both changes in distribution broadness and mean value directly affect MRI signal intensity when present in the slice selection direction. While intravoxel dephasing is often even stronger than that which occurs in the frequency- and phase-encoding directions (as section thickness usually surpasses in-plane voxel dimensions), a mean frequency shift may easily preclude most spins from refocusing.

Intravascular susceptibility changes in human brain that are associated with activation-related changes in deoxyhemoglobin concentration alter both the broadness and the mean of the frequency distribution of affected spins. Although the relative importance of respective MRI signal changes depends on a large number of unknown variables, the slice selection process is expected to be particularly sensitive as it benefits from both intravoxel dephasing and incomplete slice refocusing. These considerations should be taken into account when optimizing volume coverage in CBO-sensitive functional brain mapping. For example, multislice ap-

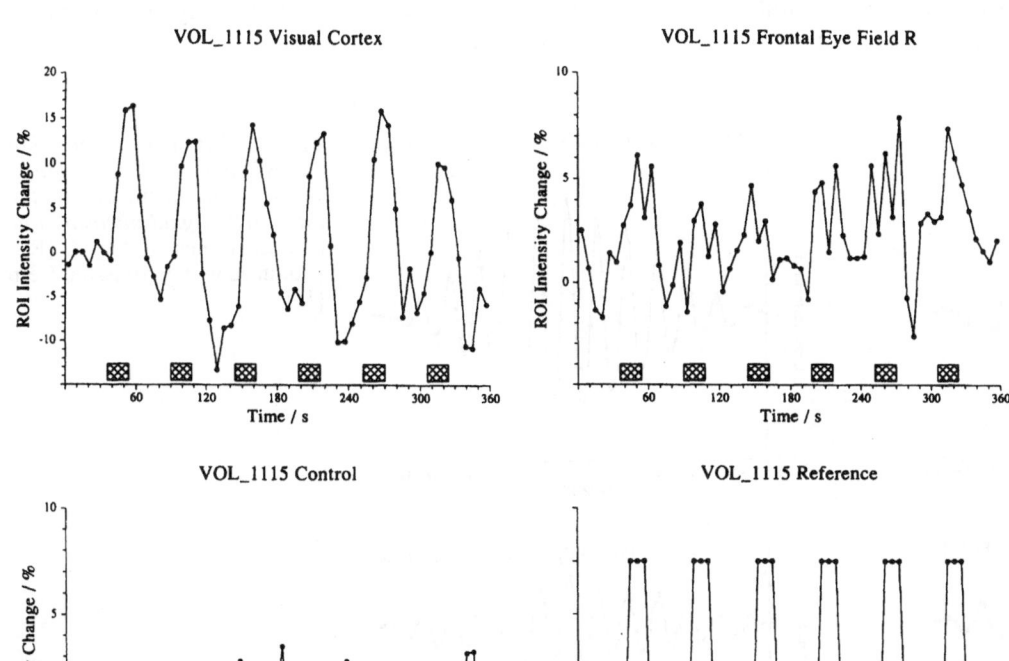

Fig. 4. *Normalized regional time courses of MRI signal intensities (6 s temporal resolution) sensitized to changes in CBO during a repetitive protocol. The protocol comprised 6 periods of 18 s of visual stimulation (cross-hatched bar). The data are representative for strong (visual cortex), weak (frontal eye field), and putatively lacking responses (centroparietal gray matter). The reference wave form used for correlational analysis is time-shifted relative to the protocol by one image (6.0 s) to account for latencies and rise times. (Reproduced with permission from [11])*

proaches are likely to be preferable over three-dimensional MRI, since both the two- and three-dimensional phase-encoding gradients at least partially compensate for magnetic field inhomogeneities by echo shifts in data space.

In contrast to the macroscopic nature of most structurally induced susceptibility differences, e.g. at air-tissue interfaces, the deoxyhemoglobin-induced magnetic field variations around the microvasculature are microscopic in nature and well below the size of a typical MRI voxel. This is not only advantageous for defining functional anatomy at high spatial resolution [6], but also helpful in reducing macroscopic susceptibility artifacts by decreasing voxel sizes. Finally, functional contrasts are also affected by the strength and shape of the imaging gradients and are sensitive to involuntary subject motion. Suitable strategies that desensitize MRI sequences with respect to motion (and flow) range from motion-compensating gradient waveforms and navigator echoes to the recording of low flip angle gradient echo images with relatively long repetition times as used here.

Data Evaluation and Functional Mapping

The definition of "activation" by analysis of the temporal and spatial characteristics of stimulus-related MRI signal alterations represents a crucial issue. Figure 4 shows representative signal time courses for a repetitive stimulation protocol as described above. The data originate from the primary visual cortex, the right frontal eye field, and an unaffected control region. Although averaging across functional states (here flickerlight versus darkness) and subsequent pixel-by-pixel subtraction of signal intensities would result in a map highlighting areas of strong responses, sensitivity can be considerably improved by exploiting the temporal characteristics of the dynamic data [10]. For example, effective strategies correlate signal time courses with either themselves (auto-correlation) or a reference vector (cross-correlation) that represents the stimulus protocol, a suitable hemodynamic model function, or any other waveform including internal signal time courses.

As shown in Fig. 5 (left column), the auto-correlation function simply asks for periodic signal fluctuations irrespective of their phase relationship to the stimulation protocol. Phase information may be preserved when computing cross-correlation functions of signal time courses (Fig. 5, right column) with a reference waveform similar to that shown in Fig. 4 (bottom right). Both sensitivity of the cross-correlation function and potential relevance of phase information are illustrated by the fact that a regional time course displaying no obvious response by auto-correlation analysis (Fig. 5, bottom left) appears weakly but clearly modulated by the stimulation protocol (Fig. 5, bottom right). However, despite a periodicity similar to that of functional responses, these correlations are phase-shifted relative to the protocol and represent inverse modulations or relative MRI signal decreases during stimulation. While such observations are not necessarily neurobiologically meaningful (e.g., hemodynamic epiphenomena), they may be important for a deeper understanding of signal physiology in functional brain studies.

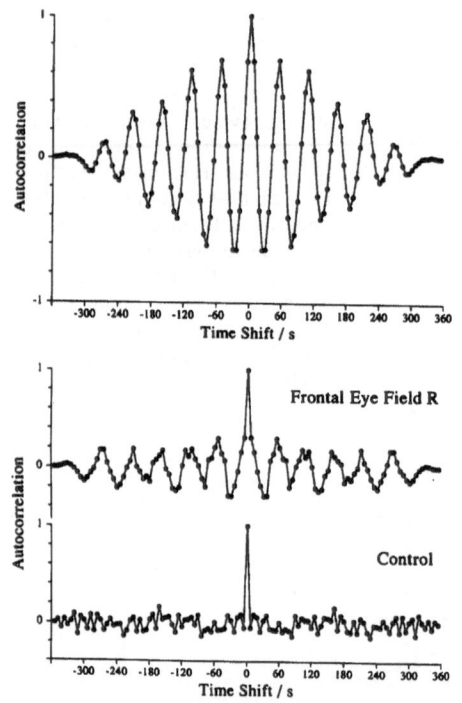

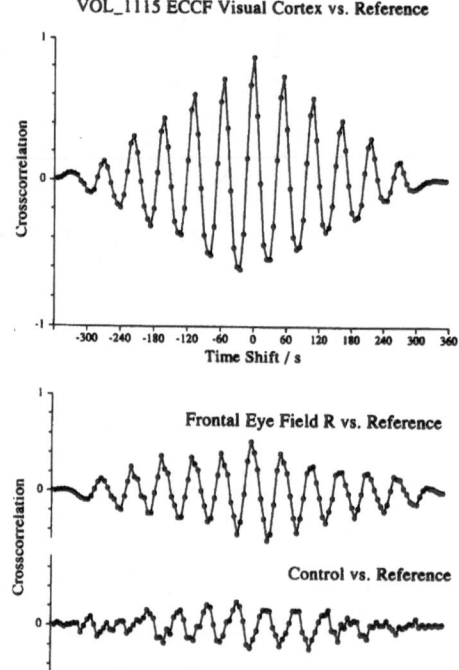

Fig. 5. *Auto-correlation (left traces) and cross-correlation functions (right traces) for the three MRI signal intensity time courses shown in Fig. 4. (Reproduced with permission from [11])*

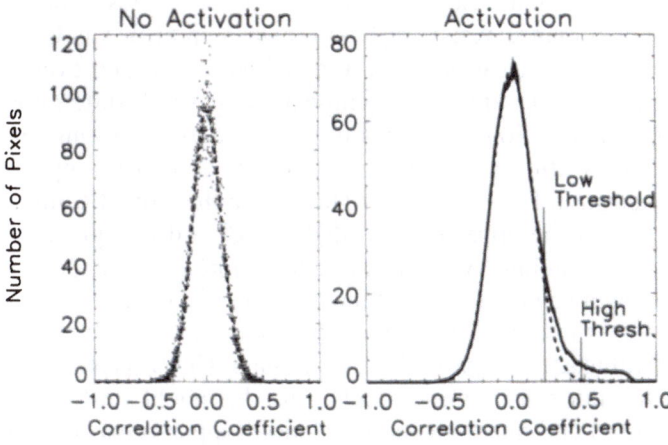

Fig. 6 *Image distributions of correlation coefficients (values of cross-correlation function at zero time shift) from an analysis of dynamic CBO-sensitive MRI data sets without and with stimulation, respectively.* Reconstruction of a symmetrized noise distribution (dashed line) identifies a sub-population of activated pixels at high positive correlation coefficients. (Reproduced with permission from [11])

Several possibilities exist to reconstruct activation maps from correlation functions or their power spectra obtained after Fourier transformation. A particularly attractive approach exploits the center maximum of the cross-correlation function (at zero time shift) as its value represents the well-known correlation coefficient. This simplest form of correlation analysis results in a map of correlation coefficients that qualify activation by the temporal response pattern rather than by the amplitudes of the dynamic MRI data set. While correlation coefficients close to zero describe signal fluctuations unrelated to activation ("correlational noise"), high positive values represent pixels with a strong temporal correlation between actual signal changes and an ideal response to the stimulus protocol as given by the reference waveform. It should be emphasized, however, that the use of fixed correlation coefficients as thresholds for defining statistically significant activation is precluded by intertrial variability.

A more flexible though still largely empirical strategy emerges from the example shown in Fig. 6 which compares distributions of correlation coefficients that were obtained from dynamic MRI data sets acquired in the absence and presence of visual stimulation. Without visual stimulation the distribution is symmetrically centered around zero and may be approximated by a Gaussian function. In the presence of activation, the distribution broadens (solid line) and turns asymmetric due to the occurrence of high positive correlations in a comparatively small number of pixels. Because the negative and central parts of the distribution are still well approxi-

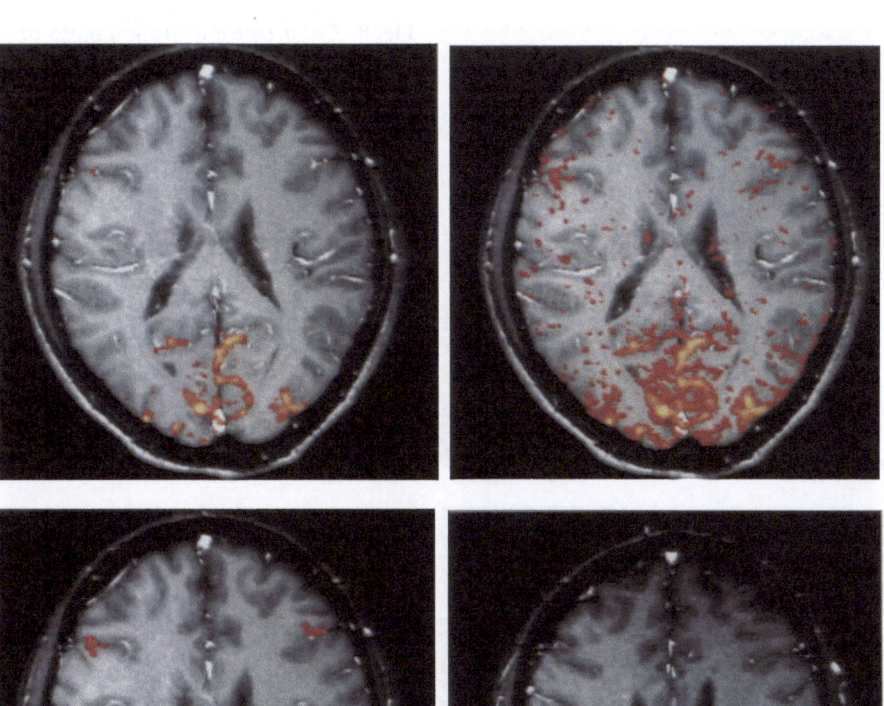

Fig. 7. *Color-coded activation maps of correlation coefficients that are noise-corrected and thresholded.* As outlined in Fig. 6 (same data). Combination of an upper threshold for specificity (*upper left*) and lower threshold for sensitivity (*upper right*) ensures both identification of activation foci and adequate response delineation (*bottom left*). Visual stimulation of the upper right (*coded in red*) and left quadrants (*coded in blue*) with persistent illumination of a central fixation field throughout stimulation and control states yields activation of anterior portions of the contralateral primary visual cortex (*bottom right*). (Reproduced with permission from [11])

mated by – though different – Gaussian functions (dashed line), invariance against intertrial differences may be achieved by introducing a symmetrized noise distribution for the whole range of correlation coefficients.

Rescaling of correlation coefficients into percentile ranks with respect to the integral of the noise distribution and selecting a high percentile rank as an upper threshold can then be used to define primary sites of activation. While a single threshold will always be subject to a trade-off between specificity (high threshold) and sensitivity (low threshold) as demonstrated in Fig. 7 (upper left and right), a comparison of both maps identifies pixels with very high correlation coefficients to be embedded within the enlarged areas of activation admitted at the lower threshold. Thus, adequate response delineation may be achieved by iteratively incorporating neighboring pixels into highly specific activation foci (Fig. 7, bottom left) provided their correlation coefficients are high enough to contribute to the positive deviation from the noise distribution.

Paradigm Design and Sensitivity

So far, most paradigms for MRI studies of brain activation employ gross differences between activated and control states such as visual stimulation versus darkness or motor performance versus rest. Although helpful in validating methodological progress in data acquisition and evaluation, such techniques may obscure more subtle differences in the functional anatomy of higher order processing that are of utmost neurobiologic interest. A first example is shown in Fig. 7 (bottom right) where flickerlight stimulation of the upper right (coded in red) and left quadrants (coded in blue) was compared to no flicker, while the paradigm included constant illumination of a central fixation field throughout activation and control states. Activation within anterior parts of the contralateral infracalcarine cortex not only revealed coding for hemifield (left versus right) and quadrant representation (upper versus lower), but also reflected retinotopic organization along the cortical band (peripheral versus central).

An even more impressive example stems from a study of color processing where we have mapped responses to selective stimulation of the parvo- and magnocellular visual pathways in calcarine and adjacent ventral occipital cortex [12]. Figure 8 demonstrates in a single subject that both color (upper left) and luminance modulation (upper right) induce widespread activation of occipital cortical areas when alternated with darkness. With steady light as a control condition, a much weaker pattern in calcarine cortex is retained for chro-

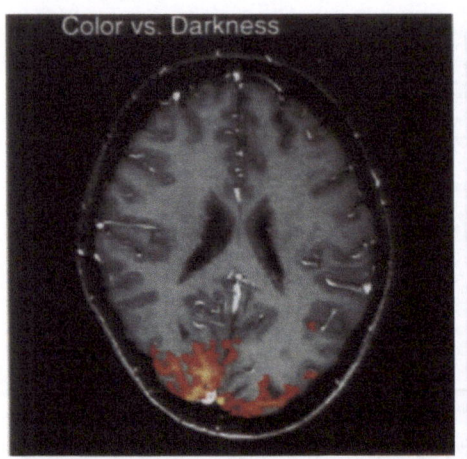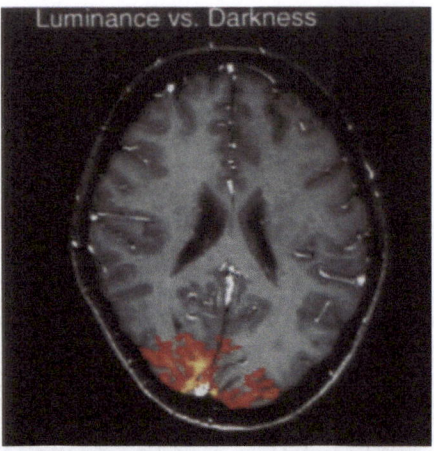

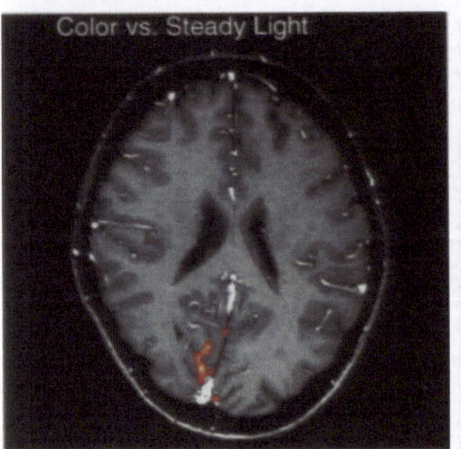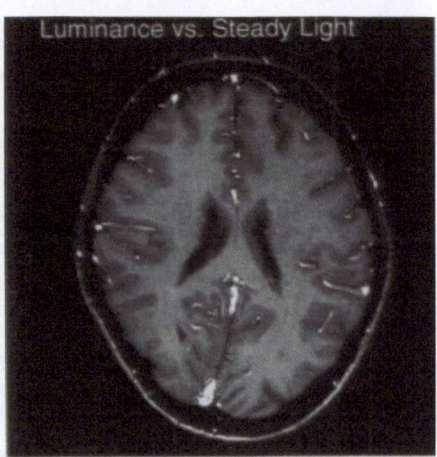

Fig. 8. *Color-coded activation maps of responses to selective stimulation of the parvo- and magnocellular visual pathways in calcarine cortex. Both color (upper left) and luminance modulation (upper right) induce widespread activation relative to darkness, whereas isoluminant steady light as a control condition results in a much weaker pattern for chromatic stimulation (bottom left) and no responses to luminance modulation (bottom right)*

matic stimulation (bottom left), whereas no responses to luminance modulation pass the conservative evaluation procedure (bottom right). Clearly, the use of refined paradigms without unspecific control conditions such as darkness not only attenuates putative contributions from arousal, attention, and cardiorespiratory changes, but also offers a more unambiguous assignment of responses to specific afferent pathways.

Finally, a recent perfusion-sensitive MRI study of finger movements versus rest concluded that the hand area of human primary motor cortex is not somatotopically arranged [13]. We addressed this issue by CBO-sensitive MRI during isolated finger movements alternated with either motor rest or a different finger task of the same hand [14]. When comparing motor performance with rest, our data confirmed substantial overlap of single finger representations along the posterior precentral gyrus. However, when directly switching between different motor tasks, an orderly pattern emerged that supports the classic concept of within-hand somatotopy in human primary motor cortex. In this case selection of a proper control condition helped to improve the sensitivity by probing predominance of task movement and thereby allowed detection of a *quantitative* rather than *qualitative* somatotopy.

Acknowledgements

A. Kleinschmidt is on leave from the Department of Neurology, Heinrich-Heine-Universität, Düsseldorf. Data analysis and figure preparation used the facilities of the Gesellschaft für wissenschaftliche Datenverarbeitung Göttingen.

References

1. Raichle ME (1987) The Nervous system. In: Mountcastle VB (ed.) Handbook of physiology, Sect. 1, Vol: 5. American Physiological Society, pp. 643-674
2. Frahm J, Krüger G, Merboldt KD, Kleinschmidt A (1996) Dynamic uncoupling and recoupling of perfusion and oxidative metabolism during focal brain activation in man. Magn Reson Med 35:143-148
3. Fox PT, Raichle ME (1986) Focal physiological uncoupling of cerebral blood flow and oxidative metabolism during somatosensory stimulation in human subjects. Proc Natl Acad Sci USA 83:1140-1144
4. Fox PT, Raichle ME, Mintun MA, Dence C (1988) Nonoxidative glucose consumption during focal physiologic neural activity. Science 241:462-464
5. Clarke DD, Sokoloff L (1994) Circulation and energy metabolism of the brain. In: Siegle GJ, Agranoff GW, Albers RW, Molinoff PB (eds) Basic neurochemistry, Raven, New York, pp. 645-680
6. Frahm J, Merboldt KD, Hänicke W (1993) Functional MRI of human brain activation at high spatial resolution. Magn Reson Med 29:139-144
7. Frahm J, Merboldt KD, Hänicke W, Kleinschmidt A, Boecker H (1994) Brain or vein – oxygenation or flow? On signal physiology in functional MRI of human brain activation. NMR Biomed 7:45-53
8. Krüger G, Kleinschmidt A, Frahm J (1996) Dynamic MRI of cerebral blood oxygenation and flow during sustained activation of human visual cortex. Magn Reson Med (in press)
9. Frahm J, Merboldt KD, Hänicke W (1995) The effects of intravoxel dephasing and incomplete slice refocusing on susceptibility contrast in gradient-echo MRI. J Magn Reson B 109:234-237
10. Bandettini PA, Jesmaniwicz A, Wong EC, Hyde JS (1993) Processing strategies for time-course data sets in functional MRI of the human brain. Magn Reson Med 30:161-173
11. Kleinschmidt A, Requardt M, Merboldt KD, Frahm J (1995) On the use of temporal correlation coefficients for magnetic resonance mapping of functional brain activation. Individualized thresholds and spatial response delineation. Intern J Imag Sys Technol 6:238-244
12. Kleinschmidt A, Lee BB, Requardt M, Frahm J (1995) Functional mapping of color processing by magnetic resonance imaging of responses to selective P- and M-pathway stimulation. Exp Brain Res (in press)
13. Sanes JN, Donoghue JP, Thangaraj V, Edelman RR, Warach S (1995) Shared neural substrates controlling hand movements in human motor cortex. Science 268:1775-1777
14. Kleinschmidt A, Nitschke M, Frahm (1996) Somatotopy in the human motor cortex and area (submitted)

In Vivo Verification of the Intravascular BOLD Effect

E.M. Haacke, S. Lai, J.R. Reichenbach, F. Hoogenraad, H. Takeichi, K. Kuppusamy, W. Lin

Mallinckrodt Institute of Radiology, Washington University, 510 S. Kingshighway, Saint Louis, MO 63110, USA

Introduction

There has been much controversy over the brain/vein debate in functional magnetic resonance imaging (fMRI). Low resolution studies create a broad pattern of signal enhancement upon brain activation which could be from brain or blurred vessels. Our goal is to validate the blood oxygenation level dependent (BOLD) model and its mechanisms in relation to blood flow and susceptibility changes. We investigate the visibility of small vessels in the brain using high spatial resolution. Flow-compensated sequences are used to obtain susceptibility information and velocity-encoded sequences to measure velocities.

Materials and Methods

1. Flow Measurements

To measure velocities in small vessels, we used a high resolution two-dimensional (2D) phase contrast (PC) sequence (slice thickness TH = 4 mm, in-plane resolution 0.55 μm × 0.55 μm) which collects two gradient echoes in an interleaved fashion. The first echo is acquired with flow compensation, the second echo with a bipolar gradient pair in slice selection to encode a specified velocity encoding value (VENC) value. Due to the available gradient strength of 25 mT/m, measurements with a short echo time (TE) of 40 ms and a VENC value as low as 1 cm/s are possible. A low bandwidth of 49 Hz/pixel was used to get a high signal-to-noise ratio (SNR). To minimize partial volume effects, the slice position was chosen perpendicular to the vessel of interest. The system was shimmed locally to avoid complex phase terms due to background field gradients. Using 4 acquisitions gave an SNR of 27:1.

A conventional finger tapping paradigm was used for the activation state in order to study flow changes in the pial draining vein(s) within the central sulcus [1]. The sequence was run for both resting and activation states. Subtracting the velocity-sensitized image from the flow-compensated one in each state showed many vessels yielding a map of small vessels. Subtraction of such a "vessel map" of the resting state from that of the activation state showed only a few vessels, demonstrating that very localized flow changes occur in association with the finger tapping task. Correspondingly, subtracting the flow-compensated image in the resting state from that in the activation state showed the same vessels, giving a very high resolution functional image.

2. Oxygenation Measurements

To extract oxygenation levels in vivo in veins phase images were acquired in the resting state using a three-dimensional (3D) FLASH sequence with first order flow compensation in all the three imaging directions. To avoid linear shifts in phase which are usually seen with asymmetric echoes, the sequence was designed to have a symmetric echo if no field inhomogeneity is present, since such linear phase shifts complicate the extraction of susceptibility and oxygenation levels. The imaging parameters were: repetition time (TR) = 135 ms, flip angle 15°, bandwidth = 98 Hz/pixel, field of view (FOV) = 256 mm × 256 mm, matrix size = 256 phase encoding steps × 512 sampling points, and 32 partitions of 1 mm thickness. Through-plane vessels larger than one pixel were chosen to minimize partial volume effects.

Three different echo times were run at 24, 48, and 72 ms, respectively, to extract constant background phase (ϕ_0), any remnant velocity terms from very tiny unshimmed gradients (G′) and the susceptibility-induced phase term itself. The value of the phase inside the vessels was fit to

$$\phi(\text{TE}) = \phi_0 + 2\pi\gamma\Delta B\text{TE} + \pi\gamma G' v\text{TE}^2 \qquad (1)$$

where γ = 42.58 MHz/T is the gyromagnetic ratio of the proton. To avoid possible ϕ_0 changes from scan to scan, the phase was normalized to that of the cerebrospinal fluid (CSF). All numerical values of ϕ_0, ΔB, and G′v were extracted for each measured vessel. The extracted

ΔB was attributed to the bulk susceptibility $\Delta \chi$ inside the vessel, which in turn was calculated from the following equation:

$$\Delta B = 2\pi \Delta \chi B_0 (\cos^2\theta - 1/3) \qquad (2)$$

where θ is the angle between the vessel and the static field. Here, θ was measured by following the spatial coordinates of the vessel in the consecutive slices in which it appeared.

Then the oxygenation level Y in the vessel was calculated from:

$$\Delta \chi (Hct, Y) = \Delta \chi_{do} Hct (1 - Y) \qquad (3)$$

where Hct is the hematocrit and $\Delta \chi_{do} = 0.18 \times 10^{-6}$ (in cgs units) is the susceptibility difference between deoxygenated whole blood and oxygenated whole blood [2]. We used Hct = 0.40 in the calculations.

3. Eliminating Signal from Blood

Two methods could be used to eliminate signal from blood. Blood signal can be dephased using a bipolar gradient or saturated using a 90° radiofrequency (RF) pulse in a thick slice adjacent to the slice being imaged. It is also possible to saturate blood from all regions around the motor cortex area with 4 saturation pulses. As a final check on the role of blood signal, both methods are applied to ensure suppression of blood signal.

Results

1. Flow Measurements

Generally, in the velocity difference images, many vessels are observed with velocities ranging from 2 cm/s to 8 cm/s through plane. The changes in velocity under activation are sometimes as large as 50% and can even reach 100%.

To demonstrate the role of flow enhanced BOLD, we first consider theoretically the signal response for through-plane flow (Fig. 1). Clearly, the signal response for blood depends on how many RF pulses it sees and the flip angle. For low flip angles, no flow (T1) effects remain and any signal changes will be BOLD alone (although still mostly from blood). For very rapid flow in the resting state, complete refreshment will occur. In the activation state, if flow increases, there will still be complete refreshment and flow will not contribute to the change in signal intensity $\Delta S = S_{act} - S_{rest}$. However, flow will give enhanced signal for BOLD and we call this "inflow enhanced BOLD".

To demonstrate this effect, Fig. 2 shows the experimental results obtained from a volunteer study. In this case a 2D FLASH sequence was used with TE = 40 and 60 ms, flip angle 90° and the TR was varied from 60 ms up to 400 ms. As one can clearly see there is a steep increase in the observed percentage signal change in the parameter regime where blood in the resting state has experienced one additional RF pulse, while blood in the

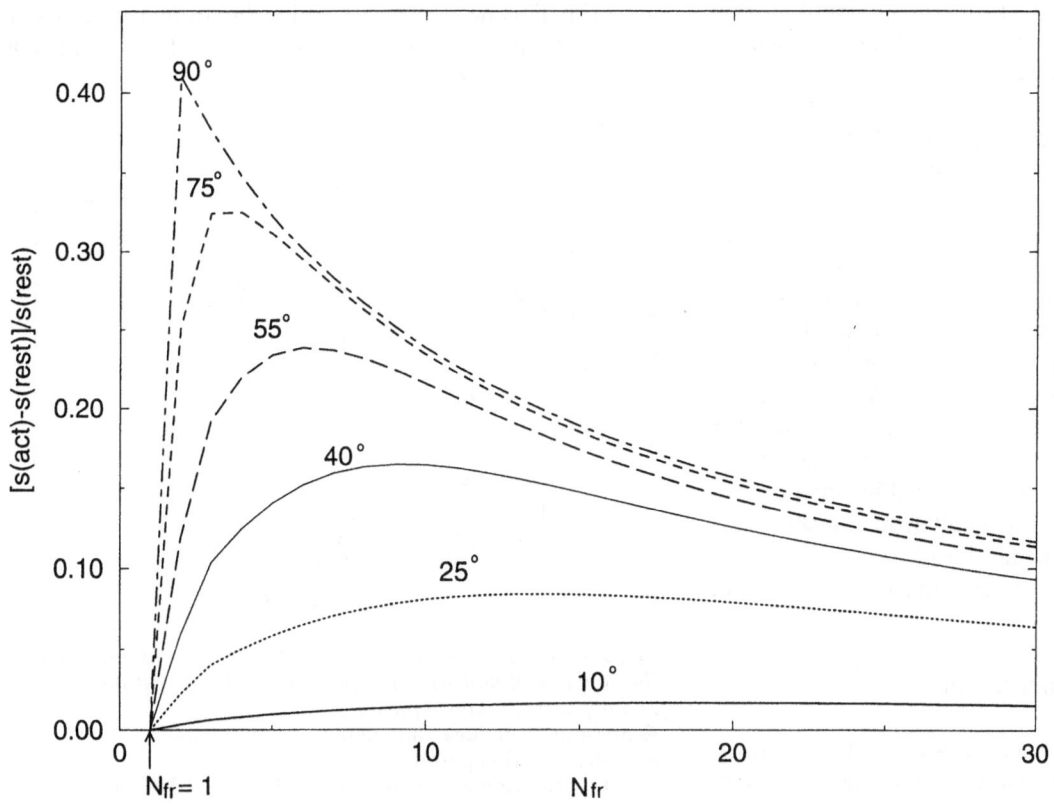

Fig. 1. Inflow effects for the relative signal change for different flip angles as a function of the number of RF pulses (N_{fr}) blood experienced in the resting state in the 2D gradient echo imaging slice. (N_{fr} = TH/(v · TR), where TH = slice thickness, v = velocity in the resting state, TR = repetition time). Plots are for through-plane flow. The flow velocity in the activation state is assumed to be 1.5v (a typical increase according to experimental results with PET and MRI), with v being the flow velocity in the resting state. Parameters used are: TR = 125 ms, T1 = 1200 ms. The plots show percentage signal change relative to the resting state. Note that when blood flows fast enough so that complete refreshment occurs ($N_{fr} < 1.0$), inflow induces no signal change

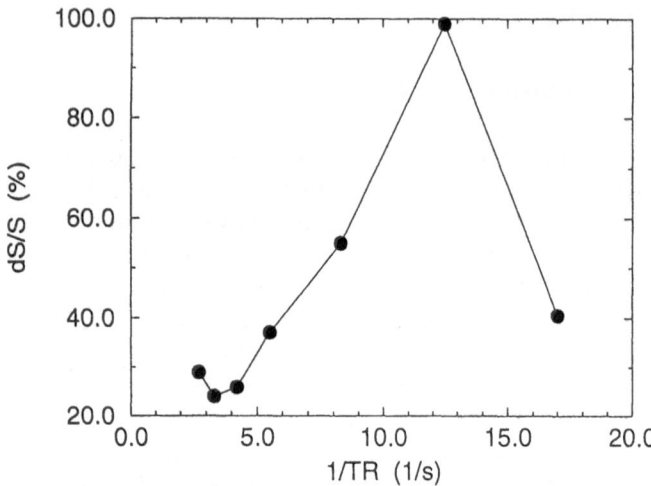

Fig. 2. *Experimental verification of the inflow-enhanced BOLD concept.* The signal changes are plotted versus the inverse of repetition time TR, which is proportional to the number of RF pulses blood experienced in the resting state

activation state has been mostly refreshed. Note the constant level of signal change of roughly 20% to 30% for TR values longer than 200 ms, which corresponds to the regime of flow enhanced BOLD mentioned above.

2. Oxygenation Measurements

We examined 14 vessels in five healthy male subjects. The value of blood susceptibility $\Delta\chi$ was found to be $\Delta\chi = 0.0328 \pm 0.0021$ ppm which leads to an in vivo value for the oxygenation level $\Delta\chi = 0.544 \pm 0.029$ averaged over the fourteen vessels. These results predict that blood signal in a vessel parallel to the static field will be 180° out of phase with gray matter at roughly TE = 60 ms at 1.5 T. The extracted $G'v$ value was found to be less than 1.0×10^{-6} T/s in all cases, proving that both shimming of the system and the flow compensation of the sequence were excellent.

At longer echo times (TE) each of the vessels appeared in the magnitude images as a bright spot surrounded by a dark ring. This can be explained by the fact that, due to the presence of paramagnetic deoxyhemoglobin the blood signal develops a phase angle deviating strongly from that of the surrounding tissues at longer echo times. Thus signal cancellation occurs for the edge voxels containing blood and brain parenchyma, while the center voxel remains visible since it contains only blood signal. (This cancellation vanishes with other increasing echo times as the phase of the blood signal once again gets closer to the phase value of brain parenchyma.)

3. Elimination of Signal from Blood

Last, in the low flip angle case we applied both saturation pulses and dephasing gradients and observed only

little signal changes in the corresponding fMRI images indicating that most signal is intravascular in nature. Figure 3 illustrates this behavior as a function of flip angle and shows the clear decrease in signal change upon application of saturation pulses. Applying only dephasing gradients did not completely eliminate the signal even for a VENC of 1 cm/s. Both together, however, basically give zero signal changes suggesting that fMRI changes are due to the blood signal itself.

Discussion and Conclusion

The results are encouraging in that the extracted values of $\Delta\chi$ and Y are consistent among different vessels in different volunteers. This confirms that with sufficiently high resolution measurements it is possible to extract in vivo oxygenation levels in blood. Care must be taken to ensure that no velocity or baseline phase contaminates the measurements and that the vessel is straight for a sufficient distance so that it can be regarded as an infinitely long cylinder. High resolution is necessary to avoid partial volume effects. For example, if veins were partially volumed, we found correspondingly smaller susceptibility values. 3D acquisitions allow the measurement of the angle θ between static magnetic field and vessel axis, which in turn makes it possible to extract $\Delta\chi$ precisely from Eq. (2). A further advantage of 3D acquisition is its high signal-to-noise ratio, which is crucial for accurate phase measurements. The successful extraction of blood oxygenation level in vivo will allow future measurements of changes in Y during brain activation [3]. This holds important implications for comparison of positron emission tomography (PET) and MR data for human studies.

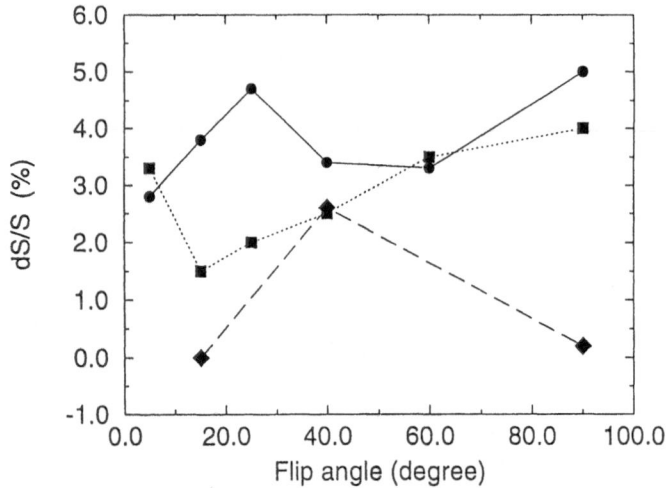

Fig. 3. *Percentage signal changes upon activation as a function of flip angle with and without application of RF saturation pulses and dephasing gradient pulses*
● no saturation pulses and dephasing gradients
■ with saturation pulses
◆ with saturation and dephasing gradients (VENC 1)

The fact that dephasing or saturation each only reduced the signal by roughly two-thirds of the original change from resting to activated state, but both together essentially eliminated the signal, suggests that slow flowing blood is not dephased even with low VENC values. One possible explanation is that capillaries and/or venules do not always have rapidly enough flowing blood and, consequently, both suppression methods are needed to eliminate the signal.

If pial venules and veins are the major contributors to fMRI signal changes, then it is critical to do high resolution measurements not only of their anatomy but also with respect to their flow and susceptibility in order to validate the BOLD model [4]. We have shown that it is possible to extract some useful flow information from small pial veins. The 3D sequences with long TE (about 60 ms) may also reveal many vessels smaller than 500 μm in size which are associated with larger draining veins [5]. In conclusion, these experiments reaffirm the major role that the blood itself plays in fMRI.

Acknowledgment

This work was supported in part by a research grant from Siemens Medical Systems (Erlagen, Germany), and by NS 06833.

One of the authors (J.R.R.) acknowledges support from the Deutsch Forschungsgemeinschaft (DFG, Re 1123/1-1).

References

1. Lai S, Hopkins A, Haacke EM, et al (1993) Magn Reson Med 30: 387
2. Weisskoff R, Kihne S (1992) Magn Reson Med 24: 375
3. Ogawa S, Lee T, Nayak A, et al (1990) Magn Reson Med 14: 68
4. Haacke EM, Hopkins A, Lai S, et al (1994) NMR Biomedicine 7: 54
5. Haacke EM, Lai S, Yablonskiy D, et al (1995) Int Imag Systems Technol (6: 153.)

Human Brain Mapping: State of the Art*

B. Mazoyer

Group d'Imagerie Neurofonctionelle, CEA-DSV, and Université Paris 7, Service Hospitalier Frédéric Joliot, 91401 Orsay, France

Introduction

Human brain mapping (HBM) is a research field that has considerably evolved over the past five years. Since the pioneering work of Paul Broca [1] and up to the 1970's our knowledge on the implementation of cognitive functions has relied on studies of patients bearing brain lesions. Not underestimating the teaching of neuropsychology, one has to acknowledge the fundamental limits of this approach such as, for example, the extreme variability between patients in the lesion site and the extent of functional recovery. Within this context, the first cerebral blood flow maps obtained under brain activation in rodents by H. Kennedy and L. Sokoloff can be considered as a milestone. Application of this method in man occured in the early 1970's using radioactive xenon and external detectors [2] but this first attempt was limited both by the limited spatial resolution of the apparatus and by the absence of reference to brain anatomy.

Fortunately, the 1980's have been a golden age for the brain imaging technology. In less than 10 years, a variety of tomographic techniques have been made available to map both the brain anatomy and various physiological correlates of brain activity. With a still improving technology, one is now able to obtain submillimetric three-dimensional (3D) images of the brain anatomy using magnetic resonance imaging (MRI), 3D cerebral blood flow maps using positron emission tomography (PET) [3], and the localisation of electromagnetic activity using electroencephalography (EEG) or magnetoencephalography (MEG) systems [4]. In addition, functional MRI (fMRI) [5] has recently emerged has a major technique for human brain mapping, providing another means to look at the metabolic correlates of human brain activity. Finally, additional techniques that will be available either in humans or in animals (optical imaging, near infrared spectroscopy, confocal microscopy) are still under development. Over the past few years, a very fast expansion of the

brain mapping research domain has become apparent, in terms of number of laboratories, publications or grants. Brain maps have been produced for a large variety of cognitive functions using the techniques previously cited but what seemed to be missing, however, was a forum where these various approaches could be confronted. This was the primary goal assigned to the First International Conference on Functional Mapping of the Human Brain (Human Brain Map 95 or HBM95).

Human Brain Map 95 Scientific Program Elaboration

The scientific program of the conference was built upon the answers to a call for abstracts sent to about 10 000 scientists belonging to a series of societies, namely the Society for Cerebral Blood Flow and Metabolism, the Society for Cognitive Neuroscience, the Society for Magnetic Resonance in Medicine, the EEG society, and European Society for Neuroradiology. Abstracts were accepted whenever they were scored above average by three members of the scientific advisory board; oral presentations were awarded to 16% of the 404 communications that obtained the highest scores.

The scientific program, that extended over three and a half days, included 6 oral sessions and 3 poster sessions on the following topics: vision, audition and somatosensory system, language, attention and mental imagery, motor system, learning and memory, and brain disorders. Since the meeting was focused on brain imaging of cognition rather than on techniques, all abstracts dealing with methodological issues were placed in a poster session, and the hottest technical issues were debated during a pre-meeting refresher course.

Human Brain Map 95 Attendance

HBM95 gathered 800 scientists from more than 30 countries. France (30%), USA (24%), and Germany (12%) were the countries with the largest representation

---

* Report on the First International Conference of Functional Mapping of the Human Brain (Human Brain Map 95) held in Paris (France) on June 27-30 1995

Table 1. Human Brain Map 95 attendance

Provenance	Attendees	
USA	**200**	
Europe	**500**	
France		250
Germany		100
England		50
Sweden, Finland, Norway, Denmark		40
Netherlands		20
Italy		15
Belgium		15
Spain		10
Japan	**40**	
Canada	**25**	
Russia and Eastern Europe Countries	**15**	
Others	**20**	
Total	**800 (students 20%)**	

(Table 1) and the European Union (EU) countries accounted for two-thirds of the total. Needless to say that such an audience was quite unexpected, even more so when considering that this meeting, the first of its kind, was held at a time close to that of other societies' meetings such as Brain 95 (Cologne, July 1995), the EPIC Conference (Kyoto, same week as HBM95) or the SM-RM (Nice, August 1995). The attendance figures demonstrate that a community has been mobilized, justify *a posteriori* the decision of having HBM95 and indicate that there exists a need for some sort of long term formal organization of this research community.

Human Brain Mapping: Topics

The sorting of the HBM95 communications [6] by topics (see Table 2) shows three main categories: cognition in normal subjects (54%), methods (28%) and cognition in brain disorders (18%). In the first category, the major topics covered by the abstracts were (by decreasing order) the motor system, vision, attention, language, learning and memory, with a smaller number of abstracts dealing with audition, the somatosensory system and emotions. In the methods category, five major topics emerged: fMRI, MEG, EEG, anatomy, pharmacology and receptor mapping. This reflects the efforts made by various groups to develop, validate and establish fMRI as a major tool in the field. For MEG and EEG, the majority of papers addressed the question of localization. In brain anatomy, a leading subtopic was that of unsupervised computerized analysis of brain MRI images. The reduced number of papers focusing on PET methods can be explained by the fact that most of the PET methods developments were presented at the Brain 95[1] meeting (see above). Interestingly, there was only a small number of papers reporting on multi-modal experiments. Finally, papers on brain disorders investigated imaging of cognition in patients with neurological diseases (epilepsy, cerebrovascular diseases and dementia) and with psychiatric diseases (mainly schizophrenia

[1] HBM95 was an official satellite of Brain 95, the XIIth international symposium of the CBFM society held in Cologne, Germany in July 1995.

Table 2. Topics of Human Brain Map 95 communications

Topics	No. Abstracts	
Cognition	**214**	
Motor system		46
Vision		39
Attention		37
Language		35
Learning & memory		27
Audition		16
Somatosensory system and emotions		14
Methods	**112**	
fMRI		25
MEG		19
EEG		18
Anatomy		16
Pharmacology		15
PET		8
Multi-modality		6
SPECT		5
Brain disorders	**78**	
Neurology		41
Psychiatry		25
Neurosurgery		12
Total	**404**	

Table 3. Human Brain Map 95 communications by countries

Provenance	No. Communications	
USA	**158**	
Europe	**185**	
Germany		64
Sweden, Finland, Norway, Denmark		35
France		29
England		27
Italy		9
Others		21
Japan	**20**	
Russia	**15**	
Canada	**14**	
Others	**10**	
Total	**404**	

Table 4. Human Brain Map 95 communications by topics and countries

	USA	D	F	UK	SW	JPN	RUS	CAN
Cognition								
Motor system	17	16	-	1	4	3	-	-
Vision	23	3	3	2	1	3	-	1
Attention & language	27	8	6	3	4	4	5	5
Learning & memory	12	3	1	5	-	1	-	3
Auditory & somatosensory	11	3	4	2	4	-	-	-
Methods								
fMRI	14	3	3	3	-	-	-	1
MEG	3	5	2	2	4	1	2	1
EEG	5	3	2	-	-	-	3	1
Anatomy	7	5	1	-	2	-	-	1
Pharmacology	5	1	1	1	3	1	-	-
PET	1	-	2	1	2	-	2	-
Multi-modality	3	1	1	-	-	-	-	1
Brain disorders	29	13	4	7	3	7	4	2

D, Germany; F, France; SW, Sweden, Finland, Norway and Denmark; JPN, Japan; RUS, Russia; CAN, Canada.

and depression) and reported the use of brain imaging techniques in neurosurgery.

The sharing of the 404 communications by the various countries is shown in Table 3. EU (45%) and USA (39%) were the two largest contributors; Germany was the leading European country (16%). Apart from the EU and the USA, only 3 countries had a significant number of contributions, namely Japan, Russia and Canada.

Crossing the two previous criteria (country and topic) reveals some disparities between the global analysis and the various topics. Table 4 shows, for example, that papers on vision came almost exclusively from the USA, while contributions on motor system were restricted to USA and Germany. In the other cognition themes, as well as in the brain disorders theme, contributions from the USA were matched by an equivalent number of contributions coming from the other countries. Similarly, for the methods topic, fMRI developments appeared to be mainly occuring in US laboratories while Germany and Finland emerged as the leading countries for MEG methodology. USA and Germany shared most of the papers dealing with brain anatomy. Note that apart from the USA, most countries seemed to focus their research on a few cognitive topics such as the motor system for Germany or attention and language for Russia.

Table 5. Human Brain Map 95 communications by techniques and topics

	fMRI	PET	MEG+EEG
Motor system	20	19	5
Vision	17	7	11
Attention & language	16	31	22
Learning & memory	4	8	5
Audition & somatosensory	5	4	16
Brain disorders	9	30	20

Human Brain Mapping: What are the Different Techniques Used For?

Since various methods are available for studying the same cognitive functions, it is relevant to investigate the relative contribution of each of them to the various topics that were addressed during the conference. This is summarized in Table 5 which shows that if fMRI and PET evenly share the investigations of the motor system, fMRI appears to be the technique of choice for studying the visual system. This result is not surprising considering the very high spatial resolution capability of fMRI. More surprising is the contribution of the electromagnetic techniques to the vision topic which can be explained by the interest in the chronometry of visual cognitive processes. PET keeps a leading position for studying high order cognitive functions such as attention, language, mental imagery, learning and memory, and also for studying brain disorders. There are several explanations for this, including the ability of PET to provide full 3D brain activation maps which allow visualization of large scale networks that may be involved in the executions of such cognitive functions. Finally, MEG and EEG dominate the domains of audition and of the somatosensory system since these techniques allow studying the timing of events in primary cortices.

Crossing the technique and country criteria reveals deep differences in the use of the different available brain imaging techniques (Table 6). Functional MRI is largely used in the USA and to a much lesser degree in Germany, while PET is used in most countries, the leading ones being the USA, Sweden, Japan and England. EEG is widely developed in the USA, Germany, Russia and France, whereas MEG is mostly implemented in the USA, Germany and Finland. Several countries use preferentially one or another of these techniques, for example, PET is mainly used in England, Sweden and Japan,

Table 6. Human Brain Map 95 communications by techniques and countries

	No. Communications						
	fMRI	PET	EEG	MEG	SPECT	Anatomy	Others
USA	61	37	14	14	9	7	16
Germany	16	6	13	11	4	6	8
France	7	6	9	3	1	1	2
England	3	11	3	4	3	-	3
Sweden	3	15	1	-	-	2	2
Japan	1	12	1	3	2	-	1
Russia	-	3	10	2	-	-	-
Canada	2	7	4	1	-	-	-
Finland	1	-	-	10	-	-	-
Total	94	97	55	48	19	16	32

MEG in Finland, and EEG in Russia. Finally, it is interesting to note that the overall contribution of PET (26%) was shortly leading that of fMRI (24%), followed by EEG (18%) and MEG (12%).

Conclusion

The Human Brain Map 95 conference has shown the existence of a community sharing, across the various imaging modalities, a common project. This community has decided on pursuing this kind of meeting: Human Brain Map 96 is to be held in Boston in June 1996 and further annual meetings are planned until year 2000. Meanwhile, an extended scientific advisory board has been appointed by this same community to investigate the kind of formal association that could provide a framework for exchange and collaboration in this rapidly growing field of research.

Acknowledgments

Human Brain Map 95 has been supported by grants from the the European Union Directorate General XII, the Direction des Sciences de la Vie du Commissariat à l'Energie Atomique, the Ministère de l'Enseignement Supérieur et de la Recherche, le Réseau Régional Cogniseine du CNRS, le Ministère de la Défense, the INSERM and the Délégation à la Recherche Clinique de l'Assistance Publique - Hopitaux de Paris.

References

1. Broca P (1863) Localisation des fonctions cérébrales siège du langage articulé. Bull Soc Anthrop Paris 4: 200-202
2. Ingvar DH, Schwartz MS (1974) Blood flow patterns induced in the dominant hemisphere by speech and reading. Brain 97: 273-288
3. Fox PT, Mintun MA, Raichle ME, Herscovitch P (1984) A non-invasive approach to quantitative functional brain mapping with ^2H-^{15}O and positron emission tomography. J Cereb Blood Flow Metab 4: 329-333
4. Wiskwo Jr JP, Gevins A, Williamson SJ (1993) The future of the EEG and MEG. Electroencephalogr Clin Neurophysiol 87: 1-9
5. Belliveau JW, Kennedy DN, Mc Kinstry RC, Buchbinder BR, Weiskoff RM, Cohen MS, Veavea JM, Brady TJ, Rosen BR (1991) Functional mapping of the human visual cortex by magnetic resonance imaging. Science 254: 716-719
6. Mazoyer B, Roland P, Seitz R (eds) (1995) Abstract Book of the First International Conference on Functional Mapping of the Human Brain. Hum Brain Mapping, (supp 1) Wiley, New York

Clinical Applications of Functional MRI

D.G. Gadian

Radiology and Physics Unit, Institute of Child Health, 30 Guilford Street, London, WC1N 1EH, UK

Introduction

There are several ways in which magnetic resonance (MR) can contribute to the investigation of brain function. Perhaps the most direct (and remarkable) way takes advantage of the fact that magnetic resonance can now be used to map activated regions of the brain. This type of magnetic resonance study, commonly referred to as functional magnetic resonance imaging (fMRI), provides the opportunity for learning a great deal about the functional anatomy of the normal brain. There are also a number of potential clinical applications of the technique.

While the above functional MRI approach has, not surprisingly, received great interest in the last few years, another magnetic resonance approach also has an important role to play in the investigation of brain function. This involves defining focal pathology by means of a number of MRI and MR spectroscopy (MRS) techniques, and relating this pathology to specific abnormalities in brain function, for example seizure activity or cognitive dysfunction.

In this article, a brief description will be given of the studies that we have carried out using both of these approaches, as part of our research programme at the Institute of Child Health and Great Ormond Street Hospital for Children. The studies to be described relate primarily to problems associated with epilepsy.

Magnetic Resonance Methods

Magnetic resonance studies were carried out at 1.5 T using a conventional Siemens whole-body system at the Great Ormond Street Hospital for Children. A standard circularly polarized head coil was used as both transmitter and receiver. For the investigation of temporal lobe epilepsy, we have developed a magnetic resonance protocol that combines visual inspection of optimized MRI scans with more quantitative imaging and spectroscopy techniques [1-5]. These quantitative methods include T2 relaxometry of hippocampal water protons [3], and ^{1}H MRS of $2 \times 2 \times 2$ cm regions within the medial temporal lobes, using the "PRESS" sequence with an echo time of 135 ms [4, 5]. Our functional MRI studies have been carried out using a "FLASH" sequence with an echo time of 60 ms [6, 7].

Results

1. Presurgical Evaluation of Patients with Intractable Epilepsy

The definition of structural and biochemical abnormalities using the above magnetic resonance techniques has played an important role in the establishment at our hospital of an epilepsy surgery programme for children with intractable epilepsy [2, 5]. One important point to emphasise is that in some cases T2 relaxometry and MRS reveal pathology that is difficult to see on visual inspection of the more conventional MRI scans. This includes the detection of bilateral pathology, even in patients with well-lateralised seizures [3-5]. Another important point is that the magnetic resonance findings need to be considered in the context of findings from a wide range of additional techniques that are used in the presurgical assessment of these patients. One of these techniques is single photon emission computed tomography (SPECT), using ^{99}Tc^m-HMPAO (hexamethyl propylene amine oxime) as a marker of regional cerebral blood flow [8]. Comparison of ictal SPECT scans with interictal SPECT scans can reveal focal increases in blood flow during the seizure process, thereby providing information about physiological changes associated with the seizures. In contrast, while the structural and biochemical abnormalities seen on MRI and MRS provide key information about the location and extent of the underlying pathology, they do not provide direct functional information. Clearly, it would be useful to examine

Recent Advances in Clinical Neurophysiology
J. Kimura and H. Shibasaki (eds.)

whether fMRI techniques can be used for such purposes. We have carried out preliminary studies showing that functional MRI can indeed be used to map the cortical activation that occurs during focal seizures [7].

In these functional MRI studies, we used our conventional clinical imaging system for the investigation of a 4-year-old boy suffering from frequent partial motor seizures of his right side. We acquired FLASH images (echo time = 60 ms) every 10 s over intervals of 10 min, and derived activation images by subtracting baseline images from those obtained during clinical seizures. These images revealed sequential activation associated with specific gyri within the left hemisphere with each of five clinical seizures, and also during a period that was not associated with a detectable clinical seizure. These preliminary studies have opened up the exciting possibility of using functional MRI to map out not only the clinical seizures themselves, but also sub-clinical or interictal events.

2. Relationship of Focal Pathology to Cognitive Dysfunction

Patients with chronic and intractable epilepsy commonly show impaired cognitive function, and a major part of our research programme involves investigations of the pathological basis for these functional deficits. Here, we briefly describe findings from two series of patients.

In one series of studies, we investigated 22 right-handed children with intractable temporal lobe epilepsy [9]. We found that left-sided pathology (as assessed by ^{1}H MRS of the medial regions of the two temporal lobes) was associated with a loss of verbal cognitive functions, whereas right-sided pathology was associated with loss of nonverbal functions. These findings are consistent with the pattern of lateralization of verbal and nonverbal functions that has been observed in adults.

We have also investigated 48 patients who had undergone surgery for relief of temporal lobe epilepsy [10]. We initiated the magnetic resonance investigations in an attempt to explain some unexpected verbal memory deficits that had been found in patients with right-sided excisions. We showed that many of these patients had damage in the unoperated temporal lobe, as assessed by T2 relaxometry of the hippocampus and by MRS measurements in the medial region of the temporal lobe. This contralateral damage is consistent with the high frequency of bilateral pathology found by MRS and T2 relaxometry in presurgical cases of epilepsy [3-5]. The presence of left temporal lobe pathology in the patients with right-sided excisions provides an explanation for these unexpected verbal memory deficits.

Discussion

These findings illustrate some of the roles that magnetic resonance can play in the investigation of functional abnormalities in patients with brain disease. The scope of functional MRI for such studies is, of course, quite extensive. For example, one important area not discussed above involves the use of functional MRI for the presurgical definition of primary cortical areas [11]. Such studies could prove to be very valuable in presurgical planning and in guiding safe resection, for example, of lesions that may be close to primary sensory or motor cortex. Similarly, there is a possibility that presurgical functional MRI studies [12] may in due course replace the invasive sodium amytal test, which is sometimes used in the presurgical work-up to determine the dominant hemisphere for speech and language functions.

However, it is important to emphasise that more conventional magnetic resonance investigations of focal pathologies and of their relationship to abnormalities in function can also make significant contributions to our understanding of brain dysfunction in disease, and in turn, of the normal functional brain anatomy. The techniques that we have been using highlight pathology that, in some cases, might otherwise have gone undetected, and this is clearly of critical importance to any study attempting to relate focal pathology to specific impairments of function.

In conclusion, magnetic resonance can contribute in a variety of ways to the investigation and understanding of brain function, not only through the techniques of functional MRI, but also through the increasing power of MRI and MRS techniques for the detection and definition of focal pathology.

Aknowledgments

I gratefully acknowledge all the colleagues involved in our research programme, which is supported by the Wellcome Trust and Action Research.

References

1. Jackson GD, Berkovic SF, Duncan JS, Connelly A (1993) Optimizing the diagnosis of hippocampal sclerosis using MRI. Am J Neuroradiol 14: 753-762
2. Cross JH, Jackson GD, Neville BGR, Connelly A, Kirkham FJ, Boyd SG, Pitt MC, Gadian DG (1993) Early detection of abnormalities in partial epilepsy using magnetic resonance. Arch Dis Child 69: 104-109
3. Jackson GD, Connelly A, Duncan JS, Grunewald, Gadian DG (1993) Detection of hippocampal pathology in intractable partial epilepsy: Increased sensitivity with quantitative magnetic resonance relaxometry. Neurology 43: 1793-1799
4. Connelly A, Jackson GD, Duncan JS, King MD, Gadian DG (1994) Magnetic resonance spectroscopy in temporal lobe epilepsy. Neurology 44: 1411-1417
5. Cross JH, Connelly A, Jackson GD, Johnson CL, Neville BGR, Gadian DG (1996) Proton magnetic resonance spectroscopy in children with temporal lobe epilepsy. Ann Neurol 39: 107-113

6. Connelly A, Jackson GD, Frackowiak RSJ, Belliveau JW, Vargha-Khadem F, Gadian DG (1993) Functional mapping of activated human primary cortex with a clinical MR imaging system. Radiology 188: 125-130

7. Jackson GD, Connelly A, Cross JH, Gordon I, Gadian DG (1994) Functional magnetic resonance imaging of focal seizures. Neurology 44: 850-856

8. Cross JH, Gordon I, Jackson GD, Boyd SG, Todd-Pokropek A, Andersen PJ, Neville BGR (1995) Children with intractable focal epilepsy: ictal and interictal $^{99}Tc^m$ HMPAO single photon emission computed tomography. Dev Med Child Neurol 37: 673-681

9. Gadian DG, Isaacs EB, Cross JH, Connelly A, Jackson GD, King MD, Neville BGR, Vargha-Khadem F (1996) Lateralization of brain function in childood revealed by magnetic resonance spectroscopy. Neurology (in press)

10. Incisa della Rocchetta A, Gadian DG, Connelly A, Polkey CE, Jackson GD, Watkins K, Johnson CL, Mishkin M, Vargha-Khadem F (1995) Verbal memory impairment after right temporal lobe surgery: Role of contralateral damage as revealed by ^1H magnetic resonance spectroscopy and T2 relaxometry. Neurology 45: 797-802

11. Jack CR, Thompson RM, Sharbrough FW, Kelly PJ, Hanson DP, Butts RK, Hangiandreou NJ, Riederer SJ, Ehman RL, Cascino GD (1994) Sensory motor cortex: correlation of presurgical mapping with functional MR imaging and invasive cortical mapping. Radiology 190: 1-8

12. Cuenod CA, Bookheimer SY, Hertzpannier L, Zeffiro TA, Theodore WH, LeBihan D (1995) Functional MRI during word generation using conventional equipment – a potential tool for language localization in the clinical environment. Neurology 45: 1821-1827

Functional Magnetic Resonance Imaging with Echo Planar Imaging*

K.K. Kwong

MGH-NMR Center, Department of Radiology, Massachusetts General Hospital and Harvard Medical School, Charlestown, Massachusetts, U.S.A.

Introduction

Functional magnetic resonance imaging (fMRI), a class of techniques that images intrinsic blood signal change with magnetic resonance (MR) imagers, has in the past 3 years become one of the most successful tools used to study cerebral blood flow and perfusion in the brain. Because changes in neuronal activity are accompanied by focal changes in cerebral blood flow (CBF), blood volume (CBV), blood oxygenation, and metabolism, these physiological changes can be used to produce functional maps of mental operations.

Intrinsic velocity contrast can be used to image MR angiography. Similarly, an early attempt was made to exploit intrinsic blood signal contrast to separate perfusion from tissue, based on the elegant assumption that flowing blood in capillaries has larger apparent diffusion coefficients than that of static tissue [1]. It is known as the intravoxel incoherent motion (IVIM) model. However, the measurement of cortical brain perfusion with the IVIM technique has been hampered by the observation that cortical gray matter is consistently located within the same voxel as cerebral spinal fluid (CSF), which has a large diffusion coefficient [2]. The IVIM model has continued to inspire and impact new experiments [3-5]. As it turns out, the application of diffusion or velocity dephasing gradients can be used to remove MR signals of flowing blood in large vessels (see below). This may play a helpful role in suppressing signals arising from vascular artifacts observed in the current crop of known MR methods of perfusion imaging.

The search for successful noninvasive MR perfusion techniques turned promising when two completely different methods of exploiting the intrinsic blood signal contrast came along in 1990-1991. The first one is a classical steady state perfusion technique first proposed by Detre et al. [6], who suggested the use of saturation or inversion of incoming blood T1-weighted signal to quantify absolute blood flow [6-10]. By focusing on T1 signal change, and hence blood flow change, and not just steady state blood flow, it was shown that one could successfully image brain visual functions associated with quantitative perfusion changes [11]. There are many advantages in studying blood flow change alone. Many confonding effects (magnetization transfer, imperfect cancellation of signals from static tissue, etc.) associated with MR absolute flow techniques can be subtracted out when one is only interested in changes. And one can obtain adequate information in most functional neuroimaging studies with information on flow change alone.

The second technique also looks at change of a blood parameter - blood oxygenation change and its associated T2* change during neuronal activity. The utility of T2* change was strongly evident in the work of Turner et al. [12] using cats with induced hypoxia. Turner et al. [12] found that during hypoxia the MRI signal from the cats' brains decreased as the level of deoxyhemoglobin rose. This result was an extension of Ogawa's earlier study [13, 14], which showed that deoxyhemoglobin lowered MR signals in veins. The new obsevation by Turner et al. [12] was that when oxygen was restored, the brain signal in a cat model climbed up and went above its baseline level. This suggested that the vascular system overcompensated, bringing more oxygen, and with more oxygen in the blood, the MR signal increased above baseline.

Based on the observation of Turner et al. [12] and the perfusion method suggested by Detre et al. [6], movies of human visual cortex activation (produced by a flickering stimulus) utilizing both the perfusion and blood oxygenation techniques were successfully acquired in May of 1991 (Fig. 1) at the Massachusetts General Hospital (MGH) using a specially equipped super-fast 1.5T General Electric machine known as an echo planar imaging (EPI) MR system [15]. An EPI gradient echo sequence sensitive to magnetic susceptibility effect and thus blood oxygenation change was used. MR signals at the visul cortex were observed to increase when the visual stimulus was turned on, confirming Turner's observation that blood oxygenation can be used to study flow change. At the same time, an EPI inversion recovery

* Reproduced with permission from Lippincott-Raven Press
Magnetic Resonance Quarterly 11: 1-20 (1995)

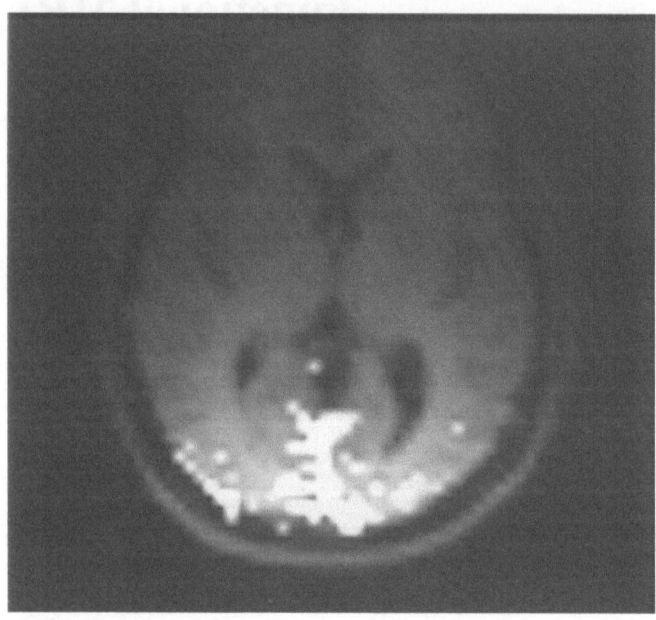

Fig. 1. *Early oxygenation sensitive functional MR image acquired at MGH on May 9, 1991 with a 5 in surface coil demonstrating activation (bright region) of the primary visual cortex (V1) upon stimulation with goggle LEDs.* MR parameters: an EPI gradient echo (GE) sequence with TR = 2.5 s, TE = 40 ms. All fMRI images (Figs. 1-13) were acquired with a SIGNA 1.5 system equipped with EPI provided by ANMR

spin echo sequence also imaged MR signal rise at the visual cortex during stimulation, obtaining a result predicted by the perfusion model of Detre et al. [6].

Visual cortex activation images (Fig. 2) using intrinsic blood contrast were first presented at the Tenth Annual Meeting of the Society of Magnetic Resonance in Medicine in August 1991 [11, 16]. Motor cortex activation images were acquired soon afterwards [11, 17]. The successful implementation of the intrinsic blood signal technique came at an opportune time for fMRI as the MR imaging of visual cortex activation had already been carried out earlier by Belliveau et al. [18] using an injection of the contrast agent Gd-DTPA. The use of a bolus of external contrast agent allows the study of change in blood volume. It acquires a precontrast and a postcontrast image, measuring two steady states of brain activation. By comparison, the noninvasive intrinsic blood contrast techniques, sensitive to blood flow and blood oxygenation, can be applied repeatedly to the same individual as often as necessary. Thus, it is ideal for the measurement of the hemodynamic time course, studying events that occur within seconds. Early model calculation showed that signal due to blood perfusion change would only be ~2% above baseline (1.5 T, echo time (TE) = 50 ms), and the signal due to blood oxygenation change was also quite small. Most studies report a 2-5%

Fig. 2. *Movie of fMRI mapping of primary visual cortex (V1) activation during visual stimulation.* Images are obliquely aligned along the calcarine fissures with the occipital pole at the bottom with a 5 in surface coil. Images were acquired at 3 s intervals using a blood oxygenation sensitive MR sequence (80 images total). A baseline image acquired during darkness (*upper left*) was subtracted from subsequent images. Eight of these subtraction images are displayed, chosen when the image are displayed, chosen when the image intensities reached a steady-state signal level, during darkness (OFF), and during 8-Hz photic stimulation (ON). During stimulation, local increases in signal intensity are detected in the medial-posterior regions of the occipital lobes along the calcarine fissurs. Upon termination of photic stimulation, an undershoot in the MR signal intensity is observed at the beginning of the OFF period

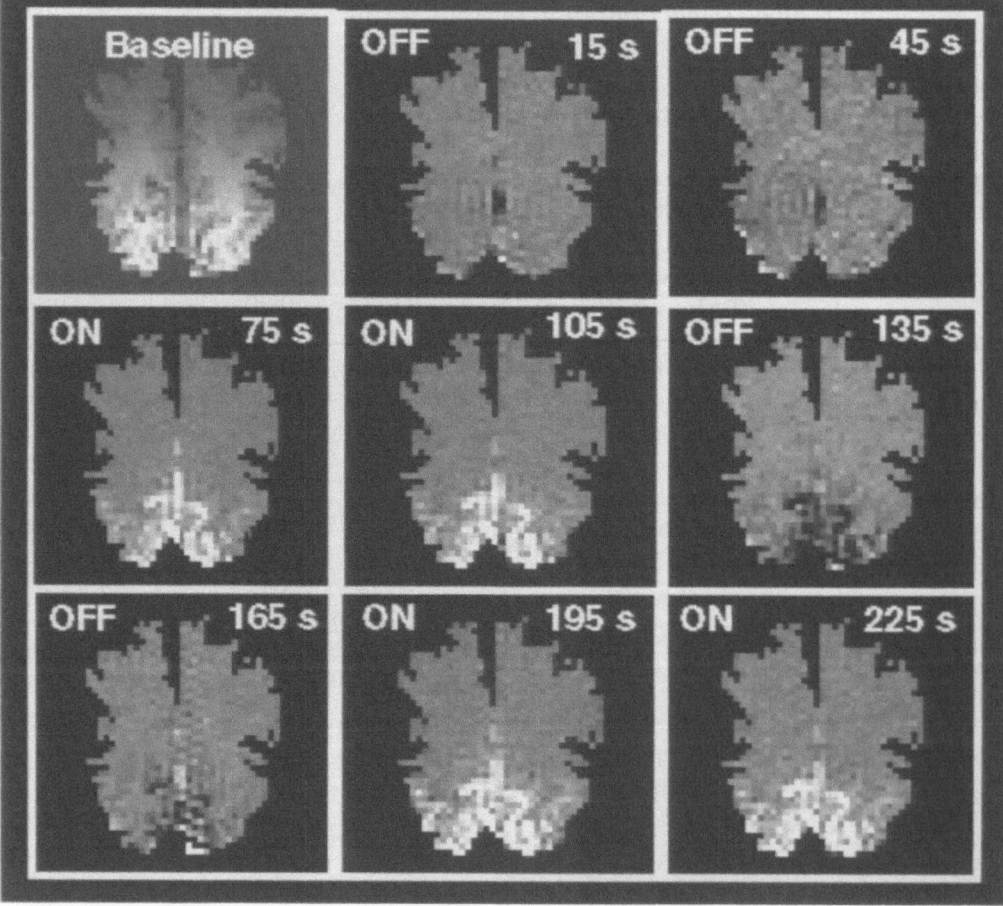

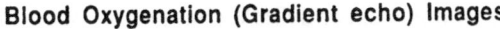

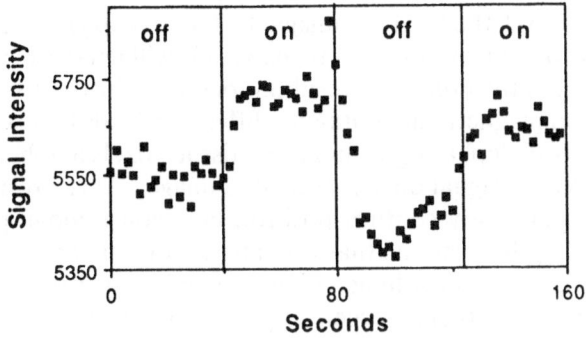

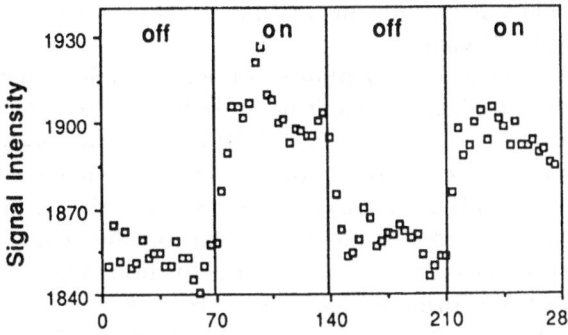

Fig. 3. *Signal intensity changes for a region of interest (~60 mm²) within the visual cortex during darkness and during 8 Hz photic stimulation.* Results using oxygenation sensitive (*top graph*) and flow sensitive (*bottom graph*) techniques are shown. The flow sensitive data were collected once every 3.5 s, and the oxygenation sensitive data were collected once every 3 s. Upon termination of photic stimulation, an undershoot in the flow sensitive signal intensity is observed. On the other hand, the undershoot in the flow sensitive signal intensity is unremarkable

signal increase at corresponding parameters. However, by imaging and measuring the difference between pre- and postactivation conditions, this 2-5% signal change is statistically quite robust and easily detectable (Fig. 3). Most subsequent fMRI sequence development has focused on increasing the detectability, reliability, and interpretability of the fMRI signal changes.

One does not need EPI to obtain fMRI images. Ogawa et al. [19] obtained visual cortex activation images on a conventional 4 T MR system. Frahm et al. [20] generated excellent fMRI images with a clinical field strength MR system. Nonetheless, as discussed in detail below, EPI is an exceptionally powerful tool for fMRI.

For the T1 perfusion method, it is impractical to collect hundreds of T1 weighted spin echo inversion recovery images with a conventional scanner. However, it is quite straightforward to collect T1-weighted, perfusion-indexed images with EPI every few seconds. The normally unwanted susceptibility sensitivity of EPI is an extra bonus for T2* imaging in fMRI. Because the paradigm to activate brain MR signal change normally requires the imaged human subjects to perform a series of

specific tasks for a number of minutes, the motion freezing image acquisition speed of EPI makes the notorious motion artifacts seen in fMRI manageable. The multi-slice whole head EPI imaging capability is an extremely important and useful tool for both exploratory and comprehensive brain mapping work. One can appreciate the difficulty of brain mapping with single slice conventional fMRI techniques. The short repetition time (TR) (<70 ms) routinely employed in conventional fMRI is highly susceptible to inflow artifacts, whereas the long TR (2 s or longer) used to acquire multi-slice EPI images turns out to be beneficial in suppressing MR signals from large vessel inflow. If we add the better signal-to-noise of EPI for images acquired in the same amount of time as with a conventional scanner, the major weakness of EPI – low spatial resolution – is an acceptable tradeoff under most conditions.

The blood-oxygenation sensitive MR signal change, coined Blood Oxygenation Level Dependent (BOLD) by Ogawa [13, 14, 21], is in general much larger than the T1-weighted MR perfusion signal change during brain activation. Since most centers doing fMRI today are only equipped with conventional MR systems and have difficulty collecting T1-weighted fMRI images, the explosive growth of MR functional neuroimaging [11, 17, 19, 20, 22-47] in the past 3 years relies mainly on the measurement of BOLD change. Recently, an interesting variation of the T1 perfusion method tagging the incoming blood has also been developed by Edelman et al. [47-49] for functional localization of brain activation. Both high-speed echo planar (EPI) and conventional MR have now been successfully employed for functional imaging in MRI systems with magnet field strength ranging from 0.5 T [51] to 4.0 T [19, 22].

EPI setups vary with different centers. At MGH, images were acquired with a whole body EPI system (Advanced NMR) [51]. At the Medical College of Wisconsin, a conventional 1.5 T General Electric scanner is equipped with an inserted three-axis balanced torque head gradient coil [52, 53] designed for rapid gradient switching. In this case, a shielded quadrature elliptical endcapped transmit/receive birdcage radiofrequency (RF) coil was used for high-sensitivity whole brain imaging. At the National Institutes of Health (NIH), a 4 T whole body imaging system fitted with shielded transverse gradient coils and a small (27 cm in diameter) z-gradient coil, which gave sufficiently large gradients and fast enough rise times to allow EPI were used [54]. To avoid RF coupling problems, a surface coil was used for RF transmission and reception.

Advances in Functional Brain Mapping

The popularity of fMRI is based on many factors. It is safe and totally noninvasive. It can be acquired in single subjects for a scanning duration of several minutes, and it can be repeated on the same subjects as many times as necessary. The implementation of the blood oxygenation sensitive MR technique is widely available. Today, with BOLD technique combined with EPI, one can acquire 20 or more contiguous brain slices covering the whole head (3×3 mm in plane and 5 mm slice thickness) every 3 s for a total duration of several minutes. The benefits of whole head imaging are many. Not only can researchers identify and test their hypotheses on known brain activation centers, they can also search for previously unknown or unsuspected sites. High-resolution work done with EPI has a resolution of 1.5×1.5 mm in-plane and a slice thickness of 3 mm. Higher spatial resolution has been reported in conventional 1.5 T MR systems [55].

In this report, a review is made of the mechanism behind the fMRI signals and the advances made in many different areas of fMRI. Such areas include understanding and compensating for artifacts specific to fMRI, postprocessing of fMRI images, the application of fMRI to areas of interest in neuroscience, some interesting new glimpses on the frontiers of studying hemodynamics and metabolic responses, and the effort to combine fMRI results with magnetoencephalography (MEG) and electroencephalography (EEG).

Mechanism

Flow-sensitive images show increased perfusion with stimulation, whereas blood oxygenation-sensitive images show changes consistent with an increase in venous blood oxygenation. Although the precise biophysical mechanisms responsible for the signal changes have yet to be determined, good hypotheses exist to account for our observations.

Two fundamental MR relaxation rates, T2* and T1, are used to describe the fMRI signal. T1 is the rate at which the nuclei approach thermal equilibrium and perfusion change can be considered as an additional T1 change. T2* represents the rate of the decay of MR signal due to magnetic field inhomogeneities and the change of T2* is used to measure blood oxygenation change.

1. T2* Changes (BOLD)

T2* changes reflect the interplay between changes in cerebral blood flow, volume, and oxygenation. As hemoglobin becomes deoxygenated, it becomes more paramagnetic than the surrounding tissue [13, 14, 21, 56], and thus creates a magnetically inhomogeneous environment. The observed increased signal on T2*-weighted images during activation reflects a decrease in deoxyhemoglobin content, i.e., an increase in venous blood oxygenation. Oxygen delivery, cerebral blood flow, and cerebral blood volume all increase with neuronal activation. Because CBF (and hence oxygen delivery) changes exceed CBV changes by two to four times [57], while blood oxygen extraction increases only slightly [58, 59], the total paramagnetic blood deoxyhemoglobin content within brain tissue voxels will decrease with brain activation. The resulting decrease in the tissue-blood magnetic susceptibility difference leads to less intravoxel dephasing within brain tissue voxels and hence increased signal on T2*-weighted images. These results independently confirm positron emission tomography (PET) observations that activation-induced changes in blood flow and volume are accompanied by little or no increases in tissue oxygen consumption [58-59].

Because the effect of volume susceptibility difference $\Delta\chi$ is more pronounced at high field strength [61], higher field imaging magnets [19, 22] will increase the observed T2* changes.

There have been a number of optical studies relevant to the physical mechanisms underlying fMRI [62-65]. Near-infrared spectroscopy (NIRS), which assesses the changes in concentration of oxy- and deoxyhemoglobin (oxy-Hb and deoxy-Hb) by changes of absorbance at different wavelengths, has been used together with T2*-sensitive fMRI to record brain activation. With NIRS subjects performing motor tasks showed an increase in oxy-Hb and total-Hb as well as a decrease in deoxy-Hb with characteristic, hemodynamically modulated temporal response (Fig. 4). Task related signal changes detected by fMRI are in agreement with changes in deoxy-Hb measured by NIRS and underline the common physiologic mechanism monitored by both techniques.

Blood oxygen saturation levels were also measured independently [66] to correlate T2*-sensitive fMRI images in cat brain during respiratory challenges. In this study, the independent blood oxygen saturation measurements were made in cats during periods of apnea, anoxia and hypercapnia using three different methods: measurement of arterial blood oxygen saturation, measurement of venous blood oxygen saturation, and using a method of spectrophometric reflectance directly from brain tissue. There is good correspondence between the fMRI results and changes in vascular oxygenation saturation for periods when the data from the spectrophotometric reflectance showed little change in blood volume. When blood volume was observed to change, the NMR results and the optical vascular oxygen saturation results diverged. This suggests that T2* is dependent on blood volume as well as on blood oxygenation.

2. T1 Change

Signal changes can also be observed on T1-weighted MR images. The relationship between T1 and regional blood flow was characterized by Detre et al. [6]:

$$\frac{dM}{dt} = \frac{M_0 - M}{T1} + fM_b - \frac{f}{\lambda} M \qquad (1)$$

Motor Stimulation

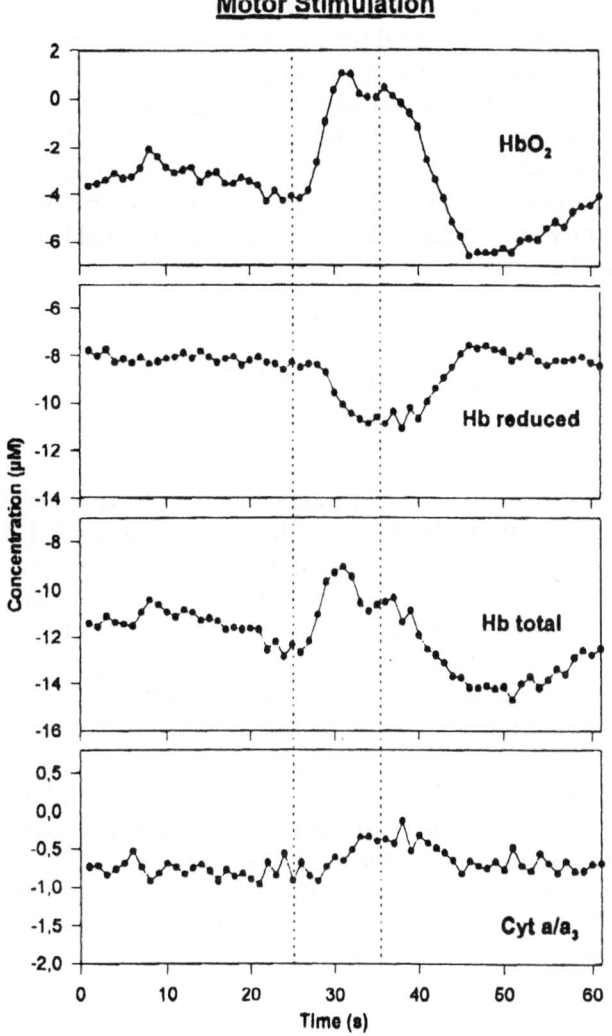

Fig. 4. *Influence of brain activation on NIRS parameters.* Brain activation was achieved by performing a finger opposition task. The NIRS parameters, HbO_2 (oxygenated hemoglobin), Hb reduced (deoxygenated hemoglobin), and Hb total (reflecting blood volume) are given in arbitrary unit (a.U.) concentration changes. (Courtesy of Dr. A. Villringer and Dr. H. Obrig)

where M is tissue magnetization and M_b is incoming blood signal. M_0 is proton density, f is the flow in ml/g per unit time, λ is the brain-blood partition coefficient of water (~0.95 ml/g). From this equation, the brain tissue magnetization M relaxes with an apparent T1 time constant $T1_{app}$ given by

$$\frac{f}{\lambda} = \frac{1}{T1_{app}} - \frac{1}{T1} \qquad (2)$$

where the $T1_{app}$ is the observed (apparent) longitudinal relaxation time with flow effects included. T1 is the true tissue longitudinal relaxation time in the absence of flow. If we assume that the true tissue T1 remains constant with stimulation, a change in blood flow Δf will lead to a change in the observed $T1_{app}$:

$$\Delta \left(\frac{1}{T1_{app}} \right) = \Delta \frac{f}{\lambda} \qquad (3)$$

Thus, the T1-weighted MR signal change can be used to estimate the change in blood flow.

The T1-weighted study can be and has been used for multi-slice functional imaging. A blood tagging method named Echo Planar MR Imaging and Signal Targeting with Alternating Radio Frequency (EPISTAR) has been developed [47-49, 67]. EPISTAR uses a proximal 180° RF tagging of inflowing arterial spins and echo planar readout of a distal slice alternating with subtracted images from similarly acquired images not preceded by the inversion pulse. Several features make this technique appealing as a method of localizing flow-related changes in local brain activity. In particular, the method is relatively insensitive to small head movements and detects flow related changes primarily on the arterial and capillary sides of circulation, without obvious contamination from venous signal.

EPISTAR, like the continuous inversion method [6], can in principle be used to estimate baseline steady state blood flow in addition to flow change. Other baseline steady state flow techniques under investigation include the subtraction of a flow-nonsensitive image from a flow-sensitive image [68, 69]. From Eq. 1, if the magnetization of blood and tissue always undergoes a similar T1 relaxation, the flow effect would be minimized. This is a condition that can be approximated by using a nonselective inversion T1 technique inverting all the blood coming into the imaged slice of interest. A flow-sensitive T1 sequence would be a slice-selective inversion pulse applied to the imaged slice. The flow nonsensitive sequence can be subtracted from the flow-sensitive sequence to provide an index of CBF without the need for external stimulation. Initial results with tumor patients show that such flow mapping techniques are useful for mapping out blood flow of tumor regions [69]. Good gray-white flow contrast (Fig. 5) can be obtained and is in good agreement with CBV maps obtained by the injection of a bolus of Gd-DTPA (Fig. 5).

From the T1 perfusion model and Eq. 1, one can derive expressions for the subtraction of signal intensity for all the perfusion mapping techniques mentioned above [69, 70]. For a flow nonsensitive image subtracted from a flow-sensitive image, the MR signal becomes

$$M_{sel} - M_{non} \approx 2M_0 \cdot TI \cdot \frac{f}{\lambda} \cdot e^{\frac{-TI}{T1}} \qquad (4)$$

where M_{sel} and M_{non} are magnetizations of the selective inversion (flow-sensitive) pulse and the non-selective inversion (flow-nonsensitive) pulse, respectively. M_0 is proton density. TI and f are the usual inversion time (TI) and flow term. One can see that the signal differences would be zero if there is no flow. With flow, the

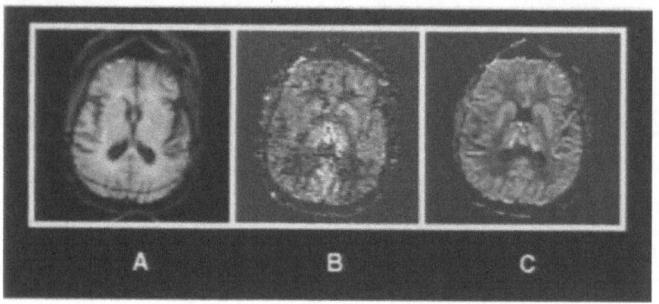

Fig. 5. Image (**B**) of a patient demonstrating good gray-white flow contrast obtained by subtracting a flow nonsensitive (nonselective inversion) image from a flow sensitive (selective inversion) image. The parameters of the EPI inversion recovery spin echo sequence were TR = 3 s, TI = 1.2 s, TE = 50 ms. Images were acquired with a quadrature head coil. Qualitatively, higher signal indicates higher flow. A cerebral blood volume (CBV) map (**C**) was obtained by fitting the time course of the injection of a bolus of MR contrast agent Gd-DTPA. T_1-weighted anatomic image of the same brain slice is shown on **A**, revealing a strong susceptibility artifact on the right side of the brain where a resection had been made. In **B**, the good gray-white flow contrast of cortical brain matches well with that of the CBV map (**C**). What is more significant, the ventricles look dark in both **B** and **C**, whereas the caudate/thalamus regions look bright due to higher gray matter flow. The good flow contrast at the deep gray regions is a strong indication that the flow contrast of B is not simply a T1-weighted effect due to the partial volume of CSF

subtracted images are weighed by flow and by proton density as well as by TI and T1 terms.

The M_0 in these equations is the M_0 of brain matter alone, and not the M_0 of mixed brain matter and CSF present at the same voxel. The CSF component has been subtracted out. It is interesting to note that Eq. 4 as a function of TI is just a gamma function commonly used to fit the kinetics of contrast agents entering and leaving the brain. This "coincidence" is not accidental. The selective, nonselective inversion method gains its signal difference from the fresh blood coming in. The kinetics of a slab of inverted blood (dark blood) coming in from the carotid, on the other hand, can here be described as an inverted gamma function [69, 70].

For continuous inversion at the neck level and assuming no relaxation of the inverted blood traveling to the imaged slice, the expression of signal intensity in the steady state has already been derived [6] as follows:

$$M_{control} - M_{inver} \approx 2M_0 \cdot T1_{app} \cdot \frac{f}{\lambda} \quad (5)$$

In comparing Eqs. 4 and 5, it can be noted that at TI = T1, which is the peak of the selective, nonselective difference, the continuous inversion technique has a theoretical advantage over the selective, nonselective inversion technique by a factor of e, if one is only interested in the subtraction of signal intensity [69]. Unfortunately, the continuous inversion technique also has a significant

problem of magnetization transfer [6], which contaminates the flow signal with a magnetization transfer signal, which is several times larger.

Within the context of the T1 model, a single shot inversion of blood at the proximal slice (e.g., EPISTAR) is similar to the selective, nonselective method, with a possible loss from relaxation of the inverted blood traveling to the imaged slice. The subtracted signal becomes smaller by a factor of $e^{-TX/T1}$

$$M_{control} - M_{tagged} \approx$$

$$2M_0 \cdot (TI - TX) \cdot \frac{f}{\lambda} \cdot e^{\frac{-(TI-TX)}{T1}} \cdot e^{\frac{-TX}{T1}} \quad (6)$$

where TX is the time it takes blood to travel from the tagged site to the imaged slice of interest. EPISTAR, however, has the advantage of visually tracking the incoming arterial flow and can time the arterial blood entry into the parenchyma. EPISTAR may also be quite insensitive to small head motion due to respiration or cardiac fluctuation. That is a good advantage when such "physiological noise" [71] appears to be a dominant source of artifacts in fMRI imaging.

Baseline CBF is useful for many clinical situations such as studies of active tumor sites or epileptic centers. On the other hand, for most of the fMRI studies where the research interest centers around brain mapping or neurological work, the more sensitive flow change techniques are more appropriate.

Problems and Artifacts in fMRI

Perhaps the biggest challenge fMRI faces is its low contrast-to-noise and contrast-to-artifact. Experimentally at 1.5 T systems, one observes an MR signal change upon brain activation to be in the order of 2-5% from baseline conditions. While the percentage change should vary somewhat depending on sequence parameters, slice thickness, etc., the optimum signal change predicted by theoretical models is normally not larger than 2% [72]. One way to increase signal-to-noise is to go to higher field strengths. Because both theoretical models and preliminary experiments point to an increase of T2* contrast-to-noise at higher field strengths [19, 22, 50, 73, 74], there is great anticipation for the new generation of 3T to 4 T machines equipped with EPI. While it is clear that BOLD contrast increases faster than system + thermal noise as field strengths increase [50, 75], a word of caution is in order as physiological noise (respiration, cardiac pulsation, brain pulsation) [71] increases substantially faster than system + thermal noise. Although preliminary data show that physiological noise may not scale with field strength as fast as "functional" signals [75], gain in functional contrast-to-noise must take into account the role of physiological noise.

1. Motion Correction

A normal fMRI study lasts several minutes while hundreds of images are acquired sequentially. Conventional fMRI gradient echo sequences have serious problems of intraimage and interimage motion artifacts. Navigator echo-based motion correction schemes are used [76, 77] to minimize the phase inconsistency among k-space lines. A data point is acquired before the application of the phase and readout gradients, and the phase of this data point is used to correct the phase of subsequently acquired k-space lines, directly minimizing k-space fluctuations. Functional images obtained with the navigator correction reduced respiration artifacts and on a 4 T scanner [76] exhibited larger gray matter regions of activation.

For EPI functional imaging which uses snapshots of the brain, interimage motion artifacts are still a serious problem. To reduce such motion artifacts, many devices have been used to provide moderate head restraint with some degree of success. Effective devices range from packing foam around the subject's head to an inflated bean bag inside a head coil. The utilization of a bite bar made of a dental mold is useful in reducing the up and down inclination head motion problem which is most common in fMRI imaging. New head position monitoring devices are continually proposed [78]. The better the head is restrained during the image acquisition, the less one has to rely on any postprocessing reregistration scheme.

A popular image registration algorithm by Woods et al. [79] aligns two image sets by minimizing the variance of the ratio of the voxels in the two image sets. It can be used to reregister a couple of image slices or a whole head volume. Several centers [80-82] have used Wood's algorithm to align their image data and showed that this has resulted in improvements in the resulting statistical maps and subsequent interpretation.

2. Brain-vein Problem and the Inflow Artifacts

One of the most famous artifacts of fMRI is known as the brain-vein problem. Basically, signals arising from large vessels can dominate signals coming from tissue. It is generally believed that microvascular changes are specific to the underlying region of neuronal activation. However, it has long been known in theoretical models that MR gradient echo (GE) is sensitive to vessels of all diameters between 10 μm and 3 mm [83-86], raising concern that macrovascular changes distal to the site of neuronal activity can be inducd [25]. Because GE sequences are most sensitive to variations in T2* and in most fMRI centers they are the only realistic sequences available, the brain-vein problem has caused great concern.

In addition, there is a nondeoxyhemoglobin related problem especially acute in conventional MR. This is the inflow problem of fresh blood that can be time locked to stimulation [35, 36, 87-90]. Such non-parenchymal and macrovascular responses can introduce error in the estimate of activated volumes. The problem is particularly acute for the short TR's (<70 ms) used in conventional gradient echo sequences.

Techniques to Reduce the Large Vessel Problems

It is not yet known how far away the draining vein carries the activation signal or whether venous blood from the activated brain site would soon be diluted by venous blood elsewhere. Some fMRI evidence currently is inconsistent with apparent activation in large distal draining veins [65]. For instance, retinotopic data [29, 45, 91] indicate no major involvement of the calcarine vein downstream from the more anterior area activated by peripheral field visual stimulation.

Most efforts have gone into devising means to separate large vessels from tissue. Lee et al. [92] examined the time course of T2*-weighted functional signals upon visual stimulation. It was shown that signals from large vessels are time-delayed compared with those from small vessels.

The other popular techniques try simply to get rid of signals from either draining veins or inflowing large vessels by exploiting the property of fast flowing blood in large vessels. Fast flowing blood signal can be removed by time of flight method or the addition of velocity dephasing gradients.

One of the simpler methods that can suppress large vessel signals but keeps the T2* sensitivity intact is the use of asymmetric spin echo (ASE) sequence which offsets the 180° pulse by a time interval [93]. ASE maintains high contrast-to-noise in fMRI. The success of ASE is most likely due to the time-of-flight effect of its spin echo component, with the flowing spins seeing the 90° but not the slice selective 180° pulse.

In the case of time-of-flight, EPI has special advantages over conventional scanners. The use of long repetition times (2-3 s) in EPI significantly reduces the brain-inflow problem. Conventional gradient echo sequences with very short TR have to rely on smaller flip angles to reduce inflow effect [87]. Based on inflow modeling [94], one observes that at an angle smaller than the Ernst angle (Fig. 6), the inflow effect drops much faster than the tissue signal response to activation [95].

To reduce inflow artifacts on a 4 T scanner, centric-reordered phase-encoding steps and interimage delays [24] had been used. A T2*-weighted Turbo-FLASH sequence [96] with a crushing gradient and a delay period between magnetization preparation and data collection had also been found useful to dephase the spins undergoing flow and diffusion.

1. Velocity Dephasing Gradients

An interesting possibility to suppress slow through-

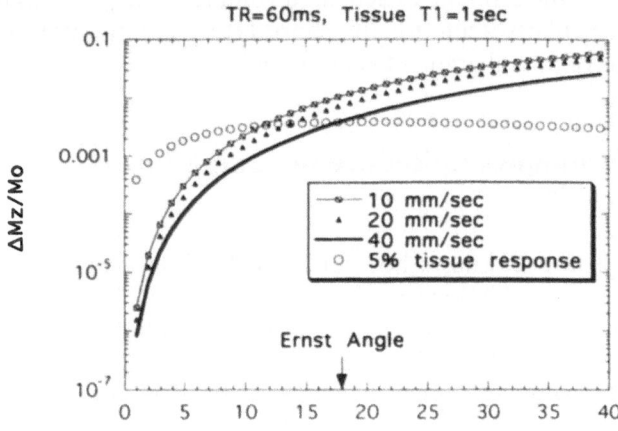

Fig. 6. *Simulated curves show that at different velocities of (10 mm/s, 20 mm/s, 40 mm/s) vessel inflow (assuming laminar flow), MR signals due to inflow drop as a function of flip angle of the radio frequency (RF) pulse.* The inflow signal is compared to a simulated tissue response of 5% signal change. MR parameters are TR = 60 ms, TE = 40 ms with a simulated tissue T1 = 1 s. It demonstrates vividly that for a flip angle smaller than that of the Ernst angle, inflow signal drops much faster than tissue signal drops

plane as well as in-plane vessel flow is to add small additional velocity dephasing gradients [95, 97-99]. Basically, moving spins lose signals while stationary spins are unaffected. Only a very small additional gradient would be sufficient. Unlike brute-force venograms, which try to visually identify vessels and potentially exclude many gray gyri regions that border the blood vessels, the use of velocity dephasing gradients can drastically reduce the presence of vessel signal and bring out the underlying tissue signal, without the need of prior knowledge of the origin, location or the cause of those vessel signals.

If one can get the maximum gradient strength of 1.73 gauss/cm (1 gauss/cm on each of the x, y, and z axes) on a 1.5 T clinical scanner, the duration of these velocity dephasing gradients does not need to be longer than 10 ms to dephase slow flow of ~1 cm/s. This can easily be accommodated by spin echo (SE) sequences or T2*-weighted ASE sequence without causing excessive loss of signal to noise.

Addition of small velocity dephasing gradients has demonstrated the drop in activation signals and a smaller region of activation (Fig. 7). It remains to be seen whether this approach will primarily affect the large and fast flowing vessels and not the response from tissues. Contrast at the activation regions with visual stimulation (Fig. 8) drops from 3% to 1.5% in ASE experiments with velocity dephasing gradients. The large drop of absolute signal is partly due to the diffusional loss of signals in CSF. The reduction of contrast-to-noise in this study makes background noise a more serious issue. With velocity dephasing, the tissue signal change is ~1.5%, and the cardiac noise level is also 1.5%. That requires the averaging of many images to bring out the underlying activation signal.

A simple calculation of the gradient strengths of the Advanced NMR EPI system suggests a way to estimate the size and duration of encoding gradients needed to dephase many vessels of concern. If we assume laminar flow, and the condition that $kV \sim \pi$ is met (where V is the average velocity and $k = 2\pi GT_aT_b$ and where γ is the gyromagnetic ratio, G is the gradient strength, and T_a and T_b are the duration and separation of the gradients, respectively), then the EPI phase encoding gradients of the Advanced NMR system can theoretically dephase

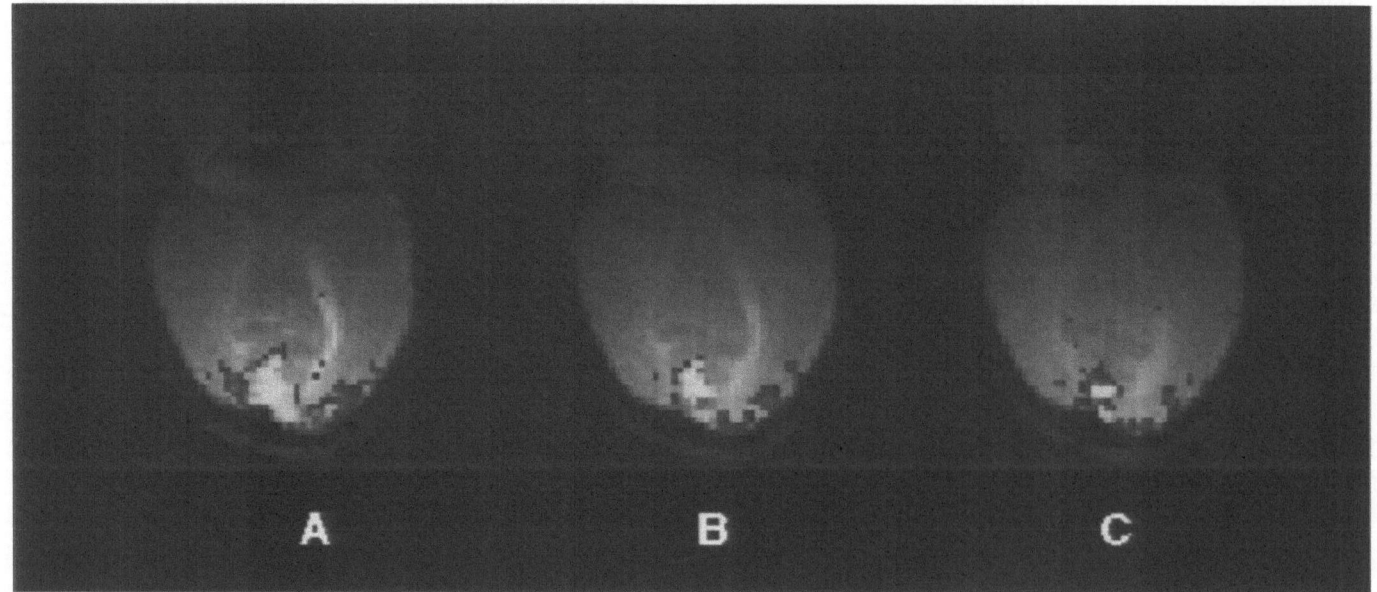

Fig. 7. *The images show that the area of activated regions (with photic stimulation) gets smaller as the velocity dephasing gradient gets stronger.* The velocity dephasing gradient strength was 1 gauss/cm. The gradient duration was 0 ms for **A**, 20 ms for **B**, and 30 ms for **C**

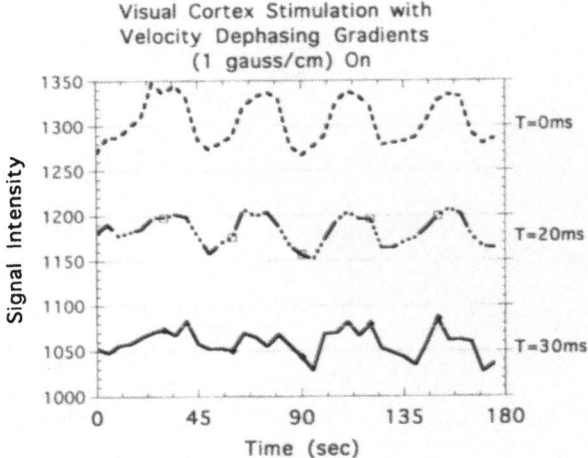

Visual Cortex Stimulation with Velocity Dephasing Gradients (1 gauss/cm) On

Fig. 8. *The curves represent time courses of MR response to photic stimulation (off-on-off-on ...), with different levels of velocity dephasing gradients turned on to remove MR signals coming from the flowing blood of large vessels.* The *top curve* had no velocity dephasing gradients turned on. The *bottom curve* was obtained with such strong velocity dephasing gradients turned on that all large vessel signals were supposed to have been eliminated. The *middle curve* represents a moderate amount of velocity dephasing gradients, a trade off between removing large vessel signals and retaining a reasonable level of MR signal to noise. The "T" values listed on the right Y-axis indicate the duration of the velocity gradients for each individual time curve

flow of V ~4 cm/s in plane. Through-plane slice selective gradients are smaller, and unwanted inflow needs additional external gradients to dephase it. The size of vessels corresponding to flow velocity of ~4 cm/s is unknown, even though such velocity is consistent with vessels with small diameter (~1 mm) [100]. We have assumed that vessels fill the full voxel. That is a conserva-

tive assumption. In practice, bright vessels are normally not observed at T1- or T2-weighted EPI spin echo sequences and the sagittal sinus is not observed to be time-locked to activation stimulus.

2. T2-weighted and T1-weighted Spin Echo Sequences

Another advantage of EPI is that an oxygenation-sensitive method such as the EPI T2-weighted spin echo (T2SE) is also available [68, 101-103]. T2SE methods are sensitive to the MR parameter T2, which is affected by microscopic susceptibility and hence blood oxygenation. T2SE methods are far less sensitive to large vessel signals [83-86]. For conventional scanners, T2SE methods take too long to perform and are therefore not practical options.

The flow model [6] based on T1-weighted sequences and independent of deoxhemoglobin are also not so prone to larger vessel artifacts as the T1 model is a model of perfusion at the tissue level.

Based on the study of volunteers, the average T2*-weighted GE signal percentage change in the primary visual cortex was 2.5 ± 0.8%. The average oxygenation weighted T2SE (TR = 3 s, TE = 90 ms) signal percentage change was 0.7 ± 0.3% (Fig. 9), and the average perfusion weighted and T1-weighted (TR = 4 s, TI = 1.1s, TE = 45 ms) MR signal percentage change was 1.5 ± 0.5% (Fig. 9). These results demonstrated that T2SE and T1 methods, in spite of their ability to suppress large vessels, are not competitive with T2* effect at 1.5 T. However, according to theoretical models, since the microscopic effect detected by T2SE scales up with field strength [73], we expect the T2SE to be a useful sequence at high field strength such as 3 or 4 T. Increasing field strength should also benefit T1 studies due to bet-

Fig. 9 A-E. *EPI T1 and T2 weighted images of the same human volunteer showing activation upon stimulation by flickering checker-board.* **A** is subtraction image showing activation at the visual cortex using the T1 weighted sequence. **B** is an EPI IRSE image (inversion recovery spin echo, TR = 4 s, TI = 1.1 s, TE = 40 ms). **C** is a conventional high resolution image. **D** is the subtraction image showing similar visual cortex activation using the T2 weighted sequence. **E** is an EPI T2SE image (spin echo, TR = 3 s, TE = 90 ms). All images are acquired with a surface coil

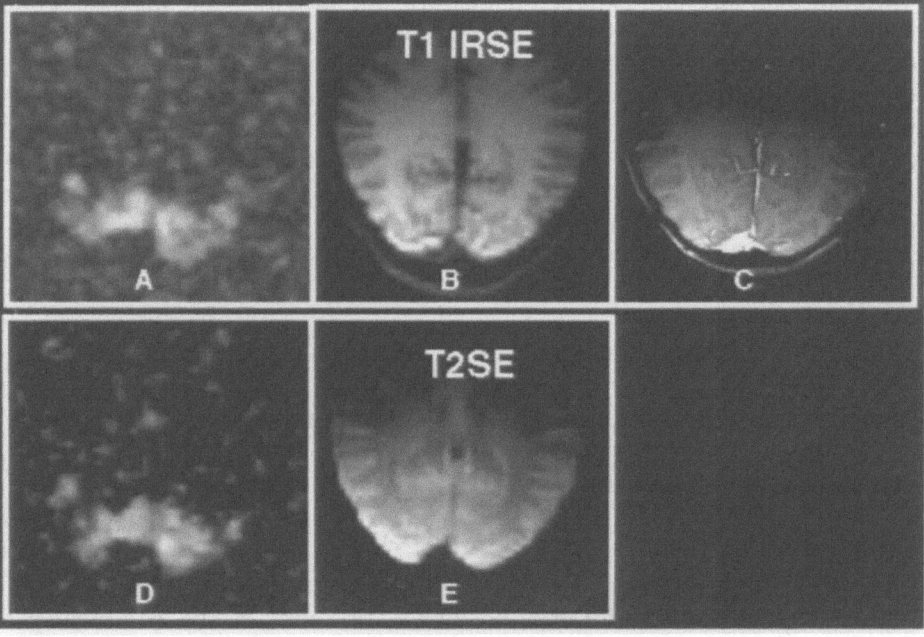

Fig. 10 A-B. *Cerebellar activation with the bending of the right elbow against a light load.* **A** demonstrates activation at the cerebellum. **B** shows activation of the primary motor cortex and the supplementary cortex of the same subject. Activation map generated uses a confidence level of p < 0.01 for statistical significance of pixels

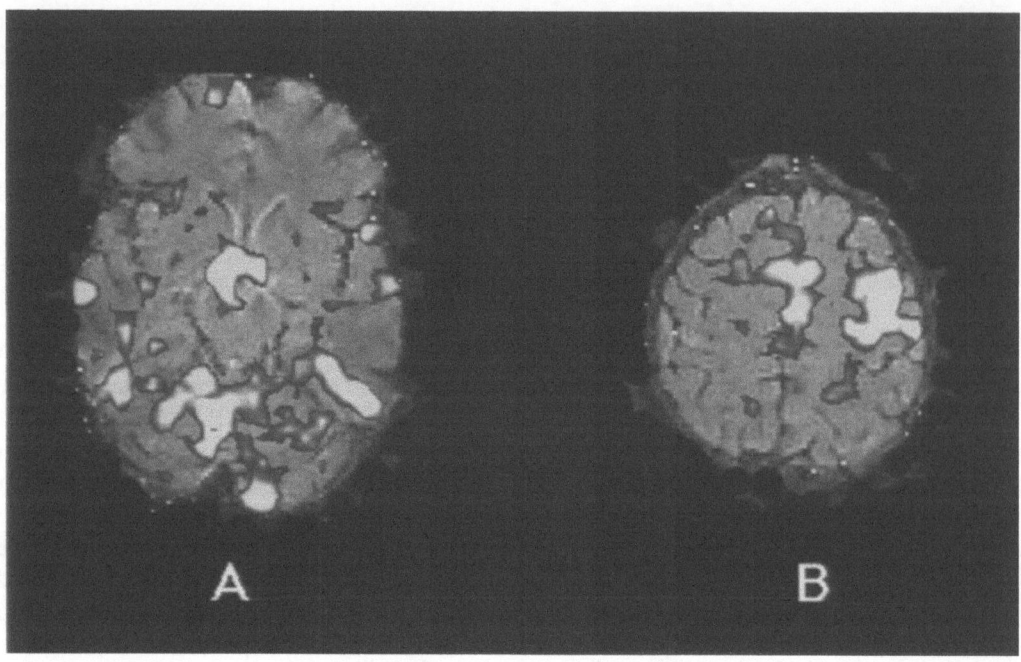

ter signal-to noise and to the fact that T_1 gets longer at higher field strength.

3. Adjusting Paradigms in fMRI

While the gradient echo sequence has a certain ambiguity, when it comes to tissue versus vessels, its sensitivity at current clinical field strength makes it an extremely attractive technique to identify activation sites. By using careful paradigms that rule out possible links between the primary activation site and secondary sites, one can circumvent many of the worries of the draining veins. A good examples is are follows. Photic stimulation activates both the primary and the extrastriate visual cortex. To show that the extrastriate regions are not just a drainage from the primary cortex, one can utilize paradigms that activate the primary visual cortex but not the extrastriate and vice versa. There are many permutations of this [104, 105]. That allows us to study the higher order functions unambiguously even if we are using gradient echo sequences. At the MGH-NMR center, the ASE sequence is routinely used as it sacrifices little T_2* sensitivity compared to the gradient echo sequence.

Image Processing Strategies

There are probably as many image processing strategies as there are centers [106] studying fMRI. The more popular analysis methods are listed.

1. Subtraction Method

The advantage of the subtraction technique is its sim-

plicity. The disadvantage is that since we are subtracting two large numbers, even a tiny movement of the head can change drastically the intensity of a boundary pixel, producing the familiar "ring" effect around the edges of the anatomy.

2. Correlation Analysis

Correlation cofficients [107-109] are calculated between the signal intensity time course of each pixel in the slice with that of an input reference function. This method has the added bonus of reducing the effect of large signal fluctuation at large vessels such as the sagittal sinus. The temporal offset of a signal can be determined via the maximum of the cross correlation function with the reference function.

3. z- and t-statistical Parametric Mapping

A ratio of signal change to the variance is due to residual fluctuations. There are many variations of the *t* test used. One version [110] used a split-half test using the first half of the data to define a small number of regions of interest, and then used the second half of the data to determine if they were stable. It was claimed that this procedure eliminated nearly all the false activations in the wrong hemisphere while note missing the true activations.

4. Nonparametric Kolmogorov-Smirnov Mapping

Since it was believed that temporal undersampling of physiological noises leads to nonnormal fMRI signal distribution, nonparametric statistical mappings such as the Kolmogorov-Smirnov statistic are used in some

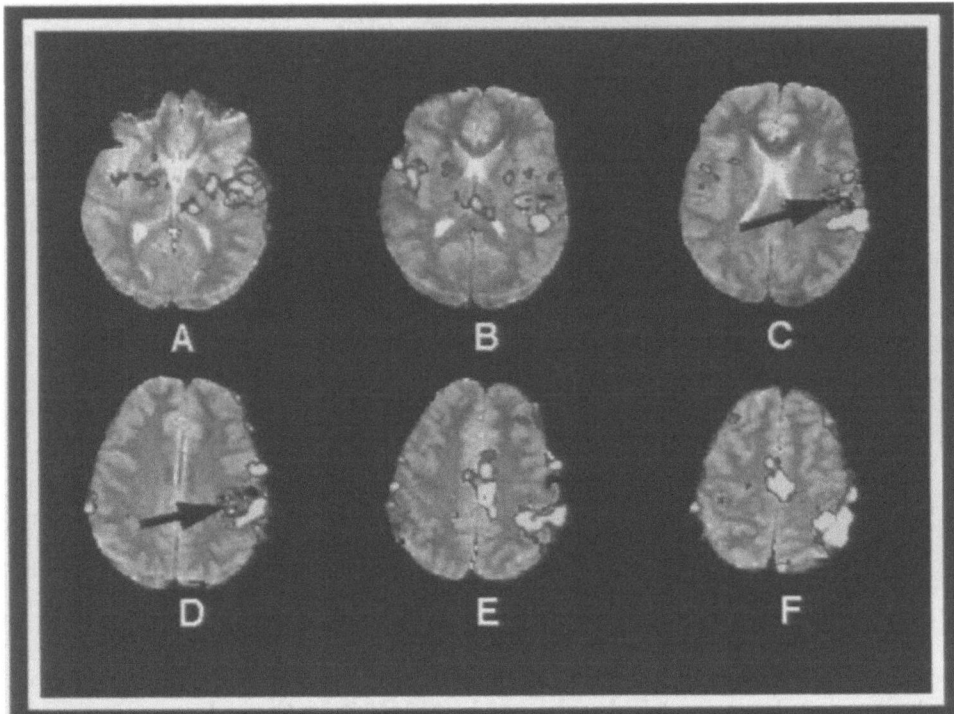

Fig. 11. A-F. *Functional MRI mapping of motor cortex for presurgical planning.* A baseline period was followed by an activation period when the patient with an arterial venal malformation (AVM) was asked to open and close his fist. Activated regions of interest (*bright regions*) are superimposed on T1-weighted multi-slice brain anatomy images. Activation map generated uses a confidence level of p < 0.01 for statistical significance of pixels. The patient's AVM is located by the black arrows in slices **C** and **D**. Activated regions in slices **C** and **D** indicate the primary motor cortex position below the AVM. The primary motor cortex and the supplementary cortex can be clearly seen on slices **E** and **F**. On both slices **A** and **B**, one observes activation at the thalamus and at the basal ganglia. (Courtesy of Dr. B. Buchbinder)

centers [111, 112]. This statistic does not rely on normality by measuring the maximum difference between the cumulative distribution functions for the sampled data during (A) experimental and during (B) control tasks.

5. Principle Component Analysis

Techniques to assess the temporal dynamics of fMRI signals are essential for the description of the synchrony of brain regions involved in cognitive processing and the relationship with behavioral observations. Principle component analysis (PCA) [111, 113] provides an objective means to identify functional components without prior definition of task blocks as is needed when using parametric and nonparametric mapping techniques. Dynamic patterns of signal change can be isolated from noise using the orthogonal set of principle components which have singular values above a significance threshold.

6. Data Clustering and Use of the Contiguity Threshold

Since coactivation of numerous contiguous voxels are expected, events of interest are considered when a contiguous region of pixels is detected, all with values above an arbitrary value [109, 112, 114-116].

7. Fourier Transform Methods

The Fourier transforms of the time responses are obtained [107] and spectral density images are made at particular frequencies. The frequency spectrum can also be filtered and have aliased frequencies rejected [117] to remove undesirable physiological fluctuations.

Application of fMRI in Brain Activation Studies

The data collected in the last three years have demonstrated that fMRI maps of the visual cortex correlate well with known retinotopic organization [29, 118, 119]. Successful studies have been carried out at higher visual regions such as motion sensitive area V5/MT [104, 105] and the face/object recognition area V4 [120]. Visual imagery has been explored [121]. The organization of motor cortex [11, 17, 28, 30, 33, 122-124] has been explored. In addition to the by-now-familiar activation of primary and supplementary motor cortex, cerebellar activation [40, 125-130] has been demonstrated (Fig. 10). Preliminary data have shown activation at the basal ganglia [131]. Activation of the deep gray matter is interesting as it may have different vascular characteristics than has the cortex. The lateral geniculate nucleus was also reported as another noncortical activation region during visual stimulation [132]. Presurgical planning work (Fig. 11) using motor stimulation [26, 133-135] has helped neurosurgeons to identify motor-sensory areas from tumors to be resected. For higher cognitive functions, several fMRI language-associated regions have been demonstrated [31, 32, 34, 44, 136-142] (Fig. 12). With either visual or auditory stimuli, language lateralization [138, 140, 143] has been demonstrated, matching results

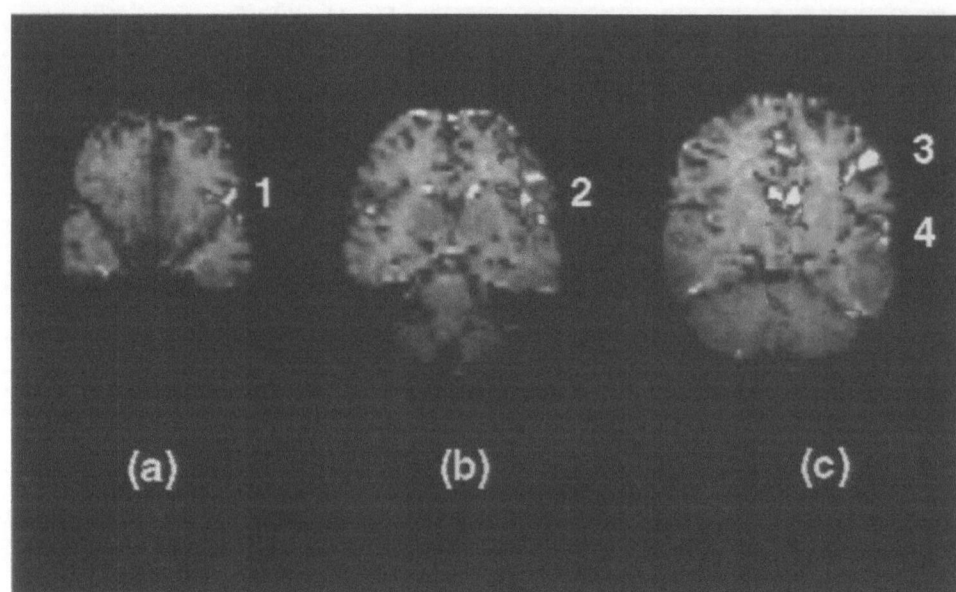

Fig. 12. *Functional data demonstrating language lateralization (EPI, gradient echo, oblique coronal slices extending to posterior sylvian fissure).* Activated language regions of interest (*bright regions 1-4*) are superimposed on T_1-weighted multi-slice brain anatomy images. Pictures of objects (airplane, cake, etc.) were projected onto a screen and shown to a subject who was then engaged in a verb generation task without overt vocalization. On slice **a**, region 1 indicates activation at area 47. On slice **b**, region 2 indicates the Broca's area. On slice **c**, region 3 indicates the pre-motor area, and region 4 indicates the Wernicke's areas. Most activated regions of interest are on the left side of the brain. Activation map generated using a confidence level of $p < 0.05$ for statistical significance of pixels. (Courtesy of Dr. R. Benson)

obtained by the standard, yet extremely invasive Wada test [144]. For memory studies, prefrontal cortex regions [145-147] have been implicated in working memory tasks. For picture encoding, fMRI also revealed significant signal intensity increases bilaterally in hippocampal and parahippocampal regions and at the temporal-occipital junction [147].

As part of the design for sleep studies and for the study of epilepsy, simultaneous functional magnetic resonance imaging and electrophysiological (EP) recording has been achieved [148, 149], requiring only minor modifications of standard EP equipment. Electrode positions included midline cephalic, biorbital and submental placements providing EEG, electro-oculographic (EOG) and electromyographic (EMG) tracings, respectively (Fig. 13). An electrode placed on the mastoid was used as a reference. The initial EP-fMRI results suggest that the method is safe and provides high quality fMRI and EP data.

Undershoots in fMRI T2* Signals: A Window to Studying Metabolism?

Note that (Fig. 3, top) with blood oxygenation sensitive MR (T_2*-weighted) technique one observes an undershoot [11, 19, 150] in signal in the primary visual cortex when the light stimulus is turned off. There has always been speculation that the undershoot might be related to metabolic events. However, it could also indicate blood volume chang. The physiological mechanism underlying the undershoot is still not well understood. Experiments (Fig. 3, bottom) also indicate that undershoot following stimulation in the flow weighted (T_1-weighted) acquisitions is not remarkable [11, 150, 151].

An equally intriguing observation that might be more tied to metabolic change is th study by proton functional spectroscopic techniques [46, 152] that demonstrated there is a signal reduction of ~0.25% ~500 ms after stimulus onset. The early signal dip can be attributed to a

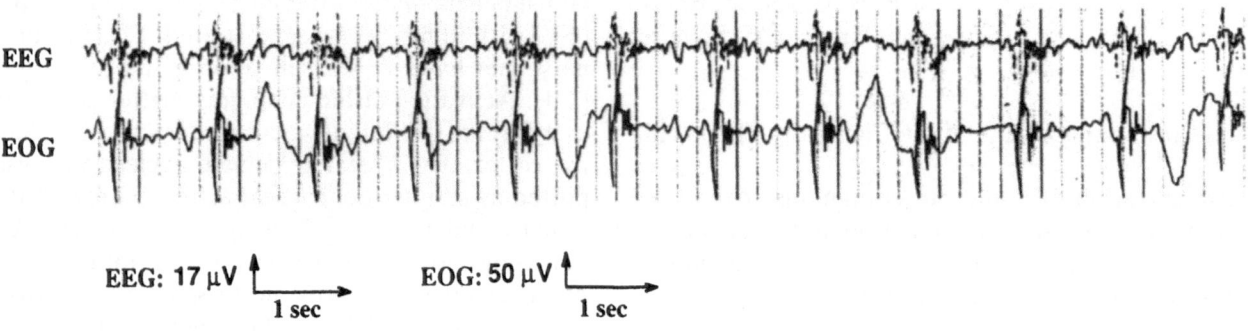

EEG: 17 μV   1 sec   EOG: 50 μV   1 sec

Fig. 13. *EEG and EOG traces acquired inside the SIGNA 1.5 T system while EPI images were acquired continuously on the subject.* The phase of the EOG signals indicates the direction of the saccade. Subjects look right and left and the full-field saccades are easily seen in the EOG tracing. Note the lack of cross-talk between the EEG and EOG data. The MRI-induced artifacts on both the EEG and the EOG tracing are small and the recovery of the EEG and EOG tracings is very rapid (Courtesy of Dr. F. Huang-Hellinger)

temporary decrease in oxygenated hemoglobin concentration. This interpretation is in accordance with optical reflectance data [65, 153]. Recently, imaging time course observed at 4 T [154] also showed a ~0.5% dip at ~2 s after goggle LED stimulus was turned on. This was also interpreted as a direct response to transient capillary changes in oxygenation and a confirmation of the BOLD effect. Right now the dip observed by spectroscopic technique appeared to occur slightly earlier than the signal drop observed by the 4 T imaging technique. Whether this is simply an experimental uncertainty or whether the two techniques point to the same phenomenon remains to be studied.

Interesting New Approaches on the Conventional Scanners for fMRI

1. High Temporal Resolution Studies

Because EPI can acquire an image every 100 ms, it is ideal for high temporal resolution studies. However, there are new, interesting methods of acquiring extremely high temporal and high spatial resolution functional images using conventional imagers [155-158]. The basic idea is to synchronize data acquisition to the repetitive stimulation. Whole images are not recorded consecutively. Instead, the sampling process is split into the recording of single Fourier lines of subsequent images. During the measurement, all Fourier line recordings are separated by the same repetition time TR. This allows precise synchronization with the external stimulus. The time resolution of this approach is determined by the time interval between two subsequent Fourier time recordings (TR < 100 ms). A total of 256 images or more could be recorded per experiment. Signal time course after 100, 300, and 700 ms visual stimulation could be obtained [155-157]. Motion artifacts during the 5 min or so of acquisition time present a potential problem.

2. Two-dimensional or Three-dimensional?

The strength of EPI in fMRI is that it can do whole head imaging. Researchers with conventional scanners have been investigating three-dimensional methods [159] since they offer a dramatic signal-to-noise ratio and cover a larger region of interest compared to two-dimensional methods. So far, at high resolution, three dimensional studies have picked up small veins activating during motor tasks. However, an interesting question has been raised as to whether two-dimensional fMRI should be chosen over three-dimensional fMRI. Frahm et al. [89] claimed that with previous studies of the effects of magnetic field inhomogeneities in FLASH sequences, the main susceptibility seemed to be due to a distortion of the refocused slice selection gradient. Any imbalance of the slice refocusing in a three-dimensional experi-

ment can theoretically be compensated for by the superimposed three-dimensional phase-encoding gradient. Whether two-dimensional or three-dimensional image acquisitions are better for fMRI is a subject of ongoing debate and investigation.

Combining Modalities: fMRI-MEG-EEG

Using EPI, one can measure hemodynamic changes associated with brain activity at a temporal resolution of ~100 ms. However, the latency of the hemodynamic response of ~2 s sets the ultimate limit on temporal resolution of any hemodynamic technique. Magnetoencephalography and electroencephalography (MEG and EEG) have much faster temporal resolution. Work has begun to combine fMRI with MEG/EEG [160-163] for improved source localization. It has been demonstrated that fMRI is sensitive to an extremely short stimulus of 33 ms [160] and allows the application of the same paradigm across fMRI and MEG/EEG studies.

Conclusion

There are many important areas related to functional studies that cannot be covered in this brief review. Such areas include new sequence developments such as the use of conventional fast spin echo [43], modified RARE sequences [164], special tailored RF sequence to increase susceptibility contrast [165], and the very successful use of spiral scan [92, 166] in conventional fMRI work. The complicated theoretical development of T2* (BOLD) contrast is only lightly touched upon [83-86, 167, 168], and there is little discussion on the rich new field of brain activation studies by MR spectroscopy such as in the study of glucose utilization [169, 170] and lactate change [60, 171-173] in the stimulation of the visual and auditory cortex.

What has been demonstrated is that fMRI is a growing field. The continuous advance of MRI mapping techniques utilizing intrinsic blood-tissue contrast promises the development of a functional human neuroanatomy of unprecedented spatial and temporal resolution.

References

1. Le Bihan D, Breton D, Lallemand D, Aubin ML, Vignaud J, Laval-Jeantet M (1988) Separation of diffusion and perfusion in intravoxel incoherent motion MR imaging. Radiology 168:497-505
2. Kwong KK, McKinstry RC, Chien D, Crawley AP, Pearlman JD, Rosen BR (1991) CSF-suppressed quantitative singleshot diffusion imaging. Magn Reson Med 21: 157-63
3. Neil JJ, Ackerman JJH (1992) Detection of pseudodiffusion in rat brain following blood substitution with perfluorocarbon. J Magn Reson 97: 194-20

4. Neil JJ, Booch CS, Ackerman JJH (1994) An evaluaition of the sensitivity of the intravoxel incoherent motion (IVIM) method of blood flow measurement to changes in cerebral blood flow. Magn Reson Med 32: 60-5

5. Henkelman RM, Neil JJ, Xiang Q-S (1994) A quantitative interpretation of IVIM measurements of vascular perfusion in the rat brain. Magn Reson Med 32: 464-9

6. Detre J, Leigh J, Williams D, Koretsky A (1992) Perfusion imaging. Magn Reson Med 23: 37-45

7. Williams DS, Detre JA, Leigh JS, Koretsky AP (1992) Magnetic resonance imaging of perfusion using spin inversion of arterial water. Proc Natl Acad Sci USA 89: 212

8. Zhang W, Williams DS, Detre JA, Koretsky AP (1992) Measurement of brain perfusion by volume-localized NMR spectroscopy using inversion of arterial spins: accounting for transit time and cross relaxation. Magn Reson Med 25: 362-71

9. Zhang W, Williams DS, Koretsky AP (1991) Measurement of rat brain perfusion by NMR using spin labeling of arterial water: in vivo determination of the degree of spin labeling. Magn Reson Med 29: 416-21

10. Dixon WT, Du LN, Faul D, Grado M, Rosnick S (1986) Projection angiograms of blood labelled by adiabatic fast passage. Magn Reson Med 3: 454-62

11. Kwong KK, Belliveau JW, Chesler DA, et al (1992) Dynamic magnetic resonance imaging of human brain activity during primary sensory stimulation. Proc Natl Acad Sci USA 89: 5675-9

12. Turner R, Le Bihan D, Moonen CT, Despres D, Frank J (1991) Echo-planar time course MRI of cat brain oxygenation changes. Magn Reson Med 22: 159-66

13. Ogawa S, Lee TM, Kay AR, Tank DW (1990) Brain magnetic resonance imaging with contrast dependent on blood oxygenation. Proc Natl Acad Sci USA 87: 9868-72

14. Ogawa S, Lee TM (1990) Magnetic resonance imaging of blood vessels at high fields: in vivo and in vitro measurements and image simulation. Magn Reson Med 16: 9-18

15. Mansfield P. Multi-planar image formation using NMR spin echoes (1977) J Physics C10: L55-8

16. Brady TJ (1991) Future prospects for MR imaging. In: Tenth Annual Meeting of the Society of Magnetic Resonance in Medicine. San Francisco, 2

17. Bandettini PA, Wong EC, Hinks RS, Tikofsky RS, Hyde JS (1992) Time course EPI of human brain function during task activation. Magn Reson Med 25:390-7

18. Belliveau JW, Kennedy Jr DN, McKinstry RC, et al (1991) Functional mapping of the human visual cortex by magnetic resonance imaging. Science 254: 716-9

19. Ogawa S, Tank DW, Menon R, et al (1992) Intrinsic signal changes accompanying sensory stimulation: functional brain mapping with magnetic resonance imaging. Proc Natl Acad Sci USA 89: 5951-5

20. Frahm J, Bruhn H, Merboldt K, Hanicke W (1992) Dynamic MR imaging of human brain oxygenation during rest and photic stimulation. J Magn Reson Imaging 2: 501-5

21. Ogawa S, Lee TM, Nayak AS, Glynn P (1990) Oxygenation-sensitive contrast in magnetic resonance image of rodent brain at high magnetic fields. Magn Reson Med 14: 68-78

22. Turner R, Jezzard P, Wen H, Kwong K, Le Bihan D, Balaban R (1992) Functional mapping of the human visual cortex at 4 Tesla using oxygen contrast EPI. In: Eleventh Annual Meeting of the Society of Magnetic Resonance in Medicine. Berlin, 304

23. Blamire A, Ogawa S, Ugurbil K, et al (1992) Dynamic mapping of the human visual cortex by high-speed magnetic resonance imaging. Proc Natl Acad Sci USA 89: 11069-73

24. Menon R, Ogawa S, Tank D, Ugurbil K (1993) 4-Tesla gradient recalled echo characteristics of photic stimulation-induced signal changes in the human primary visual cortex. Magn Reson Med 30: 380-6

25. Lai S, Hopkins AL, Haacke EM, et al (1993) Identification of vascular structures as a major source of signal contrast in high resolution 2D and 3D functional activation imaging of the cortex at 1.5T: preliminary results. Magn Reson Med 30: 387-92

26. Cao Y, Towle VL, Levin DN, Grzeszczuk R, Mullan JF (1993) Conventional 1.5 T functional MRI localization of human hand sensorimotor cortex with intraoperative electrophysiologic validation. In: Twelfth Annual Meeting of th Society of Magnetic Resonance in Medicine. New York, 1417

27. Connelly A, Jackson GD, Frackowiak RSJ, Belliveau JW, Vargha-Khadem F, Gadian DG (1993) Functional mapping of activated human primary cortex with a clinical MR imaging system. Radiology 188: 125-30

28. Kim S-G, Ashe J, Hendrick K, et al. (1993) Functional magnetic resonance imaging of motor cortex: hemispheric asymmetry and handedness. Science 261: 615-7

29. Schneider W, Noll DC, Cohen JD (1993) Functional topographic mapping of the cortical ribbon in human vision with conventional MRI scanners. Nature 365: 150-3

30. Kim SG, Ashe J, Georgopouplos AP, et al. (1993) Functional imaging of human motor cortex at high magnetic field. J Neurophysiol 69: 297

31. Hinke RM, Hu X, Stillman AE, et al. (1993) Magnetic resonance functional imaging of Broc's area during internal speech. Neuroreport 4: 675-8

32. Binder JR, Rao SM, Hammeke TA, et al. (1993) Functional magnetic resonance imaging (FMRI) of auditory semantic processing. Neurology (suppl) 2: 189

33. Rao SM, Binder JR, Bandettini PA, et al. (1993) Functional magnetic resonance imaging of complex human movements. Neurology 43: 2311-8

34. McCarthy G, Blamire AM, Rothman DL, Gruetter R, Shulman RG (1993) Echo-planar MRI studies of frontal cortex activation during work generation in humans. Proc Natl Acad Sci USA 90: 4952-6

35. Gomiscek G, Beisteiner R, Hittmair K, Mueller E, Moser E (1993) A possible role of in-flow effects in functional MR-imaging. Mag Reson Materials in Phy, Bio, Med. 1: 109-13

36. Duyn J, Moonen C, de Boer R, van Yperen G, Luyten P (1993) Inflow versus deoxyhemoglobin effects in "BOLD' functional MRI using gradient echoes at 1.5 T. In: Twelfth Annual Meeting of the Socety of Magnetic Resonance in Medicine. New York, 168

37. Hajanl JV, Collins AG, White SJ, et al. (1993) Imaging of human brain activity at 0.15 T using fluid attenuated inversion recovery (FLAIR) pulse sequences. Magn Reson Med 30: 650-3

38. Hajnal JV, Myers R, Oatridge A, Schwieso JE, Young IR, Bydder GM (1994) Artifacts due to stimulus correlated motion in functional imaging of the brain. Magn Reson Med 31: 283-91

39. Henning J, Ernst T, Speck O, Deuschl G, Feiffel E (1994) Detection of brain activation using oxygenation sensitive functional spectroscopy. Magn Reson Med 31: 85-90

40. Ellermann JM, Flament D, Kim S-G, Fu Q-G, Merkle TJ, Ugubril K (1994) Spatial patterns of functional activation of the cerebellum investigated using high field (4T) MRI. NMR Biomed 7: 63-8

41. Schad LR, Trost U, Knopp MV, Muller E, Lorenz WJ (1994) Motor cortex stimulation measured by magnetic resonance imaging on a standard 1.5 T clinical scanner. Magn Reson Imaging 11: 461-4

42. Breiter HC, Kwong KK, Baker JR, et al. (1993) Functional magnetic resonance imaging of symptom provocation in patients with obsessive-compulsive disorder versus control. In: Twelfth Annual Meeting of the Society of Magnetic Reso-

nance in Medicine. New York, 58

43. Constable RT, Kennan RP, Puce A, McCarthy G, Gore JC (1994) Functional NMR imaging using fast spin echo at 1.5 T. Magn Res Med 31: 686-90

44. Binder JR, Rao SM, Hammeke TA, et al. (1994) Functional magnetic resonance imaging of human auditory cortex. Ann Neurol 35: 662-72

45. Engel SA, Rumelhart DE, Wandell BA, et al. (1994) fMRI of human visual cortex. Nature 369: 525

46. Ernst T, Hennig J (1994) Observation of a fast response in functional MR. Magn Reson Med 32: 146-9

47. Edelman RR, Siewert B, Darby DG, et al. (1994). Qualitative mapping of cerebral blood flow and functional localization with echo-plan MR imaging and signal targeting with alternating radio frequency. Radiology 192: 513-20

48. Warach S, Sievert B, Darby D, Thangaraj V, Edelman R (1994) EPISTAR perfusion echo-planar imaging of human brain tumors. JMRI 4: S8

49. Warach S, Darby DG, Thangaraj V, Nobre AC, Sanes JA, Edelman RR (1994) Applications of EPISTAR for mapping functional changes in relative cerebral blood flow. In: Second Meeting of the Society of Magnetic Resonance. San Francisco, 72

50. Bandettini PA, Wong EC, Jesmanowicz A, et al. (1994) MRI of human brain activation at 0.5 T, 1.5 T and 3.0 T: comparisons of $\Delta R2^*$ and functional contrast to noise ratio. In: Second Meeting of the Society of Magnetic Resonance. San Francisco, 434

51. Cohen MS, Weisskoff RM (1991) Ultra-fast imaging. Magn Reson Imaging 9: 1-37

52. Wong EC, Boskamp E, Hyde JS (1992) A volume optimized quadrature elliptical endcap birdcage brain coil. In: Eleventh Annual Meeting of the Society of Magnetic Resonance in Medicine. Berlin, 4015

53. Wong EC, Bandettini PA, Hyde JS (1992) Echo-planar imaging of the human brain using a three axis local gradient coil. In: Eleventh Annual Meeting of the Society of Magnetic Resonance in Medicine. Berlin, 105

54. Turner R, Jezzard P, Wen H, et al. (1993) Functional mapping of the human visual cortex at 4 and 1.5 Tesla using deoxygenation contrast EPI. Magn Reson Med 29: 277-9

55. Frahm J, Merboldt K, Hänicke W (1993) Functional MRI of human brain activation at high resolution. Magn Reson Med 29: 139-44

56. Thulborn KR, Waterton JC, Matthews PM, Radda GK (1982) Oxygenation dependence of the transverse relaxation time of water protons in whole blood at high field. Biochim Biophys Acta 714: 265-70

57. Grubb RL, Raichle ME, Eichling JO, Ter-Pogossian MM (1974) The effects of changes in $Paco_2$ on cerebral blood volume, blood flow and vascular mean transit time. Stroke 5: 630-9

58. Fox PT, Raichle ME (1986) Focal physiological uncoupling of cerebral blood flow and oxidative metabolism during somatosensory stimulation in human subjects. Proc Natl Acad Sci USA 83: 1140-4

59. Fox PT, Raichle ME, Mintun MA, Dence C (1988) Nonoxidative glucose consumption during focal physiologic neural activity. Science 241: 462-4

60. Prichard J, Rothman D, Novotny E, et al. (1991) Lactate rise detected by ^1H NMR in human visual cortex during physiologic stimulation. Proc Natl Acad Sci USA 88: 5829-31

61. Brooks RA, Di Chiro G (1987) Magnetic resonance imaging of stationary blood: a review. Med Phys 14: 903-13

62. Vilringer A, Planck J, Hock C, Schleinkofer L, Dirnagl U (1993) Near infrared spctroscopy (NIRS): a new tool to study hemodynamic changes during activation of brain function in human adults. Neurosci Lett 134: 101-4

63. Obrig H, Kleinschmidt A, Merboldt KD, Dirnagl U, Grahm J, Villringer A (1994) Monitoring of cerebral blood oxygenation during human brain activation by simultaneous high-resolution MRI and near-infrared spectroscopy. In: Second Meeting of the Society of Magnetic Resonance. San Francisco, 67

64. Nakajima T, Fujita M, Watanabe H, et al (1994) Functional mapping of the human visual system with near-infrared spectroscopy and BOLD functional MRI. In: Second Meeting of the Society of Magnetic Resonance. San Francisco, 687

65. Turner R, Grinvald A (1994) Direct visualization of patterns of deoxygenation and reoxygenation in monkey cortical vasculature during functional brain activation. In: Second Meeting of the Society of Magnetic Resonance. San Francisco, 430

66. Jezzard P, Heineman F, Taylor J, et al (1994) Comparison of EPI gradient-echo contrast changes in cat brain caused by respiratory challenges with direct simultaneous evaluation of cerebral oxygenation via a crania window. NMR Biomed 7: 35-44

67. Edelman R, Sievert B, Wielopolski P, Pearlman J, Warach S (1994) Noninvasive mapping of cerebral perfusion by using EPISTAR MR angiography. In: First Meeting of the Society of Magnetic Resonance. Dallas, 68

68. Kwong KK, Chesler DA, Zuo CS, et al. (1993) Spin echo (T2, T1) studies for functional MRI. In: Twelfth Annual Meeting of the Society of Magnetic Resonance in Medicine. New York, 172

69. Kwong KK, Chesler DA, Weisskoff RM, Rosen BR (1994) Perfusion MR imaging. In: Second Meeting of the Society of Magnetic Resonance. San Francisco, 1005

70. Williams DS, Detre JD, Zhang W, Silva AC, Koretsky AP (1994) A survey of labeling strategies for perfusion imaging by arterial spin labeling. In: Second Meeting of the Society of Magnetic Resonance. San Francisco, 1004

71. Weisskoff RM, Baker JR, Belliveau JW, Davis TL, Kwong KK, Cohen MS, Rosen BR (1993) Power spectrum analysis of functionally weighted MR data: what's in the noise? In: Eleventh Annual Meeting of the Society of Magnetic Resonance in Medicine. New York

72. Weisskoff RM, Hoppel BE, Rosen BR (1992) Signal changes in dynamic contrast studies: theory and experiment in vivo. in: Tenth Meeting of th Society for Magnetic Resonance Imaging. Chicago, 44

73. Zuo C, Boxerman J, Weisskoff R (1992) Compartment size determines T2 relaxivity in susceptibility contrast agents: theory and experiment. In: Eleventh Annual Meeting of the Society of Magnetic Resonance in Medicine. Berlin, 866

74. McKenize CA, Drost DJ, Carr TJ (1997) The effect of magnetic field strength on signal change $\Delta S/S$ in function MRI with BOLD contrast. In: Second Meeting of the Society of Magnetic Resonance. San Francisco, 433

75. Jezzard P, LeBihan D, Cuenod C, Pannier L, Prinster A, Turner R (1993) An investigation of the contribution of physiological noise in human functional MRI studies at 1.5 Tesla and 4 Tesla. In: Twelfth Annual Meeting of the Society of Magnetic Resonance in Medicine. New York, 1392

76. Hu X, Kim S-G (1994) Reduction of signal fluctuation in functional MRI using navigator echo. Magn Reson Med 31: 495-503

77. Noll D, Schneider W (1994) Respiration artifacts in functional brain imaging: sources of signal variation and compensation strategies. In: Second Meeting of the Society of Magnetic Resonance. San Francisco, 647

78. Jezzard P, Goldstein SR (1994) A head position monitoring device for use in functional MRI studies. In: Second Conference of the Society of Magnetic Resonance. San Francisco, 648

79. Woods R, Mazziotta J, Cherry S (1992) Automated algorithm for aligning tomographic images. II. Cross-modality MRI-PET registration. J Comput Assist Tomogr 16: 620-33

80. Tyszka JM, Grafton ST, Chew W, et al (1994) Parceling of mesial frontal motor areas during ideation and movement using functional magnetic resonance imaging at 1.5 Tesla. Ann Neurol 35: 662-72

81. Jiang A, Kennedy D, Woods R, et al (1994) Motion detection and correction in functional MRI. In: Second Meeting of the Society of Magnetic Resonance. San Francisco, 351

82. Risinger R, Hertz-Pannier L, Schmidt M, Maisog JM, Cuenod CA, Le Bihan C (1994) Evaluation of image registration in functional brain MRI. In: Second Meeting of the Society of Magnetic Resonance, San Francisco, 649

83. Fisel CR, Ackerman JL, Buxton RB, et al (1991) MR contrast due to microscopically heterogeneous magnetic susceptibility: numerical simulations and applications to cerebral physiology. Magn Reson Med 17: 336-47

84. Ogawa S. Menon R, Tank D, et al. (1993) Functional brain mapping by blood oxygenation level dependent contrast magnetic resonance imaging. A comparison of signal characteristics with a biophysical model. Biophys J 64: 803-12

85. Weisskoff RM, Boxerman JL, Zuo CS, Rosen BR (1993) Endogenous susceptibility contrast: principles of relationship between blood oxygenation and MR signal change. In: Functional MRI of the brain. Society of Magnetic Resonance in Medicine. Arlington, VA, 103

86. Weisskoff RM, Zuo CS, Boxerman JL, Rosen BR (1994) Microscopic susceptibility variation and transverse relaxation: theory and experiment. Magn Reson Med 31: 601-10

87. Frahm J, Merboldt K, Hanicke W (1993) Tissue vs. vascular effects and changes of flow vs. deoxyhemoglobin? Problems revealed by functional brain imaging at high spatial resolution. In: Twelfth Annual Meeting of the Society of Magnetic Resonance in Medicine. New York, 1427

88. Duyn JH, Moonen CTW, Van Yperen GH, De Boer RW, Luyten PR (1994) Inflow versus deoxyhemoglobin effects in BOLD functional MRI using gradient echoes at 1.5 T. NMR Biomed 7:83-9

89. Frahm J, Merboldt K-D, Hanicke W, Kleinschmidt A, Boecker H (1994) Brain or vein oxygenation or flow? On signal physiology in functional MRI of human brain activation. NMR Biomed 7

90. Kim S-G, Hendrich K, Hu X, Merkle H, Ugurbil K (1994) Potential pitfalls of functional MRI using conventional gradient-recalled echo techniques. NMR Biomed 7: 69-74

91. DeYoe EA, Neitz J, Miller D, Wieser J (1993) Functional magnetic resonance imaging (FMRI) of visual cortex in human subjects using a unique video graphics stimulator. In: Twelfth Annual Meeting of the Society of Magnetic Resonance in Medicine. New York, 1394

92. Lee AT, Meyer CH, Glover GH (1994) Discrimination of large veins in time-course functional neuroimaging with spiral K-space trajectories. In: First Meeting of the Society of Magnetic Resonance (JMRI). Dallas, 59

93. Baker JR, Hopel BE, Stern CE, Kwong KK, Weisskoff RM, Rosen BR (1993) Dynamic functional imaging of the complete human cortex using gradient-echo and asymmetric spin-echo echo-planar magnetic resonance imaging. In: Twelfth Annual Meeting of the Society of Magnetic Resonance in Medicine. New York, 1400

94. Poncelet B, Weisskoff R, Wedeen V, Brady T, Kantor H (1993) Time of flight quantification of coronary flow with echo planar MRI. Magn Reson Med 30: 447-57

95. Kwong KK, Chesler DA, Boxerman JL, Davis TL, Weisskoff RM, Rosen BR (1994) Strategies to reduce macrovascular effects in fMRI. In: Second Meeting of the Society of Magnetic Resonance. San Francisco, 650

96. Hu X, Kim S-G (1993) A new T2* weighting technique for magnetic resonance imaging. Magn Reson Med 30: 512-7

97. Song W, Bandettini P, Wong E, Hyde J (1994) The effect of diffusion weighting on task-induced functional MRI. In: Second Meeting of the Society of Magnetic Resonance. San Francisco, 643

98. Boxerman JL, Weisskoff RM, Kwong KK, Davis TL, Rosen BR (1994) The intravascular contribution to fMRI signal change: modeling and diffusion-weighted in vivo studies. In: Second Meeting of the Society of Magnetic Resonance. San Francisco, 619

99. Menon RS, Hu X, Adroamu G, Andersen P, Ogawas S, Ugurbil K (1994) Comparison of spin-echo EPI, asymmetric spinecho EPI and conventional EPI applied to functional neuroimaging: the effect of flow crushing gradients on the BOLD signal. In: Second Meeting of the Society of Magnetic Resonance. San Francisco, 622

100. Caro CG, Pedley TJ, Seed WA (1974) In: Cardovascular physiology. Medical and Technical Publishers, London, Chapter I

101. Bandettini P, Wong E, Jesmanowicz A, Hinks R, Hyde J (1993) Simultaneous mapping of activation-induced $\Delta R2^*$ and $\Delta R2$ in the human brain using a combined gradient-echo and spin-echo EPI pulse sequence. In: Twelfth Annual Meeting of the Society of Magnetic Resonance in Medicine. New York, 169

102. Turner R, Jezzard P, Le Bihan D, Prinster A (1993) Contrast mechanisms and vessel size effects in BOLD contrast functional neuroimaging. In: Twelfth Annual Meeting of the Society of Magnetic Resonance in Medicine. New York, 173

103. Bandettini PA, Wong EC, Jesmanowicz A, Hinks RS, Hyde JS (1994) Spin-echo and gradient echo EPI of human brain activation using BOLD contrast: a comparative study at 1.5 T. NMR Biomed 7:12-20

104. Tootell RBH, Kwong KK, Belliveau JW, et al (1993) Mapping human visual cortex: evidence from functional MRI and histology. In: Investigative opthalmology and visual science. Annual Meeting, Sarasoto, 813

105. Tootell RBH, Reppas JB, Kwong KK, et al (1994) Coding of motion and color in human cortical area MT/V5. In: Second Meeting of the Society of Magnetic Resonance. San Francisco, 690

106. Russell DP (1994) A generalized approach to time-course data analysis of functional MRI of the human brain. In: Second Meeting of the Society of Magnetic Resonance. San Francisco, 636

107. Bandettini PA, Jesmanowicz A, Wong EC, Hyde JS (1993) Processing strategies for time-course data sets in functional MRI of the human brain. Magn Reson Med 30: 161-73

108. Friston KJ, Jezzard P, Turner R (1994) Analysis of functional MRI time-series. Human Brain Maping 1: 153-71

109. Requardt M, Kleinschmidt A, Hanicke W, Merboldt KD, Frahm J (1994) Evaluation strategies for MRI of human brain activation: individual analysis of correlational imaging and cluster detection. In: Second Meeting of the Society of Magnetic Resonance. San Francisco, 625

110. Schneider W, Casey BJ, Noll D (1993) Functional MRI mapping of individual stages of visual processing. In: Twelfth Annual Meeting of the Society of Magnetic Resonance in Medicine. New York, 56

111. Baker JR, Weisskoff RM, Stern CE, et al (1994) Statistical assessment of functional MRI signal change. In: Second Meeting of the Society of Magnetic Resonance. San Francisco, 626

112. Wu D, Lewin JS (1994) Evaluation of non-parametric statistic measures and data clustering for functional MR data analysis. In: Second Meeting of the Society of Magnetic Resonance. San Francisco, 629

113. Sychra JJ, Bandettini PA, Bhattacharya N, Lin Q (1994) Synthetic images by subspaces transforms. I: principal com-

ponents images and related filters. Med Phys 21: 193-201

114. Ding X, Tkach J, Ruggieri P, Masaryk T (1994) Analysis of time-course functional MRI data with clustering method without use of reference signal. In: Second Meeting of the Society of Magntic Resonance. San Francisco, 630

115. Xiong J, Gao J-H Lancaster JL, Fox PT (1994) Statistical analysis of spatial extent in functional MRI. In: Second Meeting of the Society of Magnetic Resonance. San Francisco, 631

116. Forman SD, Cohen JD, Mintun MA, Noll DC (1994) Improved assessment of significant change in functional magnetic resonance imaging (fMRI): use of the contiguity threshold. In: Second Meeting of the Society of Magnetic Resonance. San Francisco, 632

117. Biswal B, DeYoe EA, Jesmanowicz A, Hyde JS (1994) Removal of physiological fluctuations from functional MRI signals. In: Second Meeting of the Society of Magnetic Resonance. San Francisco, 653

118. Belliveau JW, Kwong KK, Baker JR, et al. (1992) MRI mapping of human visual cortex: retinotopic organization and frequency response of V1. In: Eleventh Annual Meeting of the Society of Magnetic Resonance in Medicine. Berlin, 310

119. DeYoe E, Neitz J, Bandettini P, Wong E, Hyde J (1992) Time course of event-related MR signal enhancement in visual and motor cortex. In: Eleventh Annual Meeting of the Society of Magnetic Resonance in Medicine. Berlin, 1824

120. Malach R, Tootell RBH, Reppas JB, et al (1994) Functional MRI reveals a candidate area V4 in human visual cortex. In: Second Meeting of the Society of Magnetic Resonance. San Francisco, 692

121. Le Bihan D, Turner R, Zeffiro T, Cuenod CA, Jezzard P, Bonnerot V (1993) Activation of human primary visual cortex during visual recall: an MRI study. Proc Natl Acad Sci USA 90: 11802-5

122. Rao SM, Binder JR, Hammeke TA, et al (1993) Somatotopic mapping of the primary motor cortex with functional magnetic resonance imaging. In: Twelfth Annual Meeting of the Society of Magnetic Resonance in Medicine. New York, 1397

123. Cao Y, Towle VL, Levin DN, Balter JM (1993) Functional mapping of human motor cortical activation by conventional MRI at 1.5 T. J Magn Reson Imaging 3: 869-75

124. Cao Y, Vikingstad EM, Huttenlocher PR, Towle VL, Levin DN (1994) Functional magnetic resonance studies of the reorganization of the human hand sensorimotor area after unilateral brain injury in the perinatal period. Proc Natl Acad Sci USA 91: 9612-6

125. Ellermann JM, Flament D, Kim SG, et al (1993) Studies of human cerebellar function using multislice nuclear magnetic resonance imaging at high magnetic field. In: Twelfth Annual Meeting of the Society of Magnetic Resonance in Medicine. New York, 1401

126. Bates SR, Yetkin FZ, Bandettini PA, Jesmanopwicz A, Estkowski L, Haughton VM (1993) Activation of the human cerebellum demonstrated by functional magnetic resonance imaging. In: Twelve Annual Meeting of the Society of Magnetic Resonance in Medicine. New York, 1420

127. Cuenod CA, Zeffiro T, Pannier L, et al (1993) Functional imaging of the human cerebellum during finger movement with a conventional 1.5 T MRI scanner. In: Twelfth Annual Meeting of the Society of Magnetic Resonance in Medicine. New York, 1421

128. Ellermann JM, Flament D, Kim SG, et al (1994) Cerebellar activation due to error detection-correction in a fisuo-motor learning task: a functional magnetic resonance imaging study. In: Second Meeting of the Society of Magnetic Resonance. San Francisco, 331

129. Kim S-G, Ugurbil K, Strick P (1994) Activation of a cerebellar output nucleus during cognitive processing. Science 265: 949-51

130. Buonocore MH, Gao L, Nordahl T, Katzberg RW (1994) Unilateral cerebral with bilateral cerebellar activation during mastication muscle tensing. In: Second Meeting of the Society of Magnetic Resonance. San Francisco, 675

131. Bucher SF, Seelos KC, Sethling M, Oertel WH, Reiser M (1994) High resolution activation mapping of basal ganglia with functional magnetic resonance imaging at 1.5 Tesla. In: Second Meeting of the Society of Magnetic Resonance. San Francisco, 332

132. Frahm J, Merboldt KD, Hanckke W, Kleinschmide A, Steinmetz H (1993) High-resolution functional MRI of focal subcortical activity in the human brain. Long-echo time FLASH of the lateral geniculate nucleus during visual stimulation. In: Twelfth Annual Meeting of the Society of Magnetic Resonance in Medicine. New York, 57

133. Buchbinder BR, Jiang JH, Cosgrove GR, et al (1994) Functional mapping of sensorimotor cortex: correlation between functional MRI, O-15 PET, and intraoperative cortical stimulation in individual subjects. American, Society of Neuro-Radiology, 162

134. Jack CR, Thompson RM, Butts RK, et al (1994) Sensory motor cortex: correlation of presurgical mapping with functional MR imaging and invasive cortical mapping. Radiology 190: 85-92

135. Howard R, Alsop D, Detre J, et al (1994) Functional MRI of regional brain activity in patients with intracerebral gliomas and AVMs prior to surgical or endovascular therapy. In: Second Meeting of the Society of Magnetic Resonance. San Francisco, 701

136. Rao S, Bandettini P, Wong E, et al. (1992) Gradient-echo EPI demonstrates bilateral superior temporal gyrus activation during word presentation. In: Eleventh Annual Meeting of the Society of Magnetic Resonance in Medicine. Berlin, 1827

137. Benson RR, Kwong KK, Belliveau JW, et al (1993) Magnetic resonance imaging studies for visual word recognition: words versus false font strings. In: 23th Annual Meeting of the Society of Neuroscience, Washington, DC, 1807

138. Binder JR, Rao SM, Hammeke TA, et al (1994) A lateralized, distributed network for semantic processing demonstred with whole brain functional MRI. In: Second Meeting of the Society of Magnetic Resonance. San Francisco, 695

139. Binder JR, Rao SM, Hammeke TA, Frose JA, Bandettini PA, Hyde JS (1994) Syllable rate determines functional MRI response magnitude during a speech discrimination task. In: Second Meeting of the Society of Magnetic Resonance. San Francisco, 327

140. Benson RR, Kwong KK, Buchbinder BR, et al (1994) Noninvasive evaluation of language dominance using functional MRI. In: Second Meeting of the Society of Magnetic Resonance. San Francisco, 684

141. Hyder F. Blamire AM, Phelps EA, Rothman DL, Shulman RG (1994) Functional magnetic resonance imaging of human prefrontal cortex during a verbal fluency task. In: Second Meeting of the Society of Magnetic Resonance. San Francisco, 685

142. Turner R, Jezzard P, Prinster A, et al (1994) Cortical regions involved in processing written English and American sign language by hearing and deaf subjects: a functional MRI study at 4 Tesla. In: Second Meeting of the Society of Magnetic Resonance. San Francisco, 683

143. Hertz-Pannier L, Gaillard WD, Mott S, et al (1994) Preoperative assessment of language lateralization by FMRI in children with complex partial seizures: preliminary study. In: Second Meeting of the Society of Magnetic Resonance. San Francisco, 326

144. Wada J, Rasmussen T (1960) Intracarotid injection of sodi-

um amytal for the lateralization of cerebral speech dominance. Experimental and clinical observations. J Neurosurg 17: 266-82

145. Blamire AM, McCarthy G, Nobre AC, et al (1993) Functional magnetic resonance imaging of human pre-frontal cortex during a spatial memory task. In: Twelfth Annual Meeting of the Society of Magnetic Resonance in Medicine. New York, 1413

146. Cohen JD, Forman SD, Casey BJ, Noll DC (1993) Spiral-scan imaging of dorsolateral prefrontal cortex during a working memory task. In: Twelfth Annual Meeting of the Society of Magnetic Resonance in Medicine. New York, 1405

147. Stern CE, Corkin S, Guimaraes AR, et al (1994) A functional MRI study of long-term-explicit memory in humans. In: 24th Annual Meeting of the Society for Neuroscience. Miami Beach, 1290

148. Ives JR, Warach S, Schmitt F, Edelman RR, Schomer DL (1993) Monitoring the patient's EEG during echo planar MRI. Electroencephalogr Clin Neurophysiol 87: 417-20

149. Huang-Hellinger FR, Breiter HC, McCormack G, et al (1994) Simultaneous functional magnetic resonance imaging and electrophysiological recording. In: Eleventh Annual Meeting of the Society of Magnetic Resonance. San Francisco, 667

150. Stern CE, Kwong KK, Belliveau JW, Baker JR, Rosen BR (1992) MR tracking of physiological mechanisms underlying brain activity. In: Eleventh Annual Meeting of the Society of Magnetic Resonance in Medicine. Berlin, 1821

151. Davis TL, Weisskoff RM, Kwong KK, Savoy R, Rosen BR (1994) Susceptibility contrast undershoot is not matched by inflow contrast undershoot. In: Second Meeting of the Society of Magnetic Resonance. San Francisco, 435

152. Henning J, Ernst T, Speck O, Laubenberger J (1993) Functional spectroscopy: a new tool for the observation of brain activation. In: Twelfth Annual Meeting of the Society of Magnetic Resonance in Medicine. New York, 12

153. Frostig RD, Lieke EE, Tso DY, Grinvald A (1990) Cortical functional architecture and local coupling between neuronal activity and the microcirculation revealed by in vivo high-resolution optical imaging of intrinsic signals. Proc Natl Acad Sci USA 87: 6082-6

154. Menon RS, Hu X, Andersen P, Ugurbil K, Ogawa S (1994) Cerebral oxy/deoxy hemoglobin changes during neural activation: MRI timecourse correlates to optical reflectance measurements. In: Second Meeting of the Societyof Magnetic Resonance. San Francisco, 68

155. Beisteiner R, Miller E, Gomiscek G, Edward V, Moser E (1994) Ultrafast high resolution functional MRI on clinical imagers. In: Eleventh Annual Meeting of The European Society of Magnetic Resonance in Medicine and Biology. Vienna

156. Beisteiner R, Gomiscek G, Edward V, Teichtmeister C, Moser E (1994) High temporal and spatial resolution in functional imaging on clinical imagers: investigating blood flow changes in the millisecond range. In: Second Meeting of the Society of Magnetic Resonance. San Francisco, 661

157. Teichtmeister C, Beisteiner R, Moser E (1994) Comparison of slow and fast GE-FMRI on a clinical imager. In: Second Meeting of the Society of Magnetic Resonance. San Francisco, 662

158. Merboldt KD, Kruger G, Hanicke W, Frahm J (1994) FLASH MRI of human brain activation using a CINE technique. An approach towards high temporal and spatial res-

olution. In: Second Meeting of the Society of Magnetic Resonance. San Francisco, 432

159. Haacke EM, Hopkins A, Lai S, et al (1994) 2D and 3D high resolution gradient echo functional imaging of the brain: venous contributions to signal in motor cortex studies. NMR Biomed 7: 54-62

160. Belliveau JW, Baker JR, Kwong KK, et al (1993) Functional neuroimaging combining fMRI, MEG and EEG. In: Eleventh Annual Meeting of the Society of Magnetic Resonance in Medicine. New York, 6

161. Sanders JA, Lewine JD, George JS, Caprihan A, Orrison WW Correlation of fMRI with MEG. In: Twelfth Annual Meeting of the Society of Magnetic Resonance in Medicine. New York, 1418

162. Beisteiner R, Gomiscek G, Erdler M, Teichtmeister C, Moser E (1994) Comparison of magnetoencephalography with functional MR imaging on the same subjects. In: First Meeting of the Society of Magnetic Resonance (JMRI). Dallas, 16

163. Ono Y, Shimizu H, Nakasoto N, Kawamura T, Fujiwara S, Yoshimoto T (1994) Evaluation of functional magnetic resonance imaging in comparison to magnetoencephalography. In: Second Meeting of the Society of Magnetic Resonance. San Francisco, 668

164. Hennig J, Hennel F, Oesterle, Speck O, Janz C, Nedelec JF (1994) Fast and robust measurement of brain activation using modified RARE-sequences with variable contrast. In: Second Meeting of the Society of Magnetic Resonance. San Francisco, 660

165. Cho ZH, Ro YM, Park SH, Chung SC, Ong R (1994) NMR functional imaging using tailored RF gradient echo sequence - a true susceptibility measurement technique. In: Second Meeting of the Society of Magnetic Resonance. San Francisco, 659

166. Noll DC, Cohen JD, Meyer CH, Schneider W (1994) Spiral K-space MR imaging of cortical activation: In: First Meeting of the Society of Magnetic Resonance (JMRI). Dallas, 25

167. Ogawa S, Lee TM, Barrere B (1993) The sensitivity of magnetic resonance image signals of a rat brain to changes in the cerebral venous blood oxygenation. Magn Reson Med 29: 205-10

168. Kennan RP, Zhong J, Gore JC (1994) Intravascular susceptibility contrast mechanisms in tissues. Magn Reson Med 31: 9-21

169. Merboldt KD, Bruhn H, Hanicke W, Michaelis T, Frahm J (1992) Decrease of glucose in the human visual cortex during visual stimulation. Magn Reson Med 22: 68-78

170. Chen W, Novotny EJ, Zhu X-H Rothman DL, Shulman RG (1994) Localized ^{1}H NMR measurement of glucose consumption in the human brain during visual stimulation. In: Twelfth Annual Meeting of the Society of Magnetic Resonance in Medicine. New York, 1528

171. Singh M (1992) Toward proton MR spectroscopic imaging of stimulated brain function. IEEE Trans Nucl Sci 39: 1161-4

172. Singh M, Kim T (1993) Time-course of lactate in the human auditory cortex during stimulation. In: Twelfth Annual Meeting of the Society of Magnetic Resonance in Medicine. New York , 1529

173. Watanabe H, Kuwabara T, Ohkubo M, Ito T, Sakai K, Yuasa T (1993) Prolonged lactate after photic stimulation in the visual cortex of patients of mitochondrial encephalomyopathy. In: Twelfth Annual Meeting of the Society of Magnetic Resonance in Medicine. New York, 1527

High Field Functional MRI in Humans: Applications to Cognitive Function

K.R. Thulborn[1,2], J. Voyvodic[1], B. McCurtain[2], J. Gillen[1], S. Chang[1], M. Just[3], P. Carpenter[3], J.A. Sweeney[2]

MR Research Center, Departments of [1]Radiology and [2]Psychiatry, University of Pittsburgh Medical Center, and [3]Department of Psychology, Carnegie Mellon University, Pittsburgh, PA 15213, USA

Introduction

Magnetic resonance imaging (MRI) technology at field strengths up to 1.5 T is mature after many years of experience by manufacturers in providing a clinically acceptable level of performance. The MRI technique is the accepted modality of choice for neuroimaging when the question of structural abnormality is raised. The development of functional MRI (fMRI) offers potential for developing clinical applications in which brain function as well as anatomy are examined [1]. The presumed mechanism on which most current fMRI is based is the increased MR signal that arises from the increased blood flow that occurs with increased neuronal activity. The increased flow, out of proportion to the tissue oxygen utilization, increases the net tissue blood oxygenation [2] thereby decreasing the magnetic susceptibility-induced transverse relaxation caused by deoxygenated blood. This has been termed blood oxygenation level dependent (BOLD) contrast [3]. Such signal changes in the microvasculature are small (1-5%), and therefore always limited by the available signal-to-noise ratio (SNR). Strategies to improve the reliability of such measurements for clinical applications would be useful. As the effect is related to magnetic susceptibility, improvements in SNR may be found at higher magnetic field strengths than currently being used clinically. The extension of the same reliable technology to higher fields to realize an increased SNR and sensitivity to this effect is now being addressed by manufacturers. The development of high-field MRI involves more than the magnet. In fact, the magnet technology is not the limiting factor as is clear from the availability of 4 T magnets for several years. Rather there are compromises in performance incurred for biological samples when the wavelength of the electromagnetic energy approaches the size of the human head or body. The signal intensity across the field of view becomes non-uniform as the wavelength approaches the size of the field of view. Similarly, the magnetic susceptibility effects of the human head are expected to become worse at higher field strengths. At very high field strengths, untoward biological effects such as headaches, disequilibrium and gustatory stimulation have been reported. Confinement of the fringe fields becomes an important siting consideration at 4 T. With these issues in mind, we have worked with three manufacturers (General Electric Medical Systems; Advanced NMR Systems, Inc.; and Magnex Scientific, Inc.) to extend the technology of a clinical scanner operating at 1.5 T to a new operating field strength of 3.0 T. This prototype scanner has the same capabilities of conventional imaging, angiography, spectroscopy and echo planar imaging as the 1.5 T scanner has. We report on the comparison in performance with respect to fMRI capabilities of the two scanners under near-identical conditions, located in the same environment.

Methods

The 1.5 T whole body Signa scanner (bore access 55 cm, General Electric Medical Systems, Milwaukee, WI) has imaging and spectroscopic capabilities of operating system Version 5.4.2 software with additional echo planar imaging capabilities (Advanced NMR Systems, Inc. Wilmington, MA). The magnet is passively shielded and has a final homogeneity of about 2 Hz over a 22 cm diameter sphere.

The 3.0 T whole body Signa scanner (bore access 55 cm, General Electric Medical Systems, Corporate Research and Development, NY) has comparable operating capabilities to the 1.5 T system from which it is derived. The magnet, manufactured by Magnex Scientific, Inc., is passively shielded and has a field homogeneity of 6 Hz over a 22 cm diameter sphere.

Comparison of fMRI performance on human subjects was made using commercial birdcage, quadrature-drive head coils supplied with each system. As relaxation constants change with field strength, T1 and T2 maps were calculated over the human head using spin echo, echo planar imaging at variable repetition time (TR) and echo time (TE), respectively. For fMRI, TE must be matched to T2* at each field strength for a valid comparison of performance. Values of T2* were calculated from gradi-

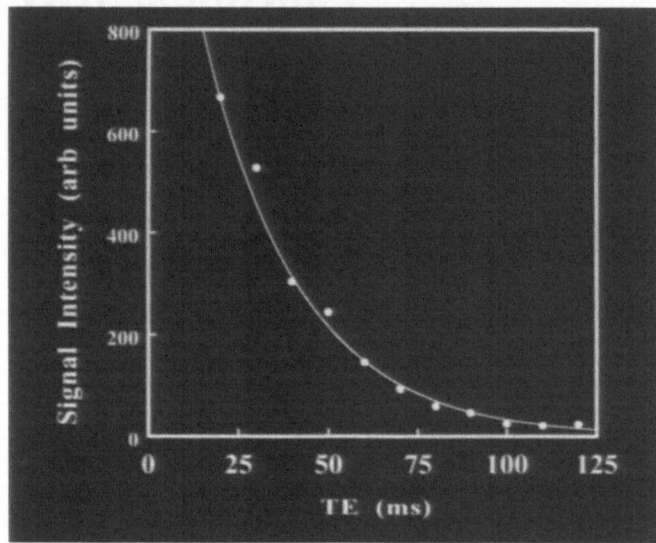

Fig. 1. *Representative data for the determination of T2* at 3.0 T on a human brain using gradient echo, echo planar imaging at variable TE.* TR = 6 s, acquisition matrix = 128 × 64, 5 mm slice thickness, 1 mm gap, axial plane

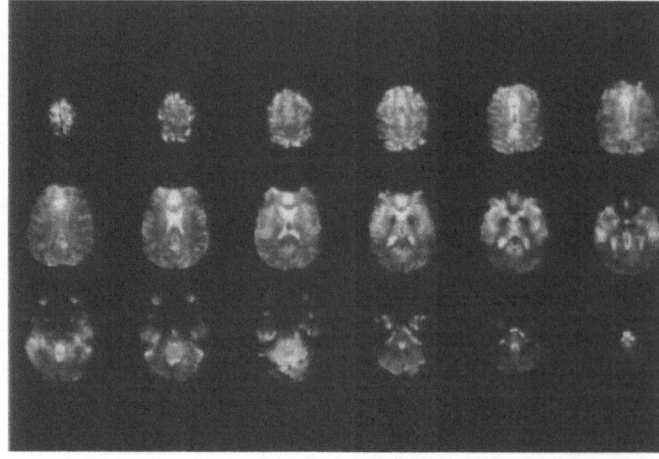

Fig. 2. *Gradient echo, echo planar images at 3.0 T covering the entire brain as used for fMRI have high SNR over most of the brain.* Artifacts from magnetic susceptibility induced field gradients are evident adjacent to the frontal and sphenoid sinuses, orbits and around the petrous bones. However most of the cerebral hemispheres, cerebellum and brainstem are accessible with minimal artifact. Acquisition parameters are given in text

ent echo, echo planar imaging at variable TE and long TR using fits of single exponential functions to the mean signal intensity in representative regions of interest (ROI) sampling multiple regions of the brain. A representative plot of the T2* measurement is shown in Fig. 1.

Functional MRI was performed with gradient echo, echo planar imaging in the axial plane as a multi-slice acquisition (TE = 25 ms at 3.0 T, TE = 50 ms at 1.5 T, single shot, full k-space, TR = 1000–4000 ms, 5 mm thickness, 1 mm gap, 128 × 64 acquisition matrix size, nominal voxel dimensions of 3 × 3 × 5 mm) using the paradigms described below. The quality of these echo planar images over the entire brain is evident in Fig. 2. The functional data were superimposed on high-resolution structural spin echo, echo planar images (TE = 100 ms, two-shot, 256 × 128 acquisition matrix size, full k-space, TR = 6000 ms, 5 mm thickness, 1 mm gap, with 1.5 mm offset for 4 overlapping series of data sets giving nominal voxel dimensions of 1.5 × 1.5 × 1.5 mm). These structural data were displayed as either a set of planar images or as three orthogonal views of the essentially three dimensional data set as shown in Fig. 3.

Neuropsychological paradigms were selected to cover both primary and higher cognitive functions appropriate for evaluating various aspects of field strength dependence of fMRI.

Test-retest reliability was investigated at 3.0 T using multiple trials of 3 cycles of a paradigm of alternating hemifield, flashing (8 Hz, 30 s) checkerboard photic stimulation interleaved with an ipsilateral sequential finger-thumb apposition motor task (50 s) described below. This paradigm is represented schematically in Fig. 4. This was performed as three separate trials separated by 10 min on the same subject. The patterns of both visual

and motor activation were compared across trials at the same t-statistic as displayed in Fig. 5. The time courses of changes in signal intensity of individual voxels from right and left visual and motor cortex are shown in Fig. 6.

The effect of field strength on detectability of functional activity was performed using a motor task of bilateral finger-thumb apposition in which the thumb was apposed to each ipsilateral digit sequentially. There were 6 cycles of alternating rest (30 s) and motor task (30 s). Activation was defined using a simple t-test com-

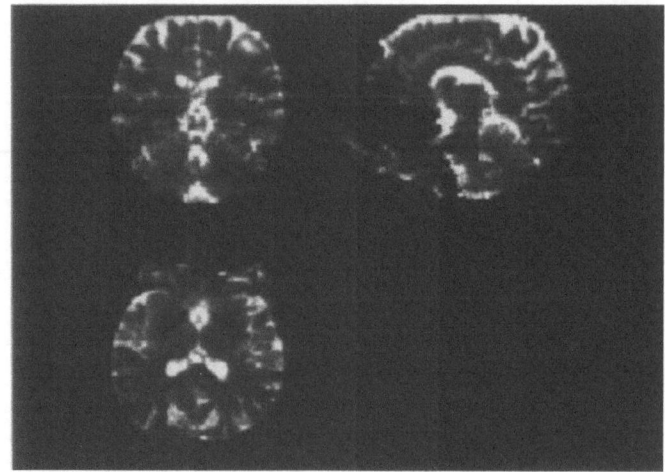

Fig. 3. *Spin echo, echo planar images at 3.0 T covering the entire brain as used for structural MRI have high SNR over most of the brain.* Artifacts from magnetic susceptibility induced field gradients are evident adjacent to the frontal and sphenoid sinuses, orbits and around the petrous bones as more evident on the gradient echo images in Fig. 2. Acquisition parameters are given in text

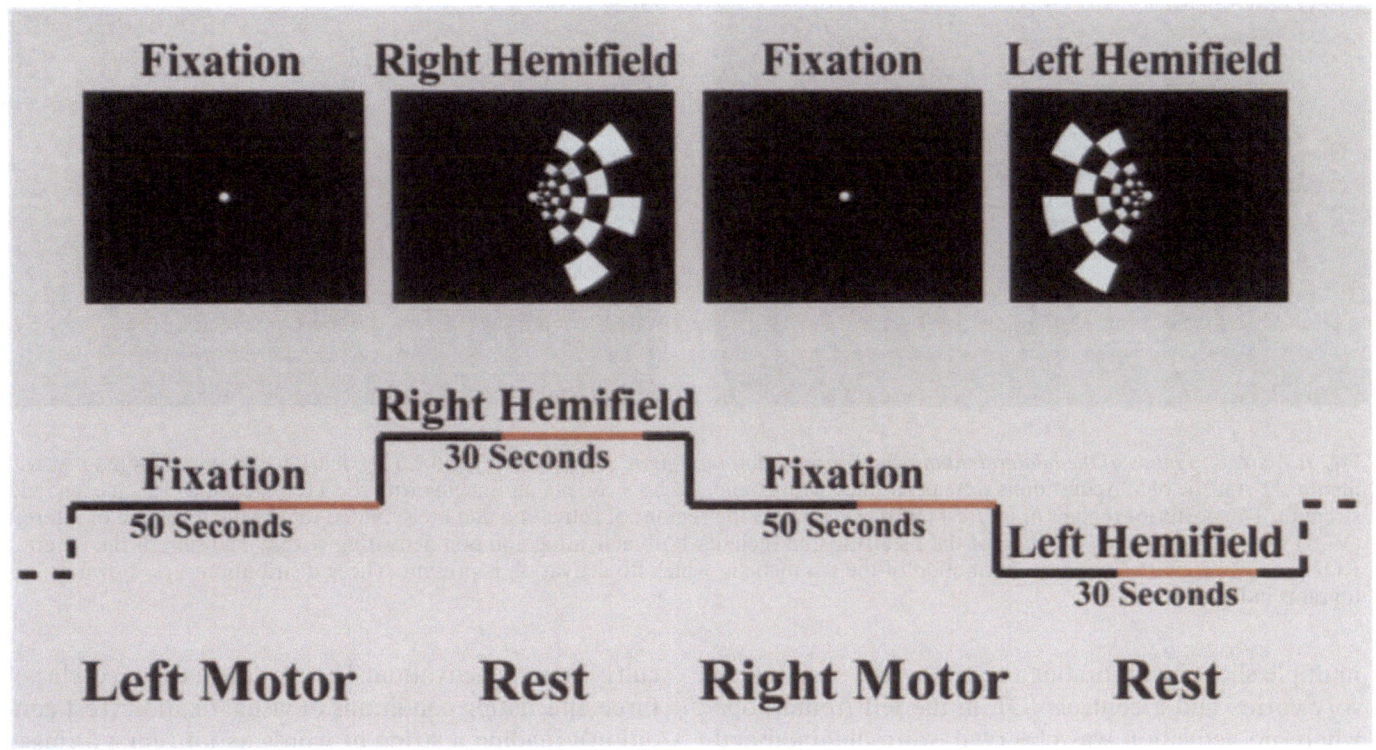

Fig. 4. *Schematic representation of temporal pattern of the visual component of the combined motor and visual activation paradigm.* An alternating hemifield, flashing checkerboard (8 Hz) is separated by visual fixation during which ipsilateral sequential finger-thumb apposition is performed

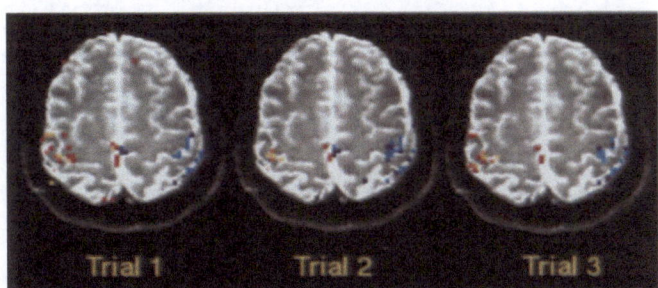

Fig. 5. *Activation maps of the combined thumb-finger apposition motor task and hemifield photic stimulation paradigm.* Images show the motor cortex (*top*) and visual cortex (*bottom*) over three trials for an individual subject. The t-statistic threshold was chosen to be identical for all trials. The patterns of activation are reproducible on a voxel by voxel basis without requiring filtering or contiguity criteria to improve statistical reliability. The motor task shows activation in the somatosensory cortex across the central sulcus because the motor task has a tactile and proprioceptive component to it in that the finger and thumb touch

parison of images acquired under these two conditions. A threshold t-statistic was chosen for the purpose of generating activation maps at each field strength, as shown in Fig. 7. No censorship of voxels was made to any location in the field of view and no contiguity criterion was imposed. This is a conservative statistical approach to such an analysis. For objective assessment of the differences between field strength, the distributions of t-statistic in a volume of interest (VOI) covering the

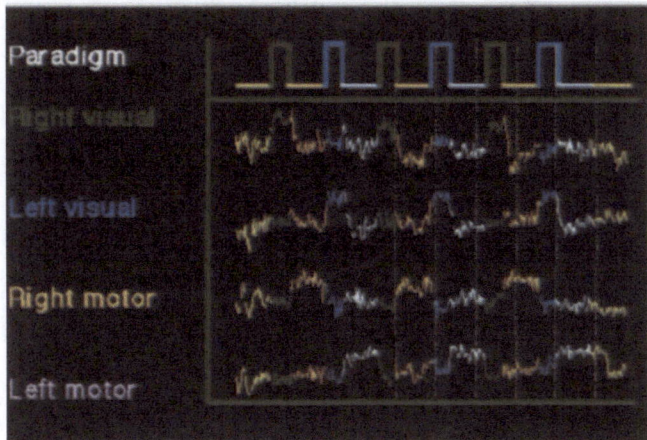

Fig. 6. *Time courses of signal intensity in single voxels selected from the right and left visual and motor regions of activation.* The SNR at 3.0 T is sufficient to identify BOLD contrast changes in single voxels in widely distributed regions of the brain

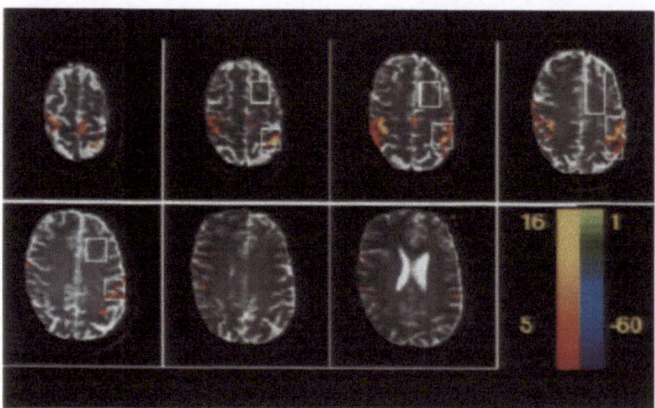
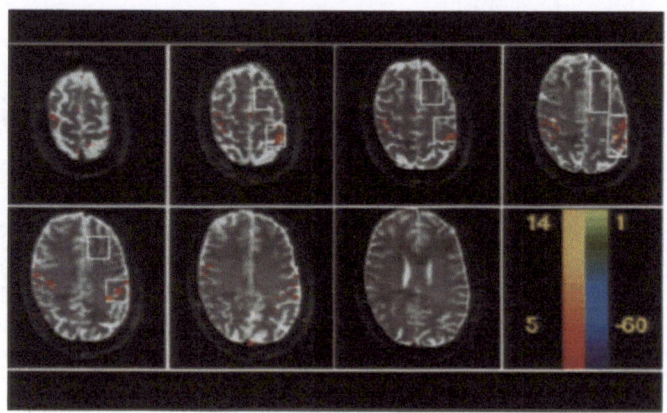

Fig. 7. *Activation maps of the bilateral thumb-finger apposition paradigm.* At 3.0 T (*left*) and 1.5 T (*right*), based on a simple t-test and identical t-statistic of 5. Acquisitions were performed with gradient echo, echo planar imaging with the TE matched to T2* at each field strength. The posterior regions of interest (ROI) encompass the regions of activation and are summed to provide a volume of interest (VOI) that samples the distribution of the t-statistic that includes both activating and non-activating voxels. The sum of the anterior ROI provides a control volume distribution of the t-statistic in which no activation is present. These distributions are shown as histograms in Fig. 8

multiple slices incorporating the motor and somatosensory cortex and a control VOI, in the left frontal lobe where no activation was observed, were obtained and compared at each field strength, as presented in Fig. 8.

Language comprehension is a higher cognitive function that can be used to examine the effects of task diffi-

culty on brain activation. The paradigm used 3 cycles of three alternating conditions of visual fixation (rest condition), reading a string of words and pushing a finger switch (active condition 1), and reading a sentence of varying difficulty that required a true/false question to be answered by pushing one of two finger switches (ac-

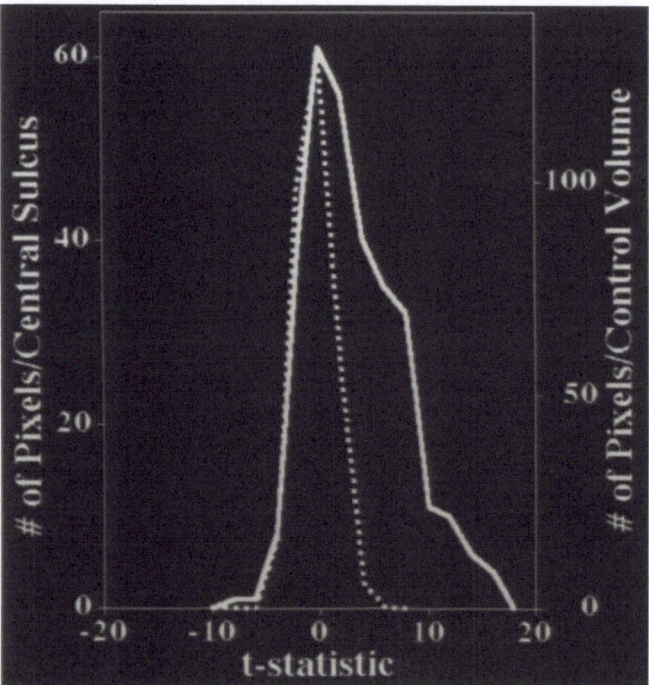
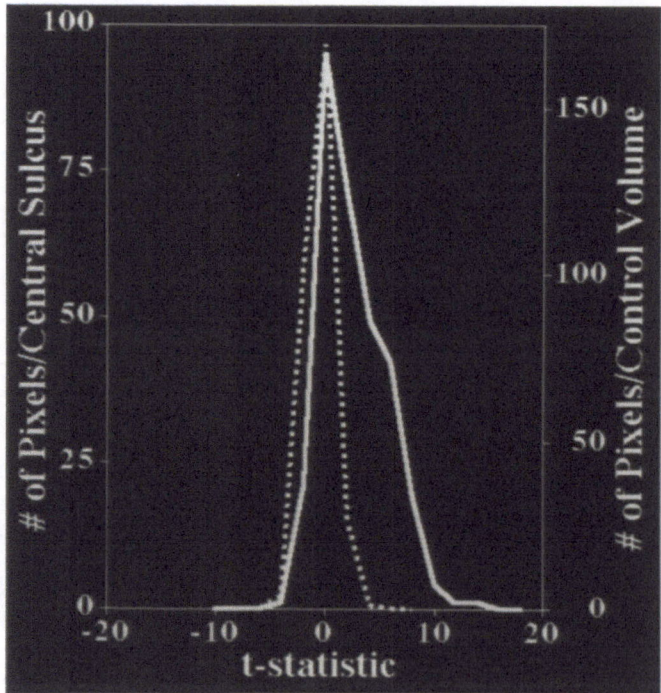

Fig. 8. *Histograms for the t-statistic.* For VOI-encompassing regions of activation (*solid line*) and no activation (*dashed line*) indicated on Fig. 7 for 3.0 and 1.5 T. The control distributions are similar at both field strengths and are symmetrically distributed about 0. The distributions for the VOI encompassing the activation are skewed as expected if activating voxels behave differently from the surrounding non-activating voxels. As the VOIs are matched in volume, the integral of the difference between the control and test VOI can be compared between field strengths. The increased integral at 3.0 T with higher t-statistics values demonstrates objectively the increased sensitivity at the higher field. The apparent bimodal nature of the distribution at high t-statistic values at 3.0 T is due to two topologically distinct regions within the VOI of motor (higher t-values) and somatosensory cortex

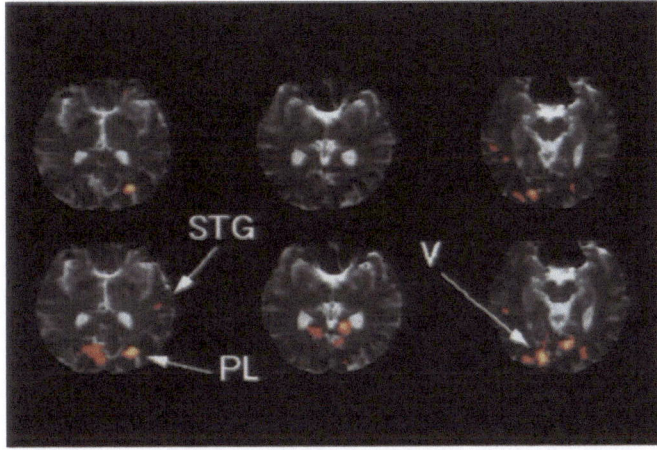

Fig. 9. *Activation maps of language comprehension for three selected contiguous images.* Superior temporal gyrus (STG), visual cortex (V) and parietal lobe (PL). Paradigm performed at 3.0 T. Sentence reading with interpretation by answering a related question is compared to visual fixation (*top images*) and word string reading is compared to visual fixation (*bottom images*). The patterns of activation are similar for the two tasks but sentence comprehension produced larger regions of activation and some new regions such as in the STG

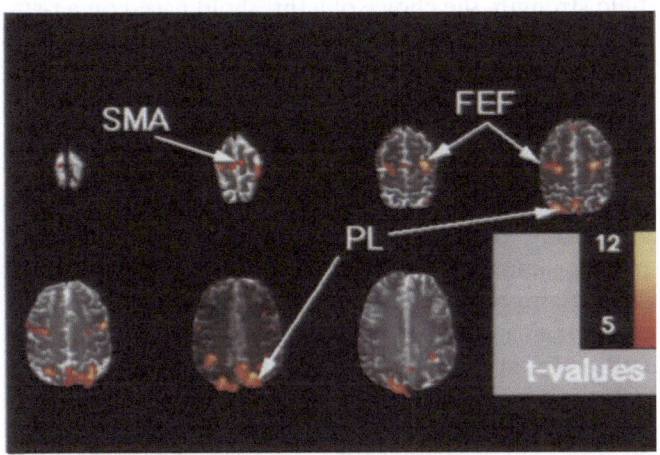

Fig. 10. *Activation map for visually-guided saccades.* At 3.0 T showing activation in frontal eye fields (FEF), supplementary motor area (SMA) and parietal lobe (PL)

tive condition 2). Activation maps for each of conditions 1 and 2 against rest were calculated using a simple t-test and choosing a threshold t-statistic. The size of the regions of activation can be compared visually in Fig. 9.

Control of eye movements is a complex but well studied neuronal pathway that is central to many cognitive functions based on visual sensory stimulation. This pathway was investigated with a visually-guided saccade (VGS) paradigm with 6 cycles of alternating visual fixation (30 s) with a randomly moving target in the horizontal plane (30 s). The activation map, shown in Fig. 10 for VGS against fixation, was calculated using a simple t-test as above.

Results and Discussion

The relaxation parameters and SNR measurements for a human brain are presented in Table 1. As expected, T1 is longer while T2 and T2* are shorter at higher field. The data were obtained using echo planar imaging and a representative data set is shown in Fig. 1. The data fits a single exponential function with acceptable accuracy. An enhancement factor of 2 in SNR is obtained for both conventional and echo planar images when compared under optimal acquisition conditions at each field strength.

As the increased T1 at higher field suggests the use of longer TR values to avoid saturation effects, greater coverage of the brain can be achieved without loss of time. The whole brain can be covered with a 4 s repeat time for fMRI, as in Fig. 2. Although magnetic suscepti-

bility artifact is present around air-bone-tissue interfaces, most of the brain is accessible to fMRI without modification of imaging strategies. Higher resolution images have less artifact as do spin echo images. These can be combined in a three dimensional display, as shown in Fig. 3, for localizing regions of activation.

Test-retest reliability is an important characteristic of the scanner-paradigm-subject performance that has been established for 1.5 T systems in many laboratories. Similar results have been achieved at 3.0 T using the paradigm represented in Fig. 4 on a voxel by voxel basis as demonstrated in Fig. 5. The time course of single voxels, shown in Fig. 6, shows that widely distributed regions of the brain are accessible within a single paradigm.

The objective comparison of fMRI sensitivity for detecting activation as a function of field strength requires appropriate acquisition conditions to equalize the relaxation weightings. As the SNR improves with increasing

Table 1. Field strength dependence of relaxation times, T1, T2 and T2*, and SNR of the human brain as measured by echo planar imaging

Parameter	Field	
	1.5 T	3.0 T
T1	900[a]	1020 ± 275
T2	85 ± 20	74 ± 18
T2*	50 ± 7	25 ± 7
SNR (spin echo EPI)[b]	102	205
SNR (gradient echo EPI)[c]	94	219

Relaxation times in milliseconds are a mean value averaged over the brain as exemplified in Fig. 1. SNR was measured with gradient echo and spin echo modes of echo planar imaging.

[a] average literature value. [b] axial plane, TR=10 000 ms, 1 NEX, TE=40 ms at 1.5 T and 40 ms at 3.0 T. [c] axial plane, TR= 6 000 ms, flip= 90°, 1 NEX, TE=50 ms at 1.5 T and 25 ms at 3.0 T.

field strength, the choice of a threshold based on a t-statistic is subjective. To avoid such biases, the distribution of t-statistics over a volume of interest that encompasses the activation has been examined by comparison to a control region. The subjective visual impression of greater volume of activation at 3.0 T from Fig. 7 is confirmed by such an analysis in Fig. 8. The activation voxels have a statistically different behavior from background that is more prominent at 3.0 T confirming the expected field strength improvement for BOLD contrast.

Cortical mapping in the frontal, temporal, parietal and occipital regions is demonstrated for the cognitive paradigms of language comprehension and eye movement control at 3.0 T, as shown in Figs. 9 and 10. In Fig. 9, there appears to be differences in volume of activation for different degrees of complexity of the tasks. Characterizing such volumes may provide a means of characterizing task performance. Clearly, such measures are dependent on the sensitivity and reliability of the method. The increased sensitivity of higher field fMRI may prove valuable in such analyses.

Conclusions

The higher field strength of the 3.0 T scanner realizes an improvement of a factor of two in SNR and delivers increased sensitivity to BOLD contrast in fMRI applications over the 1.5 T system. The system is stable with high test-retest reliability on a voxel by voxel basis. This enhanced sensitivity can be exploited in studies of both primary cortical activity and broadly distributed neuronal pathways of higher cognitive functions including language comprehension and eye movement control.

Acknowledgements

The authors acknowledge support from General Electric Medical Systems and Advanced NMR Systems, Inc.

References

1. Kwong K, Belliveau J, Chesler D, Goldberg I, Weisskoff R, Poncelet B, Kennedy D, Hoppel B, Cohen M, Turner R, Cheng H, Brady T, Rosen B (1992) Dynamic magnetic resonance imaging of human brain activity during primary sensory stimulation. Proc Natl Acad Sci USA 89: 5675-5679
2. Roy C, Sherrington C (1890) On the regulation of the blood-supply of the brain. J Physiol (London) 11: 85-108
3. Ogawa S, Lee T, Nayak A, Glynn P (1990) Oxygenation-sensitive contrast in magnetic resonance image of rodent brain at high magnetic fields. Magn Reson Med 14: 68-78

Functional MRI Brain Mapping Prior to Craniotomy or Radiosurgery: Initial Clinical Experience

P. Turski[1], B. Mock[2], M. Lowe[2], E. Baker[2], J. Sorenson[2]

[1] Department of Radiology, [2]Department of Medical Physics, University of Wisconsin Medical School, [3]Madison, WI 53792 USA

Introduction

The primary motor, sensory, visual, and language regions of the cerebral cortex can be identified using functional magnetic resonance imaging (fMRI) techniques. Identification of these cortical regions is a valuable tool for differentiating patients that may benefit from surgery from those in which focused radiotherapy (i.e. radiosurgery) is best. A variety of lesions that are located near primary cortical areas have the potential for neurologic deficit following craniotomy and surgery. Although neurologic deficits may arise from radiosurgical techniques, in general these methods have somewhat better success in treating lesions near primary eloquent cortex with minimal damage to normal brain tissue. In this investigation functional MRI applications were evaluated to provide a battery of fMRI paradigms capable of activating eloquent brain cortex adjacent to sites of various pathologic processes such as cerebral gliomas and arteriovenous malformations.

Methods

The fMRI studies were performed at 1.5 T. Four patients underwent examinations using a whole body Advanced NMR echo planar device. Six additional patients were studied using a dedicated head gradient system manufactured by Medical Advances, Milwaukee, Wisconsin. In both instances, T2*-weighted gradient echo scans were obtained employing an echo time (TE) of 50 ms and a repetition time (TR) of 1000 to 1500 ms [2].

Brain activation was achieved by employing task activation. This is accomplished by the subject either experiencing or perfoming a task for six to eight seconds followed by a rest period. The on and off states are subtracted to generate a difference image representative of variations in blood oxygen content due to activation [3].

Paradigms

1. Activation of the Primary Motor Cortex (Brodman areas 4 and 6)

The large topographical distribution of the hand on the precentral gyrus allows for a large target to be identified [4]. Thus, virtually all motor studies have been directed toward the hand region of the motor cortex. Simple hand movements result in activation predominantly of the primary motor cortex. Both primary and supplementary motor cortex can be activated by the performance of a more complex motor task. Typically, this is accomplished by the sequential application of the thumb to the fingers of the hand in a predetermined pattern [5]. This additional cognitive input apparently results in the supplementary motor activation [5, 6].

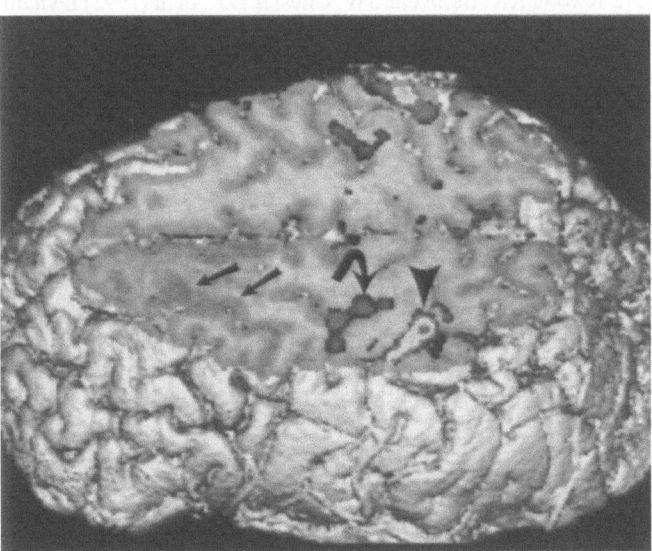

Fig. 1. *Activation of the motor cortex during complex movements of both hands.* The activation map is superimposed on a surface rendered three-dimensional (3D) image of the subject's cortex. Note the excellent geographic relationship to the precentral gyrus. The patient has a right frontal oligodendroglioma (*arrows*). The more complex motor task produces activation of the primary motor cortex (*arrowhead*) and the supplementary motor cortex (*curved arrow*). The patient's neoplasm is located anterior to the motor areas.

2. Activation of Primary Sensory Cortex (Brodman areas 1, 2 and 3)

Sensory cortex can be readily activated by stroking the hand with a brush. The subject should remain passive during the stimulation period [7].

3. Activation of Broca's Area (Brodman areas 44 and 45)

The speech area can be activated by covert or overt word production. Word generation results in the most intense activation within the inferior gyrus of the dominant hemisphere although there is also less intense activation of the contralateral inferior frontal gyrus [8].

4. Activation of Wernike's Area (Brodman area 22)

A device is needed to provide auditory input to the subjects while they are in the magnetic resonance (MR) scanner; a commercially available system equipped with headphones to exclude extraneous noise may be used. Text is read to the patient from material containing a predominance of concrete nouns. Typically, a verse from Tolstoy is used [9].

5. Activation of Primary Visual Cortex (Brodman area 17)

The visual cortex can be easily identified on fMRI exams: the presentation of a blinking checkerboard results in brisk and robust activation of the cortical regions along the banks of the calcarine fissure. High resolution fMRI studies have correlated with established retinotopic maps [10].

Discussion

In order to provide detailed presurgical maps of the cerebral cortex, a battery of functional MRI paradigms should be available. Current literature suggests that the most robust activation occurs in the primary cortical regions. In this study paradigms were selected to activate these primary cortical regions for clinical purposes. Our initial experience suggests that these paradigms can be used in cooperative patients to identify the geographic location of primary cortical tissue in relationship to a variety of pathologic processes. The most brisk activation response occurs in relationship to motor and visual stimulation. Activation of speech and language areas is more difficult, but can be achieved even with covert word production.

References

1. Belliveau JW, Kennedy DN, McKinstry RC, et al (1991) Functional Mapping of the Human Visual Cortex by Magnetic Resonance Imaging. Science 254: 716-719
2. Bandettini PA, Wong EC, Hinks RS, et al (1992) Time Course EPI of Human Brain Function During Task Activation. Magn Reson Med 5: 390-397
3. Bandettini PA, Jesmanowicz A, Wong EC, Hyde JS (1993) Processing Strategies for Time-Course Data Sets in Functional MRI of the Brain. Magn Reson Med 30: 161-173
4. Penfield W, Boldrey E (1937) Somatic and Sensory Representation in the Cerebral Cortex of Man as Studied by Electrical Stimulation Brain 60: 389-443
5. Kim SG, Ashe J, Hendrich K, et al (1993) Functional Magnetic Resonance Imaging of Motor Cortex: Hemispheric Asymmetry and Handedness. Science 261: 615-617
6. Jack, Jr CR, Thompson RM, Butts RK, Sharbrough FW, Kelly PJ, Hanson DP, Riederer SJ, Ehman RL, Hangiandreou NJ, Cascino GD (1994) Sensory Motor Cortex : Correlation of Presurgical Mapping with Functional MR Imaging and Invasive Cortical Mapping. Radiology 190: 85-92
7. Kwong KK, Belliveau JW, Chesler DA, et al (1992) Dynamic Magnetic Resonance Imaging of Human Brain Activity During Primary Sensory Stimulation. Proc Natl Acad Sci USA 89: 5675-5679
8. Hinke RM, Hu X, Stillman AR, Kim S-G, Merkle H, Salmi R, Ugurbil K (1993) Functional Magnetic Resonance Imaging of Broca's Area During Internal Speech. NeuroReport 4: 675-678
9. Binder JR, Rao SM, Hammeke TA, Yetkin FZ, Jesmanowicz A, Bandettini PA, Wong EC, Estkowski LD, Goldstein MD, Haughton VM, Hyde JS (1994) Functional Magnetic Resonance Imaging of Human Auditory Cortex. Ann Neurol 35: 662-672
10. Turner R, Jezzard P, Wen H, Kwong KK, et al (1993) Functional mapping of the human Visual Cortex at 4 and 1.5 Tesla Using Deoxygenation contrast EPI. Magn Reson Med 29: 277-279

MR Imaging in Hyperacute Stroke

A.G. Sorensen

Department of Radiology, Massachusetts General Hospital, Boston, MA, 02114, USA

Introduction

Stroke is diagnosed approximately 400000 times per year in the United States, and contributes to approximately 150000 deaths per year. While the clinical diagnosis of stroke is questionable only infrequently, intervention may depend on a more accurate assessment than clinical evaluation. Attemps to find an effective therapy for stroke have so far been limited, and many investigators believe that this is due to an incomplete understanding of human stroke, particularly in the acute stage.

The role of functional MRI (fMRI) in the evaluation of acute stroke is best understood when placed in context with what is currently understood about cerebral hemodynamics and ischemia. The relationship between cerebral blood flow and neuronal dysfunction is outlined in Table 1. The key finding in this table is that there is a level of cerebral blood flow at which neurons stop functioning but have not undergone cell death, and therefore the damage from ischemia may be reversible. This has led to the concept of an "ischemic penumbra" [1]. This penumbra has been heavily investigated in animal studies, and also in humans by means of nuclear medicine techniques [2, 3]. While the pathophysiology of the penumbra is still incompletely understood, it appears that a number of biochemical and tissue-level changes are occurring which include a mismatch of blood flow and oxygen consumption (so called "luxury perfusion"), acidosis, and anaerobic respiration [4]. One of the goals of fMRI is to visualize this penumbra, and ideally identify the difference between salvageable, non-salvageable, and undamaged tissue. Imaging of acute stoke has been undertaken with a variety of MRI techniques, including spectroscopic, diffusion, perfusion, and conventional imaging. This article will review the techniques which are now in place at some sites for use on a routine clinical basis. Foremost among these are diffusion-weighted imaging and perfusion imaging.

While assessment of acute stroke has clear clinical utility, fMRI may also be useful in the management of chronic stroke. Approximately one quarter of stroke patients hospitalized annually for stroke have recurrent disease[5]. Assessment of patient pathology after stroke may help identify patients who may benefit from intervention.

Functional MRI may also be able to contribute to clinical research into the mechanism of stroke recovery. A variety of possible mechanisms have been postulated, but determining which plays an important role in human stroke has been challenging. In 1895 and again in 1914, Von Monakow described the possible functional "shock" or dysfunction of remote intact neurons due to connectivity with neurons in the area of a stroke, which he termed "diaschisis" [6, 7]. Distinguishing between dysfunction due to diaschisis and dysfunction due to primary injury is not possible with conventional MRI studies, since the nonfunctioning remote cortex is not damaged until the affected neurons degenerate as in crossed-cerebellar diaschisis. However, recovery from diaschisis may play an important role in recovery from stroke, as most diaschisis is reversible [8]. In a clinical setting, determining which areas of cortex are dysfunctional due to primary insult and which are affected by diaschisis may play a role in therapeutic choice.

Techniques

1. Diffusion Imaging

Diffusion is the random, thermal motion of molecules (also known as Brownian motion). The quantity D is a measure of diffusion, and is typically expressed in units of an area per unit time. The D for pure water at room

Table 1. Relation between blood flow and cerebral activity

Blood flow (ml/100 g/min^{-1})	Cerebral activity
50-55	Normal
18-25	EEG flat line (loss of evoked response)
12	Membrane pump failure, cell death

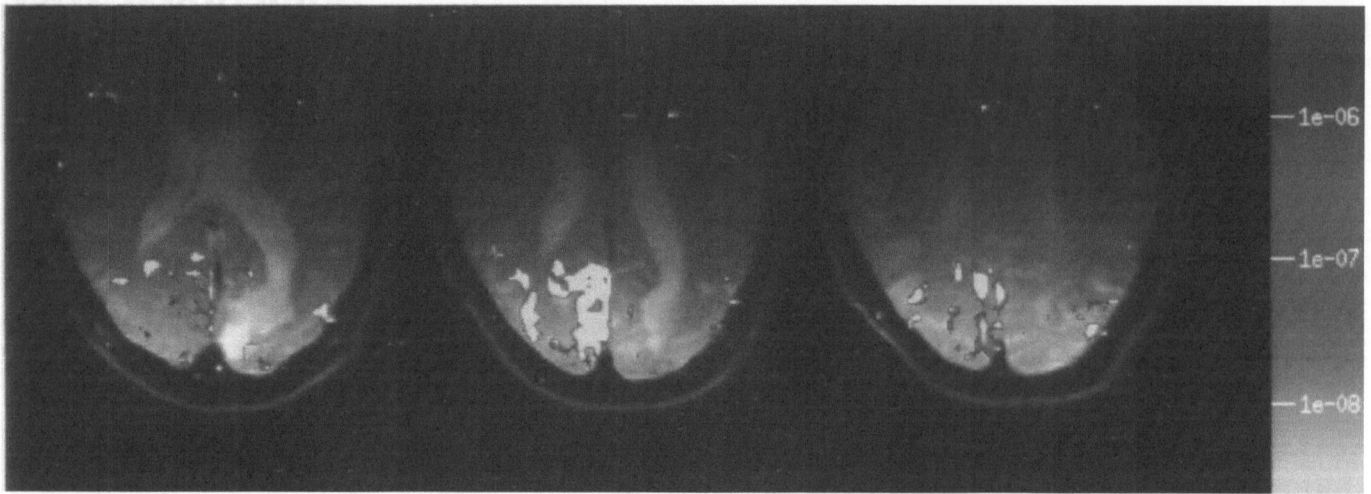

Fig. 1. *Diaschisis in chronic stroke.* A small area of tissue is affected by stroke, located in the primary visual cortex (*open arrows*). Activation mapping demonstrates that in the unaffected side there is a large area of activation, consistent with both primary, secondary, and higher centers of visual processing. However, on the affected side there is absence of activation in not only the affected primary visual cortex but also in the expected areas of activation outside the primary visual cortex, in regions known to correspond to higher centers of vision [30] (*solid arrows*). Hence a stroke in one area is demonstrated to affect distant cortex. Underlying gray-scale image: T2-weighted oblique axial spin echo image. Functional overlay: t-test p value, ranging from $p = 1 \times 10^{-5}$ to $p = 1 \times 10^{-9}$. The test was applied to 90 images acquired during full-field stimulation with LED goggles alternating with darkness

temperature, for example, is about 2×10^{-5} cm^2/s (or 2×10^{-3} mm^2/s). MR imaging can be made sensitive to intravoxel dephasing, and therefore diffusion, by the addition of gradient pulses to a standard spin echo sequence [9, 10]. MRI has provided one of the first non-invasive in vivo methods for measuring a diffusion coefficient, which is known as the apparent diffusion coefficient (ADC). While diffusion and brain function may not appear to be closely linked, numerous studies have demonstrated that the apparent diffusion coefficient changes in disease states [10-17]. Since diffusion in the brain has only recently been measurable in a clinical setting, its clinical utility and indications are still being investigated.

2. Perfusion Imaging

Magnetic resonance angiography (MRA) has demonstrated its ability to detect flow in macroscopic vasculature and is in widespread use. Perfusion imaging, on the other hand, is concerned with microscopic flow; that is, flow at the capillary level. Traditionally perfusion has been assessed using a variety of radiologic techniques, from conventional catheter angiography to positron emission tomogrpay (PET). MRI has unique features which add to its value in assessing tissue perfusion in the brain: it can be relatively sensitive to the microvasculature, it is noninvasive (requiring only an intravenous contrast injection), and it has higher spatial resolution than do most other tomographic techniques. Over the past five years this technique has demonstrated its utility in a wide variety of neuroradiologic applications; any

disease process with microvasculature alterations may potentially benefit from perfusion imaging. Clinical applications include tumor characterization, stroke, and dementia, with others under active investigation.

Susceptibility-based perfusion imaging was first proposed by Villringer et al. [18], and has been applied to a variety of clinical applications [19, 20]. The basis of this technique is imaging during the passage of a bolus of contrast agent. All three FDA-approved agents have both T1 and T2 relaxation effects. While routine clinical use of Gd-based agents depends on their T1 relaxing effects (causing increased signal intensity on T1-weighted images), perfusion imaging uses the T2 effects which dominate at higher concentrations (causing decreased signal intensity on T2-weighted images). These T2 effects cause signal loss due to susceptibility effects. The transient passage of contrast agent causes a transient signal loss. This signal loss is proportional to the blood volume in each voxel, and is similar to standard tracer experiments in nuclear medicine. Relative cerebral blood volume (rCBV) maps can therefore be generated by applying susceptibility physics and standard tracer kinetic principles.

3. Activation Mapping

As proposed as early as 1895, local cerebral hemodynamics are closely linked to local cerebral activity [21-24]. While fMRI is not yet sensitive to neuronal activity directly, cerebral hemodynamic changes can be used as a surrogate marker for cerebral activity. Hence, with task activation local changes are seen in blood volume,

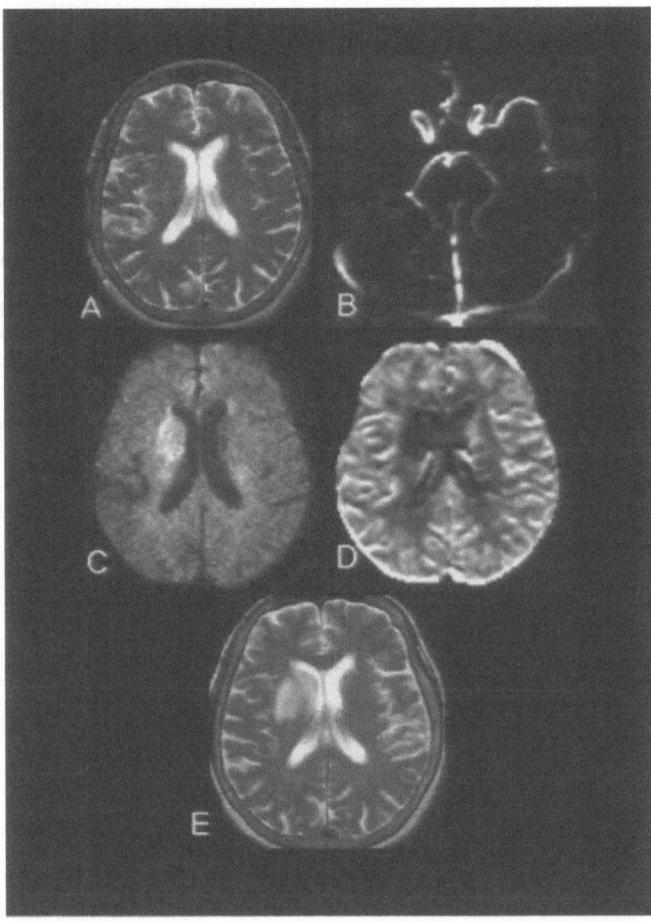

utilization in at least some parts of the cerebral cortex, with blood oxygen extraction rising only slightly with cerebral activation [25, 26]. This in turn may imply a decrease in the local concentration of deoxyhemoglobin. The oxygenation state of hemoglobin was linked to susceptibility change by Pauling in 1936 [28], and was shown by Thulborn et al. [29] in 1982 to shorten T2. Since then several groups have demonstrated that brain tissue relaxation is influenced by the oxygenation state of hemoglobin (a T2 effect) and by local tissue perfusion, a T1 effect.

Clinical Applications

Assessment of patients with acute and chronic stroke is demonstrated in Figs. 1 and 2.

Conclusions

As the availability of fMRI hardware and software increases, these techniques will continue their move into the clinical domain. The tools provided by functional MRI will allow greater insight into the pathophysiology of ischemic brain conditions. It is hoped that these improvement will in turn lead to better patient management and improved treatment and outcome.

Fig. 2 A-E. *Acute stroke.* 72-year-old female 2.5 h after last observed normal, now with left body weakness and left hemineglect. **A** T2 weighted image shows no abnormality. **B** 2D phase contrast MRA demonstrates absence of flow in the right mid cerebral artery (MCA). **C** Diffusion-weighted image shows area of abnormally low diffusion in right basal ganglia. **D** rCBV map shows decreased relative cerebral blood volume in this same area. **E** Follow-up T2-weighted image 5 days later shows infarct

References

1. Symon L (1980) Acta Neurol Scand 62: 175
2. Hakim A, Evans A, Berger L, Kuwabara H, Worsley K, Marchal G, Biel C, Pokrupa R, Diksic M, Meyer E, Gjedde A, Marrett SJ (1989) Cereb Blood Flow Metab 9: 523
3. Olsen T, Larsen B, Herming M, Skriver E, Lassen N (1983) Stroke 14: 332
4. Tomlinson F, Anderson R, Meyer F (1993) Stroke 24, 2030
5. Wolf PA, Belanger AJ, D'Agostino RB (1992) Neurol Clin 10: 177
6. von Monakow C (1914) Die Lokalistion in Grosshirn und der Abbau der Funktion durch Kortikale Herde, J.F. Bergmann, Wiesbaden
7. von Monakow C (1895) Archiv für Psychiatrie und Nervenkrankheiten 27: 1
8. Feeney DM Baron J-C (1986) Stroke 17: 817
9. Stejskal E, Tanner J (1965) J Chem Physics 42: 288
10. Le Bihan D, Breton E, Lallemand D, Grenier P, Cabanis E, Laval-Jeantet M (1986) Radiology 161: 401
11. Chien D, Buxton RB, Kwong KK, Rosen BR (1990) Comput Assist Tomogr 14: 514
12. Chien D, Kwong KK, Gress DR, Buononno FS, Buxton RB, Rosen BR (1992) Am J Neuroradiol 13: 1097
13. Hajnal J, Doran M, Hall A, Collins A, Oatridge A, Pennock J, Young I, Bydder G (1991) J Comput Assist Tomogr 15: 1
14. Hooper J, Sunder R, Rose L, LeBihan D (1990) Society of Magnetic Resonance in Medicine, Ninth Annual Scientific Meeting, New York
15. Larsson H, Christiansen P, Thomsen C, Stubgaard M, Fredriksen J, Henriksen O (1991) Society of Magnetic Resonance in Medicine, Ninth Annual Meeting, New York

blood flow, and blood oxygenation state [25, 26]. Functional MRI can detect changes in blood volume via the introduction of intravenous contrast agents, as noted in the previous section. In addition, however, fMRI techniques which are sensitive to intrinsic brain contrast mechanisms are now in widespread use. These allow direct visualization of brain activity using fMRI.

While the physiology underlying these signal changes is incompletely understood, enough is known to allow some guidance of clinical decision making and application. The signal increase appears to be secondary to changes in blood oxygenation and flow which occur during local cerebral activity. PET and other studies have shown that oxygen delivery, cerebral blood flow (CBF), and cerebral blood volume (CBV) all increase with activation, with the increase in CBF exceeding that in CBV by about a factor of two [27]. However, there is an apparent mismatch between oxygen delivery and oxygen

16. Le Bihan D, Delannoy J, Levin R (1989) Radiology 171, 853
17. Le Bihan D, Turner R, Douek P, Patronas N (1992) Am J Roentgenol 159: 591
18. Villringer A, Rosen BR, Belliveau JW, Ackerman JL, Lauffer RB, Buxton RB, Chao YS, Wedeen VJ, Brady TJ (1988) Magn Reson Med 6: 164
19. Belliveau J, Rosen B, Buxton R, Johnson K, Frazer J, Moore J, Chao Y-S, Garrido L, Lauffer R, Fisel C, Brady T (1987) Society for Magnetic Resonance in Medicine p. 7
20. Belliveau J, Rosen B, Kantor H, Rzedzian R, Kennedy D, McKinstry R, Vevea J, Cohen M, Pykett I, Brady T (1990) Magn Reson Med 14: 538
21. Sokoloff L, Reivich M, Kennedy C, Des Rosiers M, Patlak C, Pettigrew K, Sakurada O, Shinohara M (1977) J Neurochem 28: 897
22. Roy CS, Sherrington CS (1890) J Physiol (London) 11: 85
23. Posner MI, Petersen SE, Fox PT, Raichle ME (1988) Science 240: 1627
24. Petersen SE, Fox PT, Posner MI, Mintun M, Raichle ME (1988) Nature 331: 585
25. Fox P, Raichle M, Mintun M, Dence C (1988) Science 241: 462
26. Fox PT, Raichle ME (1986) Proc Natl Acad Sci USA 83: 1140
27. Grubb RL, Raichle ME, Eichling JO, Ter-Pogossian MM (1974) Stroke 5: 630
28. Pauling L, Coryell C (1936) Proc Nat Acad Sci USA 22: 210
29. Thulborn KR, Waterton JC, Matthews PM, Radda GK (1982) Biochim Biophys Acta 714: 265
30. Horton JC, Hoyt WF (1991) Brain 114: 1703

fMRI IN CURRENT CLINICAL PRACTICE

PRESTO, a Rapid 3D Approach for Functional MRI of Human Brain

C.T.W. Moonen[1], P. van Gelderen[1], N. Ramsey[2], G. Liu[1], J.H. Duyn[3], J. Frank[3], D.R. Weinberger[2]

[1]NIH In Vivo NMR Research Center, BEIP, NCRR, Building 10, Room B1D-125, Bethesda, Maryland 20892, USA
[2]Clinical Brain Disorders Branch, NIMH, NIH, 2700 Martin Luther King Jr. Avenue, S.E., Washington, DC 20032, USA
[3]Laboratory of Diagnostic Radiology Research Program, OIR, NIH, Bethesda, Maryland 20892, USA

Introduction

Ogawa et al. [1, 2] proposed in 1990 that physiological information related to neuronal activity can be incorporated in functional magnetic resonance imaging (fMRI) based on changes in the concentration of deoxyhemoglobin in blood (blood oxygenation level dependent, or BOLD effect). As compared to positron emission tomography (PET) and single photon emission computed tomography (SPECT), BOLD fMRI offers substantial advantages: minimal discomfort, no exposure to ionizing radiation and excellent spatial and temporal resolution. Several studies have now demonstrated that sensory and language functions can be mapped with fMRI.

Brain stimulation is known to lead to enhanced perfusion which, together with other physiological changes (e.g., blood volume, oxygen consumption), results in decreased deoxyhemoglobin levels in the region of neuronal activity. Because deoxyhemoglobin contains a paramagnetic iron, its magnetic susceptibility is high compared to that of oxyhemoglobin which does not contain a paramagnetic center. Therefore, the changed deoxyhemoglobin level leads to modifications in the microscopic magnetic field changes in and around the vasculature. The effects are reflected in small increases in fMRI image intensity upon activation. Although spin echo methods have been employed and have even shown advantages with respect to selectivity for capillary BOLD effect [3], the signal increases are significantly smaller than for gradient echoes under the condition of good macroscopic field homogeneity. This paper deals with gradient echo methods only.

Most fMRI methods use echo planar imaging (EPI) or fast gradient echo techniques, and repetitively scan a single two-dimensional (2D) slice or multiple slices through the brain during execution of a specific stimulation paradigm [4-9]. Several studies have now shown that, because of the small BOLD signal changes upon activation (one to a few percent at 1.5 T), other (non-BOLD) physiological effects of brain stimulation may also lead to signal changes which may be difficult to interpret unambiguously [10, 11]. For example, inflow effects should be avoided when accurate location of brain activity is needed. In addition, the small changes in BOLD fMRI necessitate careful correction for small rotations and translations between scans. Accurate registration is difficult to achieve with multislice data. A true three-dimensional (3D) sequence can avoid inflow effects and allows corrections for translation and rotation in all directions.

Conventional gradient echo methods (in particular for large volumes) require prohibitively long acquisition times for fMRI since only one k-space line is collected for each radiofrequency (RF) excitation pulse. The repetition time (TR) must be long because of the condition that TR is longer than the echo time (TE). For optimal sensitivity, all image data should in turn be acquired at long TE in order to achieve the sensitivity to deoxyhemoglobin-induced field inhomogeneity effects. Here, we use gradient echoes that are delayed beyond the next RF pulse [12-17]. This class of echo-shifted MRI results in TE > TR for a substantial gain in imaging speed. The 3D PRESTO (principles of echo shifting with a train of observations) sequence is based on a combination of echo-shifting principles together with multiple gradient echoes per RF excitation [14, 17] for a further decrease in imaging time while maintaining a high BOLD sensitivity.

Methods

All studies were performed on a 1.5 T GE (General Electric) Signa scanner using the standard GE quadrature head coil. The instrument was equipped with conventional, shielded gradients with maximum amplitude of 10 mT/m and maximum rise time of 17 $Tm^{-1}s^{-1}$. The patient protocol was approved by the intramural review board of the National Institute of Mental Health.

The 3D PRESTO technique (Fig. 1) has been described in detail recently [17], and is based on a 2D counterpart developed for tracking a bolus of contrast agent [14]. Each TR period (24 ms) contains five gradient echoes with alternating polarity of the readout gradient. Additional gradient crushers of 2 ms duration before and 3 ms after the data acquisition period were used with -3.75 mT/m and 5 mT/m strength, respectively, in all three principal directions. The additional gradient pulses were identical in each TR period and resulted in selection of the train of five gradient echoes shifted by a single TR period. The T2*-weighting varied from 29.6 ms for the first gradient echo in each TR period to 40.4 ms for the last echo. RF spoiling was used. A 65 mm thick axial slab was selected including the entire superior brain. A data matrix of $64 \times 50 \times 24$ was used in combination with a $240 \times 187.5 \times 90$ mm field of view (FOV) resulting in 3.75 mm isotropic resolution. K-space was split in five equal sections in the second dimension, each of which was encoded by one of the five gradient echoes, in linear order. The sampling frequency was 32 kHz, and the total acquisition time for a 3D data set was 5.8 s. An RF flip angle of 11° was used for optimal signal to noise ratio. At this flip angle, the T1 and spin density differences approximately cancel and no signal differences can be seen between grey and white matter.

Finger tapping stimulation paradigms were used consisting of two blocks of 8 stages of 30 s, with alternating stages of rest and stimulus. Five 3D images were collected during each stage. Anatomical images were recorded after each study using conventional inversion recovery (IR) spin echo sequences (IR 800 ms).

Data were processed off-line on Sun-SPARC workstations (Sun Microsystems, Mountainview CA) using IDL processing software (Research Systems, Boulder CO). For each activation study, the 3D raw data sets were multiplied with 25% cosine bell filters in all three directions and Fourier transformed. All images during one activation protocol were registered to the last 3D image [17]. The first scan of each series of five was discarded, since the vascular response shows a delay of a few seconds. The remaining four images obtained in each 30 s period were averaged. Statistical analysis was performed based on z_t statistics [17]. Difference images were obtained by substracting consecutive control and task scans. Mean signal changes and standard deviation were computed for each voxel. Voxels with a large variance, i.e. significantly larger than that of the total group of voxels as determined with a Chi-square test at p < 0.01, were treated as a subgroup. The standard deviation was pooled over all voxels, excluding those in the subgroup for which a separate pooled standard deviation (PSD) was computed. The number of voxels in the subgroup was always less than 1% of the total volume. The (appropriate) PSD was used to compute z-values for all voxels: $z_t = \sqrt{n} \times$ mean difference / PSD where n = number of difference volumes. A statistical threshold for z_t was determined for each subject by applying a Bonferroni correction for the total number of voxels in scanned brain tissue. Typically, a z_t-threshold of 4.4 was used for a voxel p-value of 4.5×10^{-6}, for 11 000 voxels, resulting in an omnibus p-value of 0.05 (onesided). Only positive signal changes were analysed. A bitmap was generated for voxels with a significant positive signal change, and was superimposed onto the IR images.

Results and Discussion

1. Optimum Echo Time for BOLD Gradient Echo Imaging

The optimum echo time (TE_{opt}) for BOLD fMRI with gradient echoes is between the T2* of the resting state (a) and the activated state (b). The exact value can be determined with Eq. 1, in which R_2^* is 1/T2*

$$TE_{opt} = \frac{\ln(R_2^*(b)) - \ln(R_2^*(a))}{R_2^*(b) - R_2^*(a)} \quad (1)$$

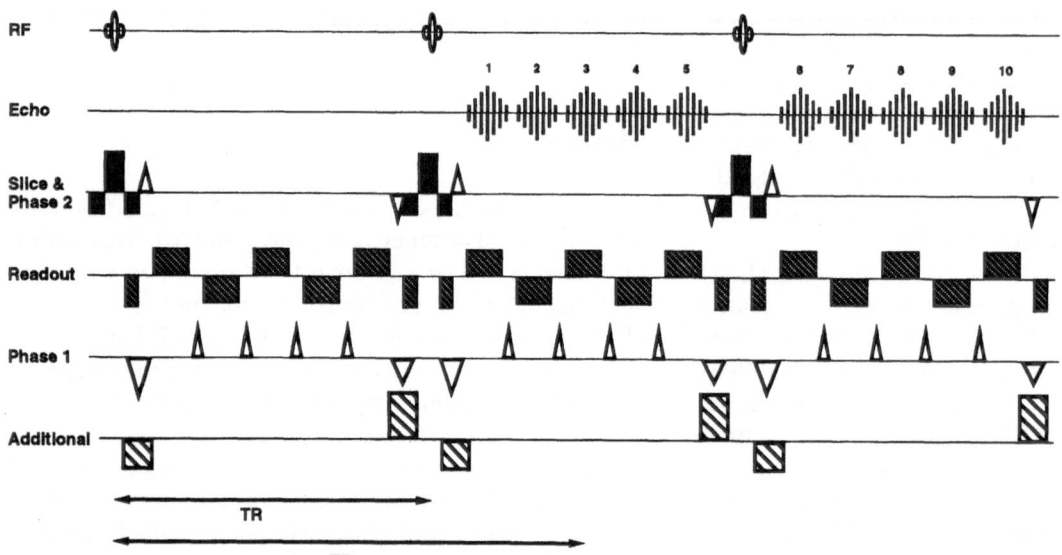

Fig. 1. *Pulse sequence for 3D PRESTO showing RF pulses, echoes, and gradient waveforms in three TR periods.* Slice selection, readout, and phase encode gradients perform the basic imaging functions, and are refocused in every TR period. The additional gradient waveforms serve to select the train of echoes shifted by one TR period. The relative surface area of the negative additional lobe prior to the acquisition period relative to that after the data acquisition is 1:2

The T2* value for a voxel is not only determined by the microscopic field heterogeneity but also by the T2 and the macroscopic field homogeneity, and can thus be expressed as

$$R_2^* = R_2^d + R_{2,mi'} + R_{2,ma'} \qquad (2)$$

where R_2^d reflects the T2 decay including diffusion effects, and $R_{2,mi'}$ and $R_{2,ma'}$ reflect the dephasing due to microscopic (mi) and macroscopic (ma) effects, respectively. The BOLD effect is predominantly in $R_{2,mi'}$ (decrease upon activation) and, to some extent, in the R_2^d term.

Figure 2 shows simulated plots of the size of the BOLD effect for different qualities of field homogeneity. It is evident that not only the size of the BOLD effect depends on the field homogeneity, but also the optimum TE becomes smaller upon decreasing field homogeneity. Since field homogeneity depends on field strength and on resolution, the TE$_{opt}$ should be determined for each case specifically. For more details, see [18].

2. Shimming Requirements for 3D PRESTO fMRI

Figure 3b shows a histogram of T2* values obtained with 3D gradient echo imaging with the same resolution (3.75 mm isotropic) as compared to the 3D PRESTO images. In addition, a histogram of T2* values is given for an isotropic resolution of 1.88 mm (Fig. 3a). Note that only the automatic GE shimming routine was used consisting of first order gradient adjustment only. The histogram shows a mean T2* value of 70 ms and 75 ms for 3.75 and 1.88 mm resolution, respectively, with a rather narrow distribution (17 and 18 ms SD, respectively). This means that for the PRESTO at 1.5 T we have approximately equal sensitivity to BOLD effect in all voxels, and that we are generally dealing with a situation as depicted in the third graph (from the top) in Fig. 2 without special shim-

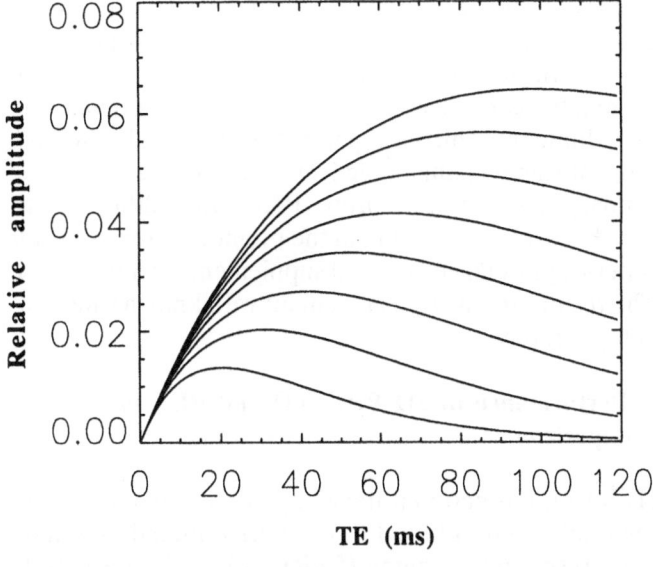

Fig. 2. *Simulated plot of the size of the BOLD effect as a function of echo time for different values of shimming.* From *top* curve to *bottom* curve, T2* (b) values of 90, 80, 70, 60, 50, 40, 30 and 20 ms were used, respectively, for increasingly poor field homogeneity

ming efforts. From the third graph in Fig. 1 it can be seen that even though TE$_{opt}$ is greater than 75 ms, at 35 ms close to 80% of the maximum BOLD effect is reached. Despite the fact that the mean T2* value is similar for 3.75 and 1.88 mm resolution, it can be seen from Fig. 3 that the number of voxels with a T2* value below 50 ms is increased for 3.75 mm resolution. These voxels were located primarily in the left and right superior cortex.

3. Performance of 3D PRESTO in Simple Finger Tapping

A simple sequential thumb-finger opposition paradigm was used to test the performance of the 3D PRESTO

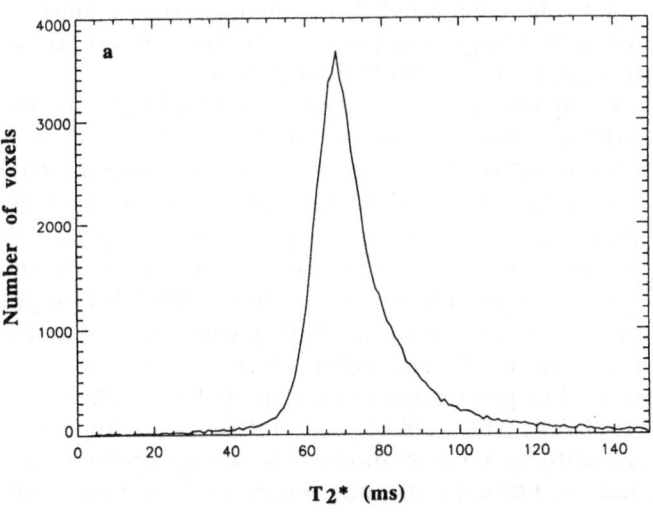

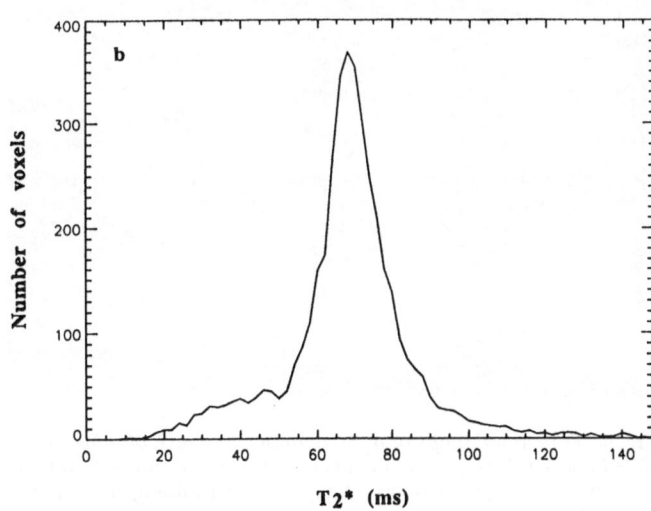

Fig. 3a. Histogram of the number of voxels with indicated T2* value of 1.88 mm resolution. **b** Histogram of the number of brain voxels with indicated T2* value for 3.75 mm resolution from the same volume as in **a** All brain voxels were taken into account from a thick superior slab comprising more than 50% of the total brain volume

method in ten volunteers. The results have been described in detail [17]. Here, we give only a short summary. Significant signal changes were found in the region around the contralateral central sulcus for both hands in all volunteers. Thirty six percent of the voxels with significant signal change ("activated") were located in the primary sensorimotor cortex (PSM). In addition, "activated" voxels were found in the premotor area, anterior superior parietal cortex, and supplementary motor area. The results are in close agreement with known functional topography.

4. Performance of 3D PRESTO and PET in a Direct Comparison

$H_2^{15}O$ PET functional imaging is based on changes in regional cerebral blood flow (rCBF). Functional magnetic resonance imaging (fMRI) is based on a variety of physiological parameters as well as on rCBF. Therefore, cross validation of 3D fMRI is important. We studied nine normal subjects with both techniques [19]. The subjects repeatedly performed the same simple thumb-finger opposition task. After image reconstruc-

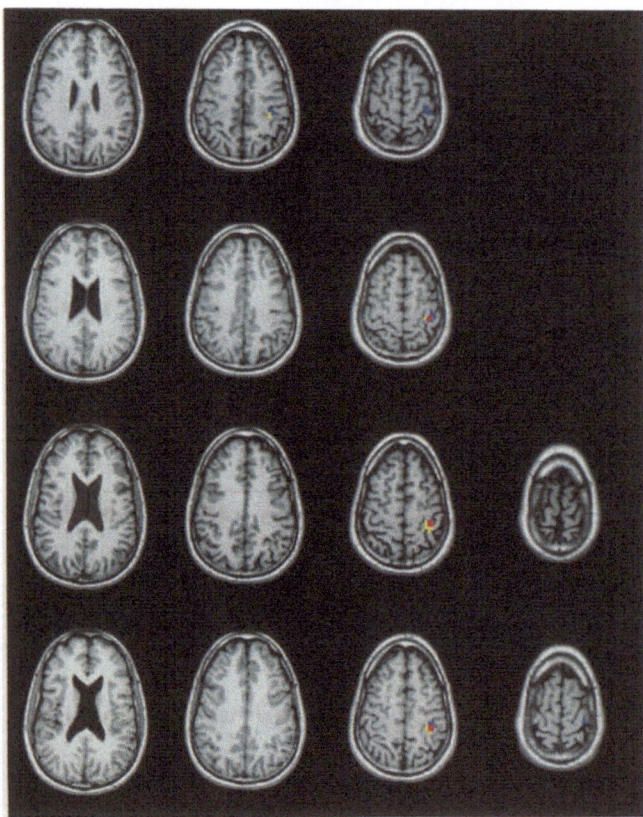

Fig. 4. *Functional maps of a finger opposition task obtained with fMRI and PET.* Regions of activation are superimposed on high resolution anatomical images. Images are in radiological orientation. Coloured voxels represent significant positive signal changes (p < 0.05 Bonferroni corrected) in fMRI only (*green*), PET only (*yellow*) or both fMRI and PET (*red*). The volumes are presented as 14 slices

tion, all of the volumes were registered to each other for each individual subject. For statistical purposes the PET and the fMRI volumes were filtered to match the data sets for voxel size and for smoothness. Figure 4 shows an example in one volunteer demonstrating the close correspondence between the results obtained with both techniques. Within-subject statistical analysis revealed significant activated signal changes in contralateral primary sensorimotor cortex (PSM) in all subjects with fMRI and with PET. With both methods, 78% of all activated voxels were located in the PSM. Overlap of activated regions occurred in all subjects (mean 43%, SD 26%). The sizes of the activated regions in PSM with both methods were highly correlated (rho = 0.87, p < 0.01). The mean distance between centers of mass of the activated regions in the PSM for fMRI versus PET was 6.7 mm (SD 3.0 mm). The average magnitude of signal change in activated voxels in this region, expressed as z-values adapted to time series (z_t), was similar (fMRI 5.5, PET 5.3). The results indicate that positive BOLD signal changes obtained with 3D PRESTO fMRI are correlated with rCBF, and that sensitivity of fMRI can equal that of $H_2^{15}O$ PET.

The topographical agreement between PET and fMRI also has implications for the question of whether large blood vessels make up a significant part of fMRI results. Differences were seen between foci of signal change in PSM, although less than the FWHM (full width at half maximum). However, there was no consistency in the direction of this spatial difference. A more superior location of signal changes could be expected if BOLD effects were dominated by draining veins, which travel from the center outward (to the superior sagittal sinus). The size and shape of the activated regions did not appear similar to the size and shape of draining veins, and the clusters of significant voxels in the PSM rarely extended to the surface of the brain where the major veins are located. These findings argue against the notion that large draining veins are the primary source of signal change in 3D PRESTO fMRI.

Compared to other reports on BOLD effects, the fMRI signal changes we observed are rather small. This is the result of the combination of smoothing the data (over 2 times the original voxel size), and the relatively small size of the activated region. Smoothing was required to match both methods for spatial resolution. Typically, signal changes in unblurred PRESTO images are on the order of 1.5%-3% [17], which is comparable to EPI at 1.5 T. The difference in signal change expressed as percentage of baseline (PET 33.1% versus PRESTO fMRI 1.0%) is not a reflection of differences in sensitivity of the methods, as is shown with the z_t-map analysis. For experimental designs utilizing single-subjects statistics, sensitivity is particularly affected by the scan-to-scan stability (expressed here as pooled standard deviation, PSD).

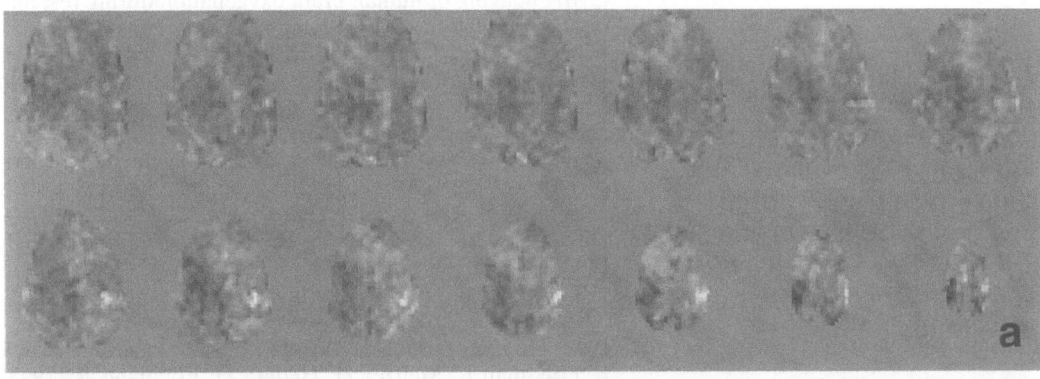

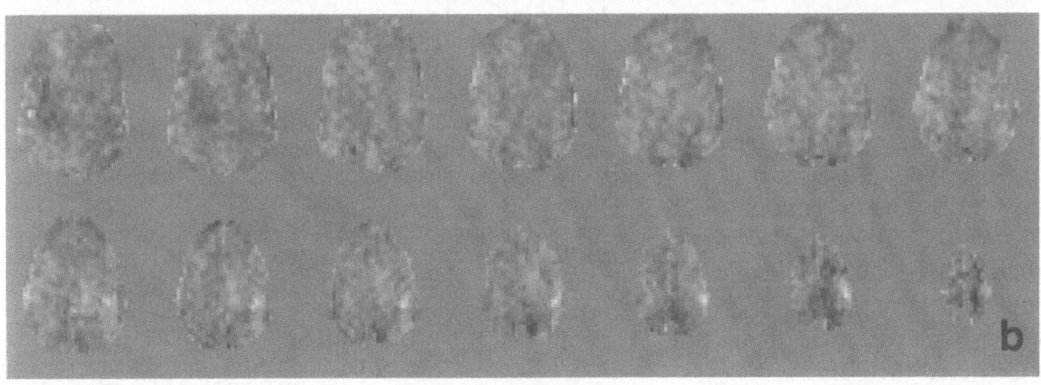

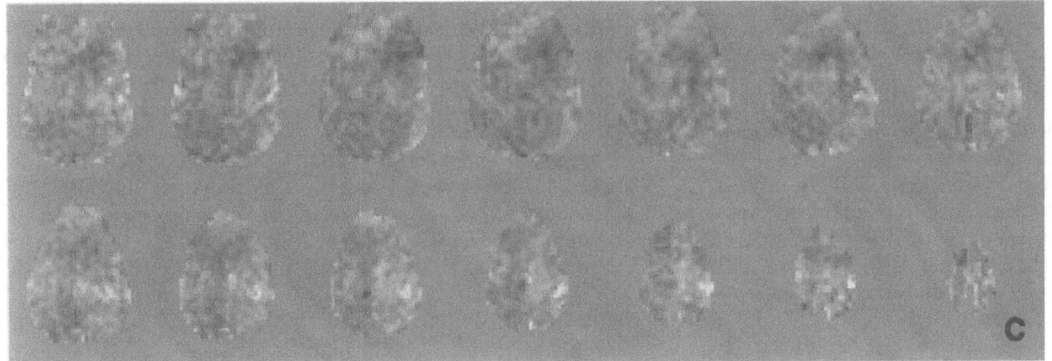

Fig. 5. *Three z_t-maps from one subject.* Each map is displayed as 14 slices (inferior to superior, radiological orientation). Greyscale ranges from –6 (*black*) to 6 (*white*).
Maps **a** and **b** were obtained in the same experimental session. Map **c** was obtained on a different day

5. Reliability of PRESTO Functional Mapping as Studied with a Test-retest Approach

A test-retest study was performed on eleven normal subjects again using the same thumb-finger opposition paradigm [20]. During one session, two series of functional scans were acquired. Nine subjects were tested once more on a different day. Each individual motor trial was analyzed separately, with a conservative z_t-based method. All studies for each volunteer were registered to a single volume scan for proper registration between the fMRI sessions. Figure 5 gives an example of the close correlation between the 3D z_t maps obtained with 3D PRESTO from one volunteer at different times. In 90% of all studies significant signal change was found in the contralateral PSM. Overall, 0.20% of all voxels (total about 11 000) in the scanned volume reached significance, and approximately 60% of the positive signal changes were located in

the PSM. Comparisons within and across sessions yielded similar results; there was a 80%-91% overlap of activated voxels in the PSM, and the distance between centers of PSM activation voxels was less than the spatial resolution. No difference was found in the magnitude of significant signal change between series. The results indicate that activation in sensorimotor cortex correlated with oppositional finger movement is reliably mapped with 3D PRESTO fMRI.

6. Hardware Requirements for 3D PRESTO

The results described in this paper were obtained with a conventional clinical 1.5 T scanner with shielded gradients with maximum amplitude of 10 mT/m and maximum rise time of 17 $mTm^{-1}s^{-1}$. The recent advent of faster gradients or higher magnetic fields is expected to lead to further improvements in the PRESTO performance.

Conclusion

A rapid 3D functional MRI imaging approach, the 3D PRESTO technique, has been developed and rigorously tested with a simple finger-tapping stimulation protocol on a conventional 1.5 T clinical scanner. These initial results show that (a) functional mapping with 3D PRESTO gives results that conform to the known functional topography, (b) 3D PRESTO fMRI is highly reproducible, and (c) there is a remarkably close correspondence between 3D PRESTO and PET data.

Acknowledgments

The authors thank G. Sobering and Y. Shiferaw for technical assistance and P. Théveaz for making his 3D registration software available to us. We acknowledge B. Rawlings for help in the design of the statistical parametric mapping. We thank B. Kirkby, K. Berman, J. Van Horn and G. Esposito for their help in the PET studies and K. Tallent, V. Mattay, and R. Sexton for their assistance with the fMRI studies. This work was performed in the In Vivo NMR Research Center at the NIH.

References

1. Ogawa S, Lee TM, Nayak AS, Glynn P (1990) Oxygenation-sensitive contrast in magnetic resonance imaging of rodent brain at high magnetic fields. Magn Reson Med 14:68
2. Ogawa S, Lee TM, Ray AR, Tank DW (1990) Brain magnetic resonance imaging with contrast dependent on blood oxygenation. Proc Natl Acad Sci USA 87:9868
3. Boxerman JR, Hamberg LM, Rosen BR, Weiskoff RM (1995) MR contrast due to intravascular magnetic susceptibility perturbations. Magn Reson Med 34:555
4. Kwong KK, Belliveau JW, Chesler DA, Goldberg IE, Weiskoff RM, Poncelet BP, Kennedy DN, Hoppel BE, Cohen MS, Turner R, Cheng H, Brady TJ, Rosen BR (1992) Dynamic magnetic resonance imaging of human brain activity during primary sensory stimulation. Proc Natl Acad Sci USA 89:5675
5. Ogawa S, Tank DW, Menon R, Ellerman JM, Kim S, Merkle H, Ugurbil K (1992) Intrinsic signal changes accompanying sensory stimulation: functional brain mapping using MRI. Proc Natl Acad Sci USA 89:5951-5955
6. Bandettini PA, Wong EC, Hinks RS, Tikofsky RS, Hyde JH (1992) Time course EPI of human brain function during task activation. Magn Reson Med 25:390
7. Frahm J, Bruhn H, Merboldt K, Hänicke W (1992) Dynamic MR imaging of human brain oxygenation during rest and photic stimulation. J Magn Reson Imaging 2:501
8. Kim SG, Ashe J, Hendrich K, Ellermann JM, Merkle H, Ugurbil K, Georgopoulos AP (1993) Functional magnetic resonance imaging of motor cortex: hemispheric asymmetry and handedness. Science 261:615
9. Schneider W, Noll DC, Cohen JD (1993) Functional topographic mapping of the cortical ribbon in human vision with conventional MRI scanners. Nature 365:150
10. Duyn JH, Moonen CTW, de Boer RW, van Yperen GH, Luyten PR (1994) Inflow versus deoxyhemoglobin effects in "BOLD" functional MRI using gradient echoes at 1.5 T. NRM Biomed 7:83
11. Lai S, Hopkins A, Haacke EM, Li D, Wasserman B, Buckley P, Friedman L, Meltzer H, Hedera H, Friedland R (1993) Identification of vascular structures as a major source of signal contrast in high resolution 2D and 3D functional activation imaging of the motor cortex at 1.5 T: Preliminary results. Magn Res Med 30:387
12. Moonen CTW, Liu G, van Gelderen, Sobering G (1992) A fast gradient-recalled MRI technique with increased sensitivity to dynamic susceptibility effects. Mag Reson Med 26:184
13. Liu G, Sobering G, Olson AW, Van Gelderen P, Moonen CTW (1993) Fast Echo-Shifted Gradient-Recalled MRI: Combining a short repetition time with variable T2* weighting. Magn Reson Med 30:68
14. Liu G, Sobering G, Duyn J, Moonen CTW (1993) A functional MRI technique combining principles of Echo-Shifting with a train of observations (PRESTO). Magn Reson Med 30:764
15. Moonen CTW, Barrios F, Zigun JR, Gillen J, Liu G, Sobering G, Sexton R, Woo J, Frank J, Weinberger D (1994) Functional Brain MR Imaging based on bolus tracking with a fast T2* sensitized Gradient-Echo Method. J Magn Reson Imaging 12:379
16. Duyn J, Moonen CTW, Mattay VS, Sexton RH, Barrios FA, Sobering GS, Frank FA, Liu G, Weinberger DR (1994) 3-Dimensional functional imaging of human brain using echo-shifted FLASH. Magn Reson Med 32:150
17. Van Gelderen P, Ramsey NF, Liu G, Duyn JH, Frank JA, Weinberger DR, Moonen CTW (1995) Three dimensional functional MRI of human brain on a clinical 1.5 T scanner. Proc Natl Acad Sci USA 92:6906
18. Van Gelderen P, Duyn JH, Liu G, Moonen CTW (1994) Optimal T2* weighting for BOLD-type functional MRI of human brain. Indian Academy of Sciences, Chem Sci 106:1617
19. Ramsey NF, Kirkby BS, Van Gelderen P, Berman KF, Duyn JH, Frank JA, Mattay VS, Van Horn JD, Esposito G, Moonen CTW, Weinberger DR (1994) Functional mapping of human sensorimotor cortex with 3D BOLD fMRI correlates highly with $H_2^{15}O$ PET rCBF. J Cereb Blood Flow Metab (in press)
20. Ramsey NF, Mattay VS, Van Gelderen P, Frank JA, Moonen CTW, Weinberger DR (1995) Test-retest reliability of 3D fMRI with PRESTO. Hum Brain Mapping (in press)

Clinical Diffusion Imaging on a Standard MR System: Diagnostic Usefulness Compared with Conventional MRI

P. Reimer[1], G. Schuierer[1], M. Deimling[2], E. Müller[2], P.E. Peters[1]

[1] Institute of Clinical Radiology, Westfalian Wilhelms-University Muenster, [2]Siemens AG, Erlanger, Germany

Introduction

Magnetic resonance imaging (MRI) has the ability to show and measure molecular diffusion. Molecular diffusion is the result of the thermal (Brownian) random translational motion involving all molecules. The interest in molecular diffusion is motivated by potential new approaches to characterize lesions based on their molecular mobility such as in the evaluation of stroke. There has been some controversy whether MRI could measure microscopic effects within a macroscopically moving environment and reports have been restricted to dedicated scanners or coils. The clinical breakthrough of diffusion MRI has been delayed by many problems encountered with the implementation of diffusion MRI on clinical scanners [1]. Clinical diffusion MRI requires careful selection of hardware and a variety of technical parameters. The purpose of our work is to evaluate the clinical value of diffusion-weighted magnetic resonance (MR) imaging in patients with brain tumors and infarcts using a commercially available scanner.

MR Imaging

All imaging studies were performed on a commercially available 1.0 T Magnetom Impact (Siemens AG) equipped with a 15 mT/m gradient system without additional hardware or software changes. A standard circular polarized head coil was used for all studies. The routine protocol (5 mm slice thickness) consisted of axial proton density weighted (PDW), T2-weighted (FSE) and T1-weighted spin echo (SE) sequences with complete anatomical coverage of the brain before administration of contrast material. Following i.v. administration of either gadopentetate dimeglumine or gadodiamide at 0.1 mmol/kg body weight, axial T1-weighted SE was repeated in the same slice position and coronal T1-weighted SE was acquired only post-contrast. All T1-weighted sequences were scanned with overlapping sections.

1. Diffusion Imaging

A modified CE-FAST (Contrast-enhanced Fourier-acquired steady-state technique, PSIF) sequence optimized for diffusion imaging was used. The sequence offers a free choice of sections (1-64), section thickness, matrix (64-256, both for frequency- and phase-encoding), orientation of the diffusion-encoding gradient, and number of signal averages (NSA). The unipolar diffusion-encoding gradient is controlled by the duration of the gradient (0-18 ms) at a constant gradient strength. A section thickness of 5 mm, a repetition time (TR) of 30-35 ms, a flip angle of 50°, and a field of view (FOV) of 230 mm was used for all studies. Acquisition time directly varied with matrix and NSA because sections were scanned in a sequential mode.

2. Volunteers

Imaging parameters were optimized to obtain best achievable image quality in 10 consented volunteers. The orientation (axial, coronal, and sagittal) of images and the orientation of the diffusion gradient, its duration, and NSA were varied. The matrix was 128×128 at a FOV of 230 mm. Diffusion images were scored for the presence of diffusion effects (0 = no effects – 5 = strong diffusion weighting/effects) and artifacts (0 = severe artifacts – 5 = no artifacts).

Optimal image quality was achieved with 8-16 NSA and a gradient duration of 6-12 ms. Diffusion effects were visible along white matter tracts. Measurements with the diffusion-encoding gradient oriented in the body axis (z-axis) were degraded by severe motion artifacts. The x- and y-axes should be prefered to avoid motion artifacts due to brain pulsation.

3. Patients

A series of 40 patients (n = 20 with brain tumors and n = 20 with infarcts) was examined and correlated with conventional MRI. Imaging parameters were kept con-

Table 1. Infarcts-Comparison with Diffusion MRI

	Scores	
Image Modality	Ischemia	Edema
PDW FSE	0.03 ± 0.47	0.09 ± 0.48
T2 FSE	0.13 ± 0.49	0.03 ± 0.40
Plain T1	0.17 ± 0.65	0.34 ± 0.60
T1 + Gd	0.47 ± 0.62	0.23 ± 0.57

stant as follows: TR 35 ms, 256×256 matrix, 230 mm FOV, 5 mm sections, and 8 ms gradient duration (x or y orientation). Diffusion images were evaluated for diffusion effects (0 = no effects – 5 = strong diffusion weighting/effects) and artifacts (0 = severe artifacts – 5 = no artifacts). Diffusion and conventional images were com-

paratively analyzed in subgroups for patients with tumors or infarcts. Imaging modalities were compared by analyzing whether diffusion imaging provided specific information (tumors: solid/cystic/edematous components; infarcts: ischemia/edema) compared to conventional MRI (equal = 0, worse = -1, or better = +1 than conventional MRI for individual pulse sequences) or additional information (equal = 0, worse = -1, or better = +1 than conventional MRI for individual pulse sequences).

The data show that diffusion MRI offers additional information in the assessment of patients with infarcts older than 24 h (Table 1 and Fig. 1). The value of this sequence for the work-up of acute (< 24 h) or hyperacute infarcts (< 6 h) has not been determined yet, because we could not scan patients within this phase.

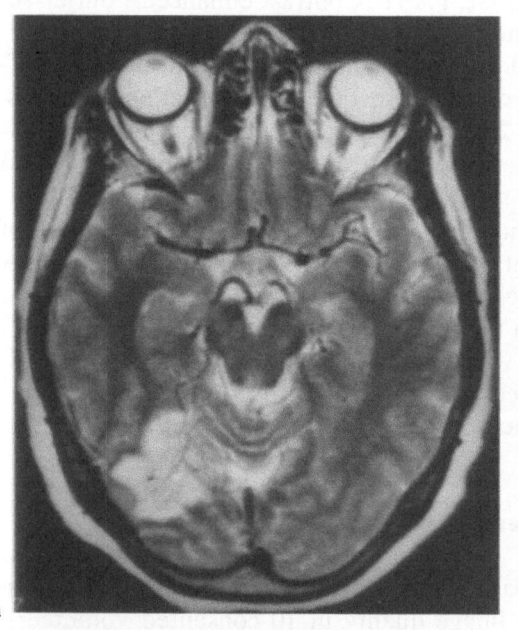
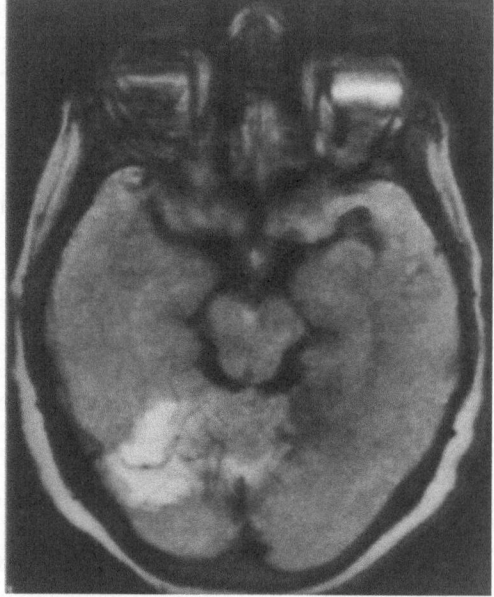
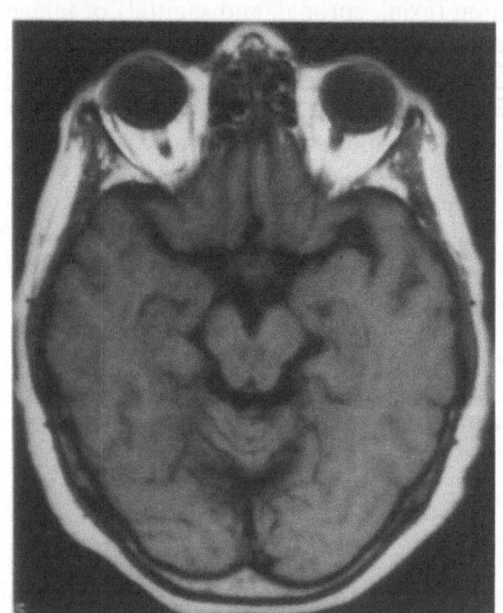
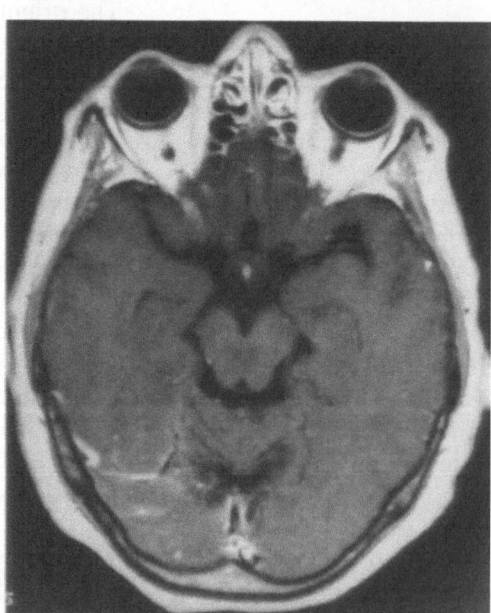

Fig. 1a-d. *Cerebral infarct* MR images (**a** T2 FSE, **b** Diffusion, **c** T1 SE - Gd, and **d** T1 SE + Gd) of a patient with a four-weeks old cerebral infarct in the right pca territory show the demarcated infarct with high signal intensity on PD/T2-weighted FSE images. Discrete signal changes are visible on the plain T1 image with subtle enhancement postcontrast. The diffusion image shows moderate artifacts with a clear demonstration of the infarcted area

Table 2. Tumors – Comparison with Diffusion MRI

	Scores	
Image Modality	Solid Tumor	Cystic Tumor
PDW FSE	0.45 ± 0.58	0.37 ± 0.49
T2 FSE	0.40 ± 0.53	0.17 ± 0.45
Plain T1	0.74 ± 0.51	0.74 ± 0.50
T1 + Gd	-0.15 ± 0.60	0.51 ± 0.51

Assessment of solid and cystic components of brain tumors was improved compared to plain MRI (Fig. 2). Gadolinium-enhanced MRI is clearly superior in the assessment of solid tumor components as demonstrated by the scores (Table 2).

Patients with tumors demonstrated fewer artifacts (0 = severe artifacts – 5 = no artifacts) than did patients with infarcts (2.97 ± 0.98 vs. 3.4 ± 0.79). This is easily explained by fewer motion artifacts of patients with tumors compared to patients with infarcts. Diffusion-effects (0 = no effects – 5 = strong diffusion effects) were therefore better visible in patients with tumors than in patients with infarcts (3.17 ± 0.92 vs. 2.56 ± 1.07).

Discussion

The main drawback of spin echo techniques for diffusion MRI is their long total acquisition time [2]. Furthermore, long TE times are required to get decent dif-

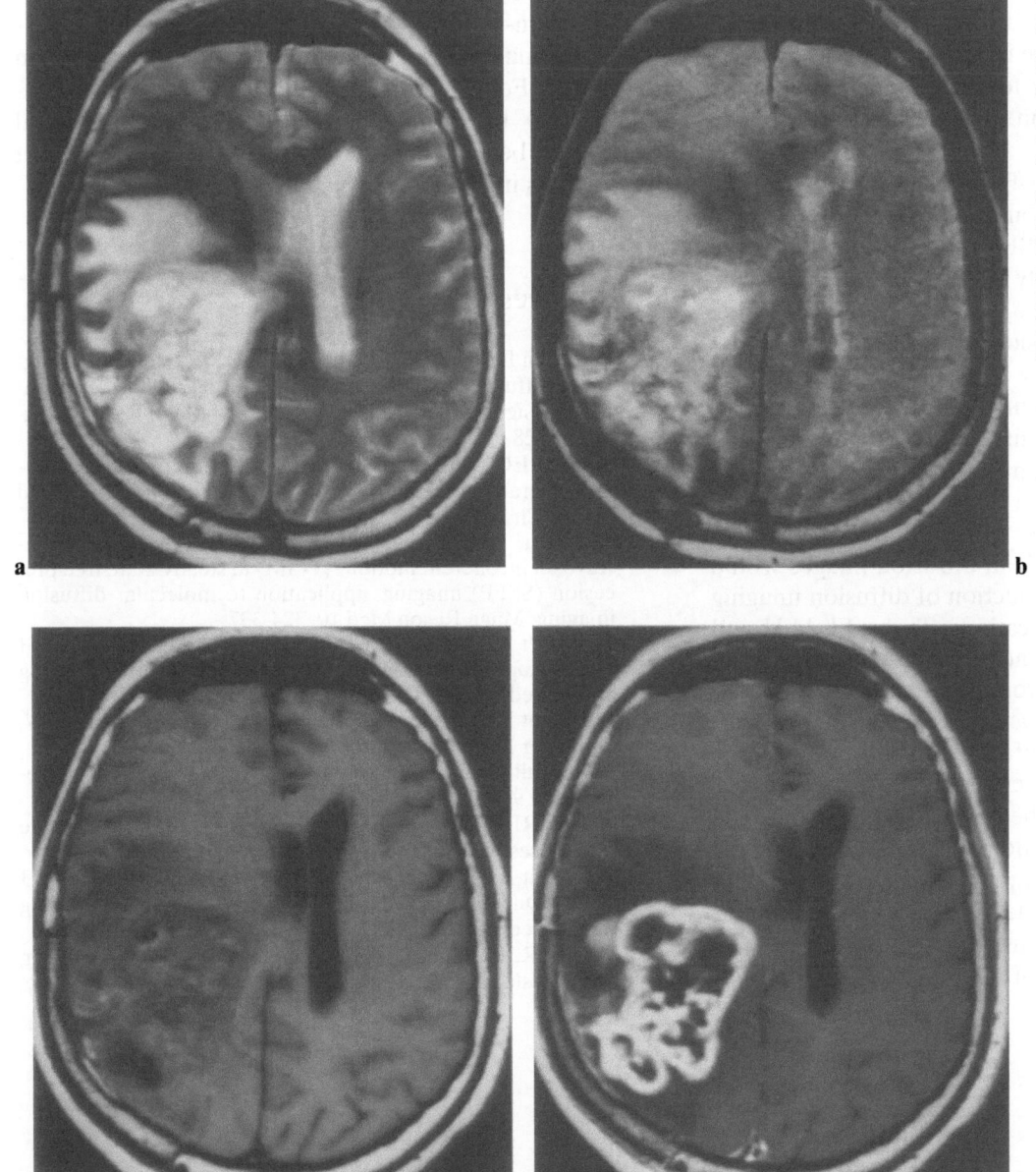

Fig. 2a-d. *Glioblastoma multiforme* MR images (**a** T2 FSE, **b** Diffusion, **c** T1 SE - Gd, and **d** T1 SE + Gd) of a patient with a biopsy-proven glioblastoma multiforme show tumor compression of the lateral ventricle with a midline shift to the left. The tumor consists of cystic and solid components and is surrounded by massive edema. All tumor components are demonstrated by diffusion imaging, however, the solid component is best seen by the contrast enhanced T1-weighted SE image

fusion effects with conventional gradient coil sets resulting in low signal-to-noise (S/N). Averaging to improve S/N or using longer TR times to minimize T1 saturation effects increase the acquisition time (> 10 min). However, long acquisition times increase the chance for patient motion, to which diffusion MRI is sensitive. Therefore, the use of fast imaging techniques is desirable to obtain diffusion images of sufficient quality. SSFP (steady-state free precession) based sequences with small flip angles can be sensitized to diffusion with the addition of gradient pulses. The theoretical analysis of diffusion effects in such sequences is complex with the main problem being that T1- and T2-effects are no longer decoupled from diffusion effects as in a spin echo approach. The CE-FAST approach has been described as a suitable SSFP scheme for diffusion purposes [3 - 5]. The sensitivity to diffusion is obtained by adding a gradient pulse before the readout gradient. Diffusion effects have been known to be larger than from spin echo equivalents because of the contribution of multiple echo paths to the signal formation [6]. Despite its speed, the CE-FAST sequence remains vulnerable to motion artifacts and the clinical benefit for diffusion imaging has not yet been demonstrated [1].

We used a modified CE-FAST scheme (PSIF) with sequential slice acquisition and free choice of technical parameters. The current PSIF version necessitates the acquisition of approximately 10 sections at a 256×256 matrix within < 10 min with a section thickness of 5 mm. This approach offers diffusion-weighted images of decent quality and is clinically applicable (Figs. 1 and 2). However, the results also demonstrate the need for further technical improvements and faster acquisition schemes especially in patients with infarcts. A second disadvantage is that diffusion maps can not be easily calculated from these data.

Faster techniques with clean diffusion images would accelerate the clinical introduction of diffusion imaging as a tool for dedicated indications. Turbo-FLASH and Turbo-Steam based sequences have been proposed, however, both need more work to improve their quality [7] Acquisition speed is crucial, because irregular motion leads to misleading artifacts. The addition of large gradients to current schemes as demonstrated in our volunteer study sensitizes the sequences to motion. The best way to prevent motion artifacts is to use a single-shot technique. Echo planar imaging (EPI) with the collection of all data in less than 100 ms eliminates artifacts caused by biologic motion. EPI is sensitized to diffusion by adding a pair of large compensated gradi-

ents before data acquisition. Because motion artifacts are reduced, diffusion coefficients can be determined with higher accuracy [8].

Improved gradient coils and amplifiers will further improve diffusion imaging. It is generally advantageous to use large stable gradients applied for a short time rather than weak gradients for a longer time [1]. Gradient amplifiers should not be used near maximum power because of potential instability. We experienced substantial artifacts from the patient table with vibrations during maximum gradient power. Both limiting gradient power and adding rubber blocks under the table helped to improve image quality. Prevention of patient motion is achieved by comfortable positioning within the magnet and use of cushions. The brain itself is subject to pulsations by large blood vessels and flow of cerebrospinal fluid (CSF) within the ventricular cavities. The best solution would be to use single-shot techniques such as echo planar imaging.

Diffusion-weighted MRI on standard scanners is feasible and may be especially utilized for early detection of stroke. Follow-up studies in tumor and infarct patients may be performed without contrast material which may become important with the upcoming budget restrictions in health care systems worldwide.

References

1. Le Bihan D, Turner R, Moonen CTW, Pekar J (1991) Imaging of diffusion and microcirculation with gradient sensitization: Design, strategy, and significance. J Magn Reson Imaging 1: 7-28
2. Stejskal EO (1965) Use of spin echoes in a pulsed magnetic-field gradient to study anisotropic, restricted diffusion and flow. J Chem Phys 43: 3597-3603
3. Le Bihan D, Turner R, MacFall JR (1989) Effects of intravoxel incoherent motions (IVIM) in steady-state free precesion (SSFP) imaging: application to molecular diffusion imaging. Magn Reson Med 10: 324-337
4. Merboldt KD, Hanicke W, Gyngell ML, Frahm J, Bruhn H (1989) Rapid NMR imaging of molecular self-diffusion using a modified CE-FAST sequence. J Magn Reson 82: 115-121
5. Merboldt KD, Bruhn H, Gyngell ML, Frahm J, Hanicke W, Deimling M (1989) MRI of "diffusion" in the human brain: new results using a modified CE-FAST sequence. Magn Reson Med 9: 423-429
6. Buxton RB (1993) The diffusion sensitivity of fast steady-state free precession imaging. Magn Reson Med 29: 235-243
7. Merboldt KD, Hanicke W, Bruhn H, Gyngell ML, Frahm J (1992) Diffusion imaging of the human brain in vivo using high-speed STEAM-MRI. Magn Reson Med 23:179-192
8. Turner R, LeBihan D (1990) Single-shot diffusion imaging at 2.0 Tesla. J Magn Reson 82: 115-121

fMRI of the Brain with Medium Field Strength Units

M. Gallucci[1-2], C. Micheli[1], G. P. Cardone[2], G. B. Minio Paluello[2], M. Castrucci[2]

[1] Department of Radiology, Ospedale Santa Maria di Collemaggio, University of L'Aquila, 67100 L'Aquila, Italy
[2] Department of Radiology, Istituto di Ricovero e Cura a Carattere Scientifico, S. Raffaele Hospital, via Elio Chianesi 33, 00144 Roma, Italy

Introduction

In the last decade, magnetic resonance imaging (MRI) has played the main role in the study of diseases affecting the central nervous system (CNS). The main limitations of the first commercial units were predominantly represented by long acquisition times and low spatial resolution. The dramatic technological developments of the 1990's have made it possible to overcome these limitations by selectively enhancing each parameter influencing the magnetic resonance (MR) signal, and have paved the way to functional studies with medium field units.

The theoretical principles at the basis of the two main techniques employed for the study of cerebral cortical function (perfusional MRI or contrast agent bolus techniques, and "BOLDc" techniques) are based on magnetic susceptibility [1-3].

The techniques exploit the modification of the relaxations times due to local changes of the magnetic field mostly evident on the T2. T2 relaxation time is constituted by two main components: the real spin-spin relaxation time (T2), related to the interactions among protons forming the examined sample, and the T2* relaxation time, which represents the changes induced on the relaxation time itself by the external magnetic field inhomogeneity. Thanks to the different acquisition techniques, inhomogenities can be reduced or enhanced in order to obtain predominantly T2 or T2*-weighted images.

The most common and clinically used application employs paramagnetic contrast agents. The gadolinium chelates, in fact, are able to represent microscopic changes of the magnetic field which surrounds the chelate itself due to the presence of free electrons within the most peripheral orbitals of the gadolinium atom. When passing through the vessel tree, the contrast agent bolus accelerates the dephasing phenomena and modifies the T2* of the tissue surrounding the vessels itself; this results in a signal intensity decrease of the MR images. Likewise, there are endogenous substances, such as deoyhaemoglobin, which produce similar paramagnetic effects. If present at the right concentration inside the vessel, the deoyhaemoglobin produces a signal intensity decrease on the T2*-weighted sequences.

It must be pointed out that magnetic susceptibility is proportional to the square of the intensity of the applied static magnetic field [4]. It also depends on the type of employed sequences. The current availability of sequences which are extremely sensitive to the T2*, such as gradient echo (GE) and gradient echo with echo planar data sampling technique, in particular, makes it possible to observe minimal changes of the T2* even with medium field units (0.5 T).

Perfusional Studies

The passage of exogenous paramagnetic contrast agent (gadolinium, dysprosium or iron chelates) can be detected with particular MR techniques (T2*-weighted sequences) and analyzed as manifestations of the regional cerebral blood flow (rCBF) and the regional cerebral blood volume (rCBV) [1, 5, 6]. The contrast agent, even though remaining within the vessel, is able to influence the magnetic field surrounding the vessel and produce a dramatic T2 decrease in the interstitial protons. A fundamental condition for detecting these changes is the employment of sequences highly sensitive to magnetic susceptibility and extremely short acquisition times. Therefore, T2*-weighted sequences with acquisition times not exceeding 2 s are needed and are acquired in series on the same slices in a time interval not inferior to 1 min.

In our studies, GE echo planar T2*-weighted sequences (repetition time (TR) = 1000 ms, echo time (TE) = 50 ms, flip angle 40°, number of exicitation (NEX) = 1, 2 min acquisition time) were employed. The same 4 slices were acquired 40 times in a total acquisition time of min 26 s. A rapid (3-5 s) i.v. (usually anterobrachial) double-dose contrast agent bolus injection was performed. Generally, the contrast agent reaches the pulmonary circle eight seconds after injection, and fills the cerebral arterial vascular bed in 10-15 s. Subse-

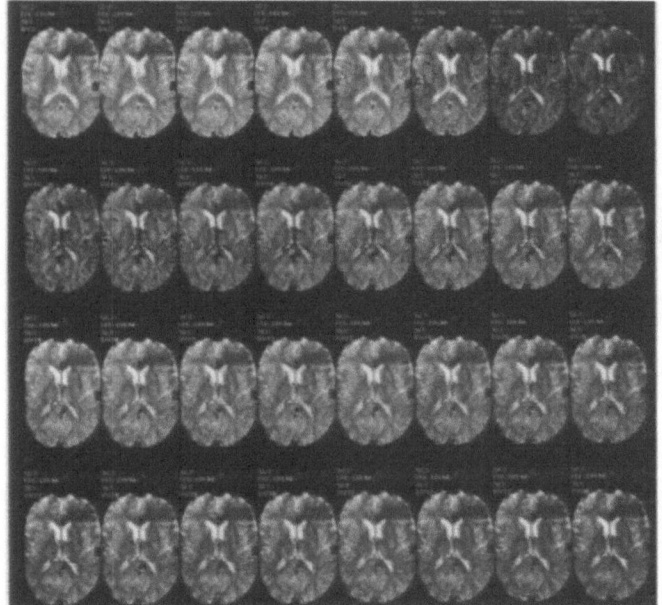

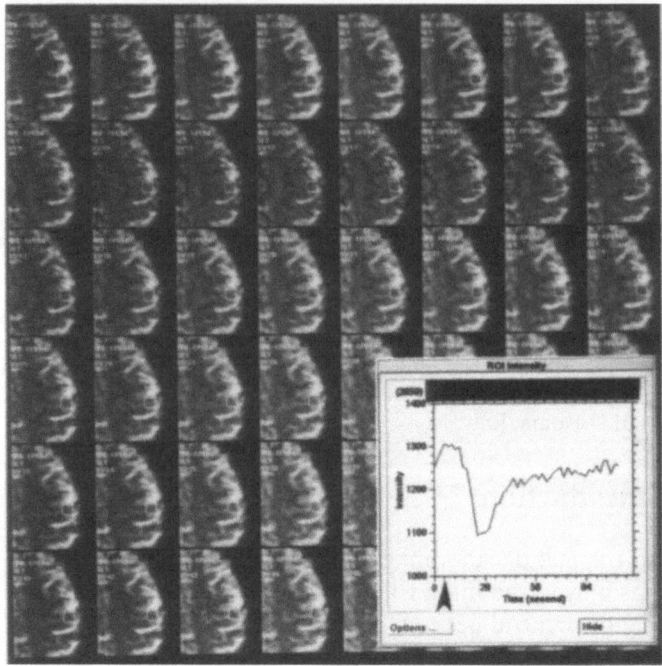

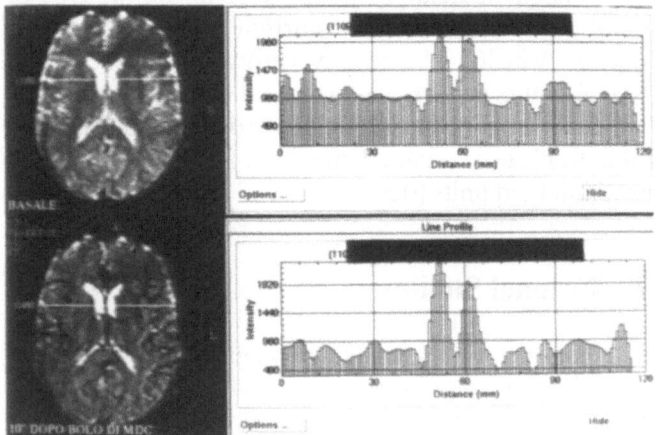

Fig. 1. a-c. *Contrast agent bolus technique.* Normal subject. **a** 32 of the 60 sequential images obtained with gradient echo-echo planar technique (1.5 min acquisition time each image). **b** Signal intensity-time curve obtained on the cortical ROI. The *arrow* indicate the starting injection time. The negative peak of the curve appears 10-15 min later. **c** *Above:* basal situation. *Below:* 1 min after injection end histogram shows a 50% signal drop of the cerebral mainly cortical tissue, expression of rCBF

quently, the contrast agent passes into the venous circle and is diluted in the systemic blood flow. At this point, it cannot be detected any more. The decrease in signal intensity induced by the first contrast agent pass through the cerebral tissue is closely related to the blood flow, since it is proportional to the contrast agent concentration within the vessel. The variation in the "signal intensity versus time" curve depends on the "contrast agent concentration versus time" curve, which, in turn, can be converted into rCBV (Fig. 1). There is a linear correlation between the signal change $\Delta (1/T2) = R2$ and the rCBV variation. Moreover, it has been proven that signal changes in each voxel are proportional to the blood volume per voxel and comparable to the changes observed in nuclear medicine tracer studies [2, 3, 7]. The graphic representation of the signal intensity versus time curve on specific cortical areas, then, is the direct expression of the blood volume versus time curve.

Experimental studies on animals showed linear corre-

lation among pCO_2 increase, signal intensity decrease on T2*-weighted sequences and rCVB increase. Similar studies performed on human volunteers showed signal intensity and rCBV changes in cortical areas consequent to specific sensory and motor stimulations. In particular, stimulations. In particular, stimulation studies of the visual cortex detected variations of about 48% of the blood volume in the pericalcarine cortex [8-10]. The main experimental clinical applications were made to investigate hypoperfusional and ischemic areas [1] (Fig. 2), and penumbra.

The described technique is quite interesting and easily repeatable, since it provides macroscopic signal intensity changes easily detectable even with medium-low field strength units. The technique proposed by us allowed optimal visualization of the contrast agent bolus passage even with a 0.5 T unit. Our images, obtained from 22 normal volunteers and 14 patients affected by cerebral ischemia, were comparable to images provided by a 1.5 T unit. Due to the lower sensitivity property of the low field unit, this technique proved to be less sensitive; however, the artifacts produced by magnetic susceptibility, chemical shift, motion (cerebrospinal fluid (CSF), vascular pulsation) and phase shift were less evident, making 0.5 T images competitive with the 1.5 T ones. In conclusion, we believe that perfusional studies

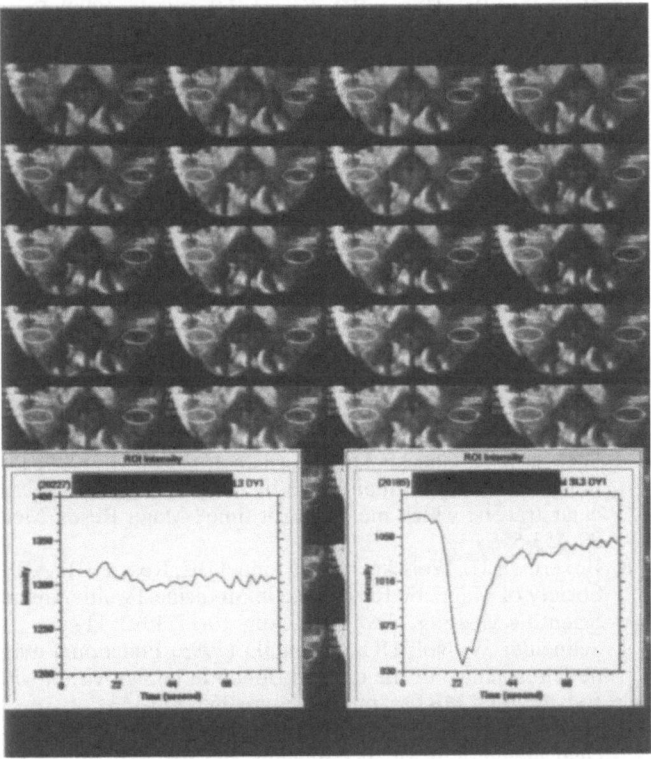

Fig. 2. a-b. *Contrast agent bolus technique in patient with acute temporo-parieto-occipital ischemia.* **a** The signal intensity-time curves obtained on symmetrical (regions of interest) ROIs of the same size on both hemispheres are extremely different. The ROI on the right-hand side does not show any signal change after contrast agent passage, proving absence or dramatic reduction of rCBF and rCBV. In the contralateral hemisphere, note the curve typical of a regular blood supply. **b** In the same case, sequential rCBV maps clearly show lack of perfusion in the ischemic area

can be perfomed even with commercially available medium field units.

BOLDc Technique

The BOLDc (blood-oxygenation level dependent contrast) technique is based on the observation of contrast agent changes linked to blood oxygenation levels. This is because deoxyhaemoglobin has a lower $T2^*$-weighted signal than does oxyhaemoglobin. Positron emission tomography (PET) studies show that in the areas of cortical activation induced by sensory and motor stimulation there is a 30%-50% increase in the rCBF and rCBV. This increase exceeds the regional oxygen need due to the cortical activation. Therefore, a local increase of oxygenated blood concentration results. All things considered, the resulting oxyhaemoglobin/deoxyhaemoglobin ratio is high; thus, a signal intensity increase on $T2^*$-weighted sequences can be hypothesized [1, 11, 12]. For this mechanism, 8-10 s for "stimulation onset-rCBV increase" and "stimulation end-restoration of normal rCBV" are needed. These latency times, assessed with

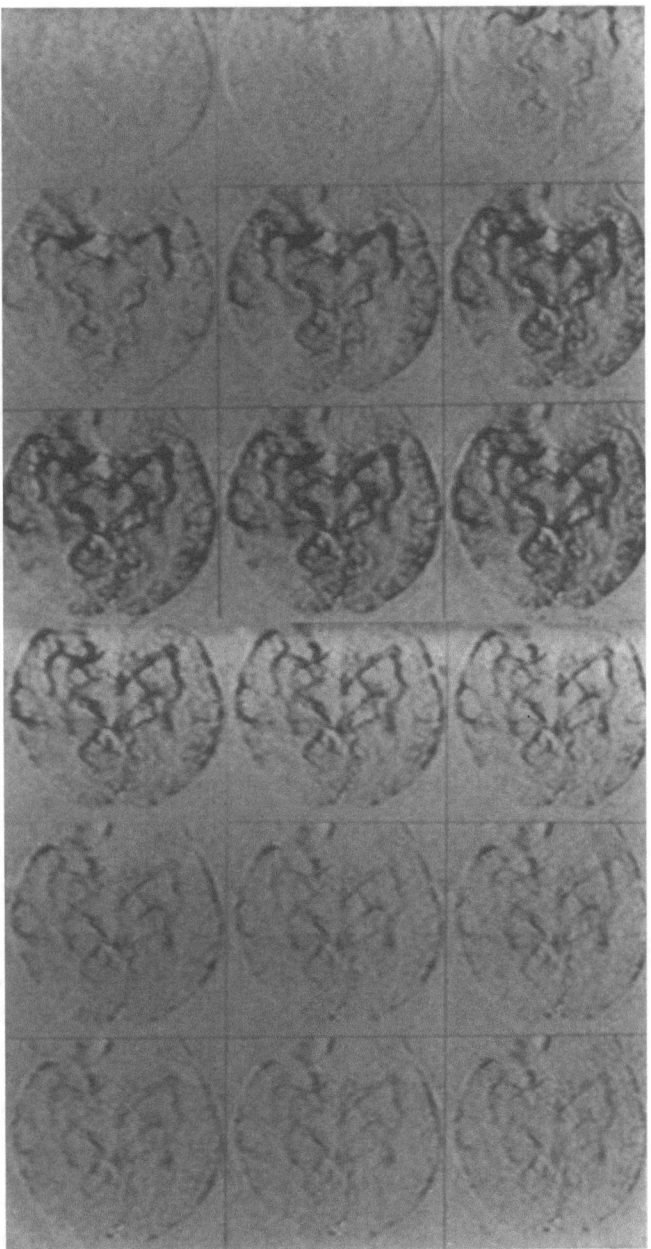

PET, are confirmed with BOLDc studies. It is therefore important that MR examination be started 8-10 s after the stimulation onset. The employment of sequences more sensitive to the $T2^*$ (gradient echo, echo planar) makes it possible to observe signal changes on the order of 5%-20% in the activated areas. Based on the evaluation of 14 healthy volunteers with motor activation task of the right or left hands upon simple movements of wrist flexion and extension, our experience shows that reliable studies can be carried out even at medium field strength (0.5 T) employing gradient echo sequences and data sampling with echo planar technique. In our studies, GE echo planar $T2^*$-weighted sequences were employed (TR = 3000 ms, TE = 40 ms, flip angle 90°, 1 NEX), acquisition time 1 min 30 s, alternatively ac-

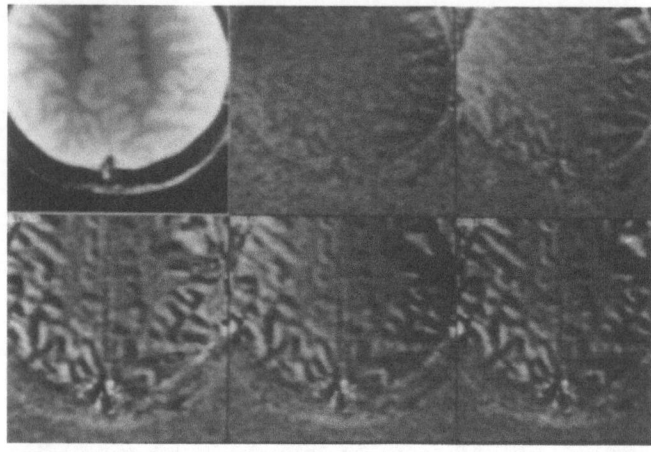

Fig. 3. *BOLDc technique with activation test of the motor area due to simple movements of the left hand (opening and clenching of the fist).* Basal image and derived images. Scarce visualization of signal difference in the subtracted images (about 3%)

quired during activation and rest. In these cases, however, the detectable signal differences varied from 3 to 5% (Fig. 3).

Since the BOLDc technique is a non traumatic procedure, it is beginning to be widely applied. Despite its complex application (long examination times with the patient absolutely motionless, proper and absolute patient collaboration to perform complicated tests, impossibility to directly assess the results, subsequent statistical studies required), interesting data comparable to those reported in the neurophysiological literature have already been provided. Functional correlations were made on motor, visual and auditory functions. Applications in the pathological field, mainly focused on the study of the vicarious functions, have already been reported in literature [14-18].

Our experience suggests that with the employment of appropriate techniques it is possible to use medium magnetic field units for functional studies. In our opinion, however, even though perfusional studies are easy and promising, the BOLDc techniques presents more limitations, mostly related to the very low signal intensity differences. Therefore, it is more effective if employedon high field strength units.

References

1. Sorensen GA, Rosen B (1996). Functional MRI of the brain. In: Atlas SW (ed) MRI of the brain and spine, 2nd edn. Lippincott-Raven, Philadelphia, 1501-1545

2. Belliveau JW, Rosen BR, Kantor HL, et al. (1990) Functional cerebral imaging by susceptibility-contrast NMR. Magn Reson Med; 14: 538-546

3. Rosen BR, Belliveau JW, Vevea JM, Brady TJ (1990) Perfusion imaging with NMR contrast agents. Magn Reson Med; 14: 249-266

4. Gomori JM, Grossman RI Goldberg H, et al. (1985) Intracranial hematoma: imaging by highfield MR. Radiology; 157: 87-93

5. Villringer A, Rosen BR, Belliveau JW, et al. (1988) Dynamic imaging with lanthanide chelates in normal brain: contrast due to magnetic susceptibility effects. Magn Reson Med; 6: 164-174

6. Fisel CR, Ackerman JL, Buxton RB, et al. (1991) MR contrast due to microscopically heterogeneous magnetic susceptibility: numerical simulations and applications to cerebral physiology. Magn Reson Med; 17: 336-347

7. Weisskoff R, Chesler D, Boxerman J, Rosen B (1993) Pitfalls in MR measurement of tissue blood flow with intravascular tracers: which mean transit time? Magn Reson Med; 29: 553-558

8. Boxerman JL, Weisskoff RM, Hoppel BE, Rosen BR (ABS) Society of Magnetic Resonance in Medicine Twelth Annual Scientific Meeting, New York, Aug. 10-17, 1993: 117

9. Schneider W, Noll DC, Cohen JD (1993) Functional magnetic resonance of the cortical ribbon in human vision with conventional MRI scanners. Nature 365: 150-153

10. Shulman RG, Blamire AM, Rothman DL, et al. (1993) Nuclear magnetic resonance imaging and spectroscopy of human brain function. Proc Natl Acad Sci USA 90: 3127-3133

11. Ogawa S, Lee TM, Nayak AS, Glynn P (1990) Oxygenation-sensitive contrast in magnetic resonance image of rodent brain at high magnetic fields. Magn Reson Med; 14: 68-78

12. Turner R, Le Bihan D, Moonen CT, Despres D, Frank J (1991) Echo-planar time course MRI of cat brain oxygenation changes. Magn Reson Med; 22: 159-166

13. Kwong KK, Belliveau JW, Chesler DA, et al. (1992) Dynamic magnetic resonance imaging of human brain activity during primary sensory stimulation. Proc Natl Acad Sci USA; 89: 5675-5679

14. Beltramello A, Viola G, Borsato A, et al. (1995) Magnetic resonance imaging of the brain. Functional rationale and magnet applications for clinical use. Rivista di Neuroradiologia 8: 345-370

15. Aronen H, Gazit I, Pardo F, et al. (ABS) Multislice MRI CBV imaging of the brain tumors: a comparison with PET studies. Society of Magnetic Resonance in Medicine. Twelth Annual Scientific Meeting, New York, Aug. 10-17, 1993: 119

16. Jack C Jr, Thompson RM, Butts RK, et al. (1994) Sensory motor cortex: correlation of presurgical mapping with functional MR imaging and invasive cortical mapping. Radiology; 190: 85-92

17. Gueckel F, Brix G, Schmiedek P, Piepgras A, Becker G, Koepke J (ABS) Assesment of cerebrovascular reserve capacity in patients with cerebrovascular disorders by using dynamic susceptibility contrast-enhanced MR imaging and the acetazolamide stimulation test. RSNA, 81th Annual Scientific Meeting, Chicago, 25 Nov. 1 Dec. 1995: 168

18. Righini A, De Vitiis O, Prinster A, et al. (1995) Functional magnetic resonance: primary motor cortex, localization in patients with brain neoplasm. Rivista di Neuroradiologia 8: 371-381

Localization of Primary Motor Cortex in Patients with Frontal-parietal Neoplasms: an fMRI Study

A. Righini[1], O. de Divitiis[2], A. Prinster[3], D. Spagnoli[2], I. Appollonio[4], L. Bello[2], P. Scifo[3], G. Tomei[2], R. Villani[2], F. Fazio[3], M. Leonardi[1]

[1] Neuroradiology and [2] Neurosurgery Departments, IRCCS Ospedale Maggiore-Policlinico, Milan, Italy - [3] INB-CNR, IRCCS HS Raffaele, Milan, Italy - [4] Neurology Department, Ospedale S. Gerardo, Monza, Italy

Introduction

Functional magnetic resonance imaging (fMRI), which uses BOLD (blood oxygenation level dependent contrast) technique, allows the identification of physiologically activated brain areas by means of a local and transient magnetic resonance (MR) signal increase [1]. The physical and physiological bases of the observed signal changes are not totally understood. The most accepted theory associates a local decrease in deoxyhemoglobin concentration within the venous microcirculation with the MR signal increase detected during brain activation [2].

Functional MRI has been applied extensively to the study of primary and supplementary motor cortex in normal volunteers using either simple or complex activation tests [3, 4]. These investigations have substantially confirmed the location of such eloquent areas previously shown by radiotracers and electrophysiology studies. Moreover, it has been shown that in normal subjects the localization of some functional areas does not always correspond to the known anatomical references [5]. In patients with brain masses the situation can be even more complicated. Neoplasms compressing or infiltrating the cerebral cortex often alter the normal anatomy so that usual anatomical landmarks cannot be easily identified. Functional MRI could be a useful tool during surgical planning for depicting the spatial relationship between the neoplasm and the eloquent cortical areas which should be spared. Moreover, the results of mass effect on brain functional anatomy have not yet been extensively studied in vivo [6]. Functional MRI investigation of the location and the morphology of motor areas in such patients could offer new insights about adaptive functional and structural changes in response to local brain insults. Very few examples of motor activation fMRI studies which use echo planar scanning technique have been reported on brain tumor patients [7, 8].

The aims of the present study were: (a) to test fMRI's ability to localize the hand primary motor cortex in patients with brain neoplasms using a conventional scanner; (b) to compare within the same subjects the location and morphology of the activated motor areas in the affected hemisphere with those of the contralateral ones.

Subjects and Methods

Seventeen right handed patients of mean age of 46.5 ± 15.9 years (11 males and 6 females) were studied (Table 1). Among them, sixteen had frontal-parietal intra- and extra-axial tumors and one had a frontal arteriovenous malformation. Histology revealed five glioblastomas, three astrocytomas, four meningiomas, one cavernous angioma, three single metastases, one arteriovenous malformation (AVM). At standard neurological examination, motor performance of the contralateral hand ranged from normal to slight impairment of finger dexterity. The subjects were scanned using a 1.5 T MR unit (Magnetom 63 SP, Siemens, Erlangen, Germany) equipped with conventional unshielded gradients (10 mT/m). Each patient's head was positioned within the standard head coil and restrained with foam padding. T1-weighted spin echo images for anatomical localization were acquired. The fMRI study was based on a series of FLASH images (repetition time (TR) = 63 ms, echo time (TE) = 40 ms, flip angle = 10°, matrix = 128 × 128, field of view (FOV) = 240 mm, slice thickness = 5 mm, acquisition time = 11 s); the small flip angle was chosen in order to minimize signal changes associated with the inflow effect [9, 10]. Two or three contiguous slices parallel to the bicommissural plane were acquired through the level of frontal-parietal cortex. Each patient was requested to perform a finger tapping task with the hand contralateral to the lesion or, when slight impairment of finger dexterity was present, a simpler repetitive flexion – extension of the last four fingers. The same task was repeated with the other hand. Each subject was requested to perform the motor task as quickly as possible. During each trial, three movement periods were alternated with three rest periods. Patients who showed gross brain motion by cine-mode evaluation were not

Table 1. Patient Summary

Patient #	Initials	Age	Sex	Lesion type
1	R.D.	47	F	Right frontal meningioma
	R.D 2 weeks after surgery	"	"	"
2	D.M.	40	M	Right frontal astrocytoma
3	S.M.[a]	63	M	Right frontal metastasis
4	N.G.[a]	67	M	Right frontal metastasis
5	A.M.	49	M	Right frontal AVM
6	P.L.[a]	64	M	Right frontal glioblastoma
7	S.L.[a]	45	F	Right frontal parietal glioblastoma
8	T.R.	32	M	Right frontal glioblastoma
9	T.M.[a]	65	M	Right parietal metastasis
10	B.F.	54	F	Right frontal glioblastoma
11	D.C.	20	F	Right frontal parietal astrocytoma
12	G.N.	14	F	Multiple angiomas
13	M.P.	54	M	Left frontal-parietal meningioma
	M.P. 2 months after surgery	"	"	"
14	B.R.	53	F	Left parietal meningioma
	B.R. 6 months after surgery	"	"	"
15	S.G.	24	M	Right frontal posterior meningioma
16	R.R.	46	M	Left parietal astrocytoma
17	B.M.	54	M	Left parietal glioblastoma
	B.M. 5 months after surgery	"	"	"

[a] Subjects excluded because of motion artifacts

considered for further analysis. Images were transferred to a Sparc 10 work station (Sun Microsystems, Mountain View, CA). Pseudo-color activation maps were then calculated by Z_score method and superimposed on high resolution images (Imview software, v. 3.3.2 by P. Jezzard, NIH, Bethesda, MD). Signal intensity time courses for those pixels or clusters of pixels with Z_scores above the chosen cut off value (1.5-2.2) were plotted to visually check their correspondence to task pattern. The percentage of signal increase over the baseline was then calculated for the largest cluster of activated pixels present in each hemisphere.

Four patients (without clinically detectable residual motor deficit) were also studied after surgery at two weeks, or at two, five or six months.

Results

Five patients were excluded because of gross motion artifacts. In all other patients, areas of significant signal increase were detected either on the center or on the posterior edge of the precentral gyrus (Fig. 1). These areas had a spot-like appearance, and no substantial side to side differences in shape and extension could be observed (Fig. 2). Only in one patient the global extension of the activated areas was found to be definitely larger in the affected hemisphere than in the contralateral one (Fig. 3). There was not a significant difference (p = 0.43, paired t-test) between the percentage of activation in the lesioned hemisphere (4.1 ± 1.1 SD) and in the contralateral one (5.0 ± 0.9 SD). In some cases the activated areas were well separated from the neoplasm. In some others they were visible on the border between tumoral and normal tissue (Fig. 2). No activated pixels were identifiable within the neoplasm borders as detectable by spin echo and T2*-weighted images. However, activation signal was clearly present within edematous parenchyma (Fig. 4). When mass effect was remarkable, the activated areas in the affected hemisphere were clearly displaced with respect to the contralateral ones.

In two of the four cases studied after surgery, the activated areas returned to a more bilaterally symmetric position (Fig. 5). In spite of good motor performance, another patient scanned after surgery showed no activation on the lesioned hemisphere. This probably arose because of large magnetic susceptibility artifacts associated with hemosiderin deposits.

Discussion

Functional MRI localization of primary motor area using a conventional scanner can be performed also in patients with brain tumors, although with a lower success rate than in normal volunteers studies mainly because of subject compliance problems. Areas of significantly increased signal are detectable even in cortex where normal anatomical patterns are lost.

The percentage of signal increase we observed in both affected and healthy hemispheres is similar to that reported for normal subjects in motor activation gradient echo fMRI studies [11]. No significant side to side difference in percentage of activation signal was found. These results are not surprising since no significant motor impairment was present in our patients and no substantial difference in motion rate was noticed between the two hands. However, compared with motor activa-

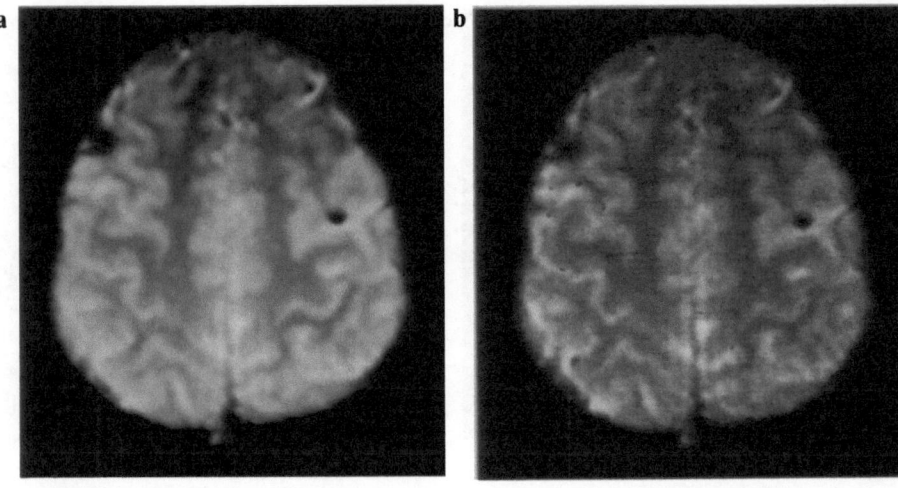

Fig. 1a-b. *Patient with multiple cavernous angiomas (# 12 in Table 1).* **a** axial T2*-weighted scan depicts a left frontal angioma. **b** the pseudocolor activation map has been superimposed on the previous image. Some significantly activated pixels are located on the precentral gyrus

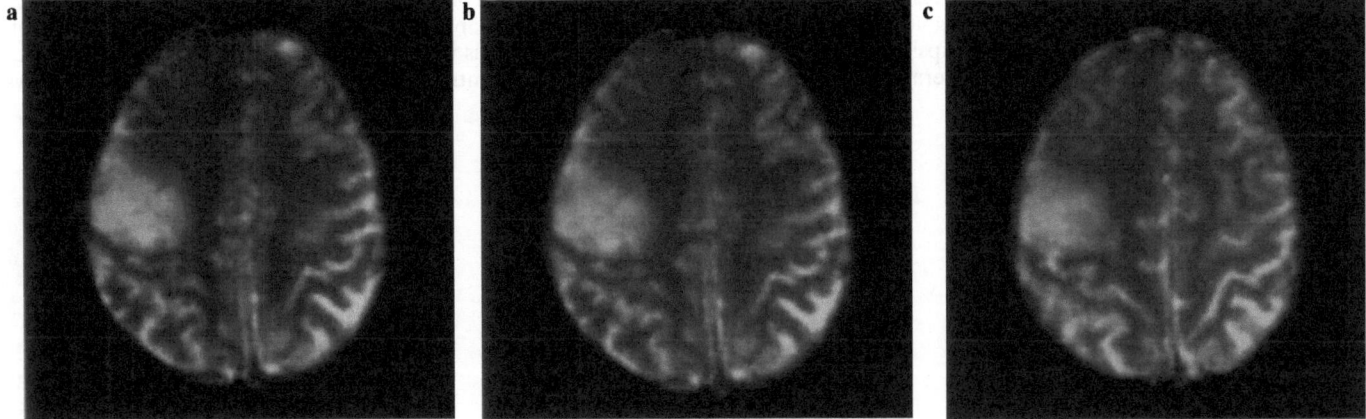

Fig. 2a-c. *Patient with a low grade right frontal astrocytoma (# 2 in Table 1).* This patient had suffered some left superior limb partial motor seizures. Activation maps are superimposed on T2*-weighted images. Sections in **a** and **b** are at the same level (the one in **c** is contiguous but more cranial). During left side motor task no activation is visible in **a** whereas in **b** some spotlike activated areas on the posterior edge of the precentral gyrus are associated with the right hand movement. Activated pixels during left side motor task can be seen only on the more cranial section (**c**) as the neoplasm had displaced the functional areas superiorly. Moreover, the latter are very close to the tumoral infiltrating tissue. However, no significant side to side differences in shape and extension of the activated areas are noticeable

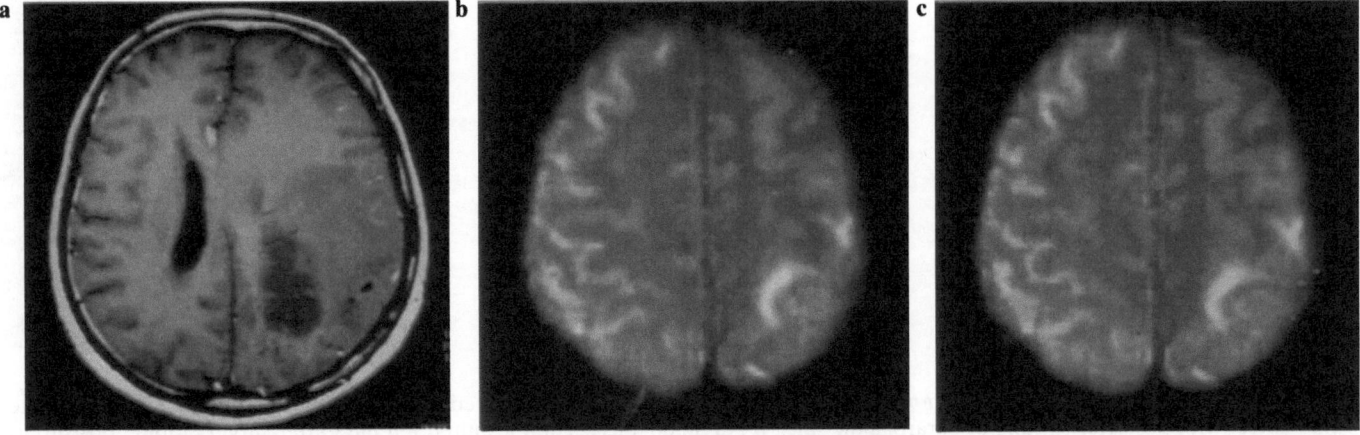

Fig. 3a-c. *Patient with left parietal astrocytoma (# 16 in Table 1)* **a** The main part of the tumor and the associated conspicuous edema and mass effect with gyral effacement. **b** The activation map for the left hand task is superimposed on a more cranial T2*-weighted section: significantly activated areas are located on the posterior edge of the precentral gyrus. **c** The corresponding activation map for the right hand is showed: on this side the activated areas have a clearly broader extension. Hyperintense signals from edema can be seen in the gyri. At surgery this patient presented a remarkably edematous cortex with vein engorgement

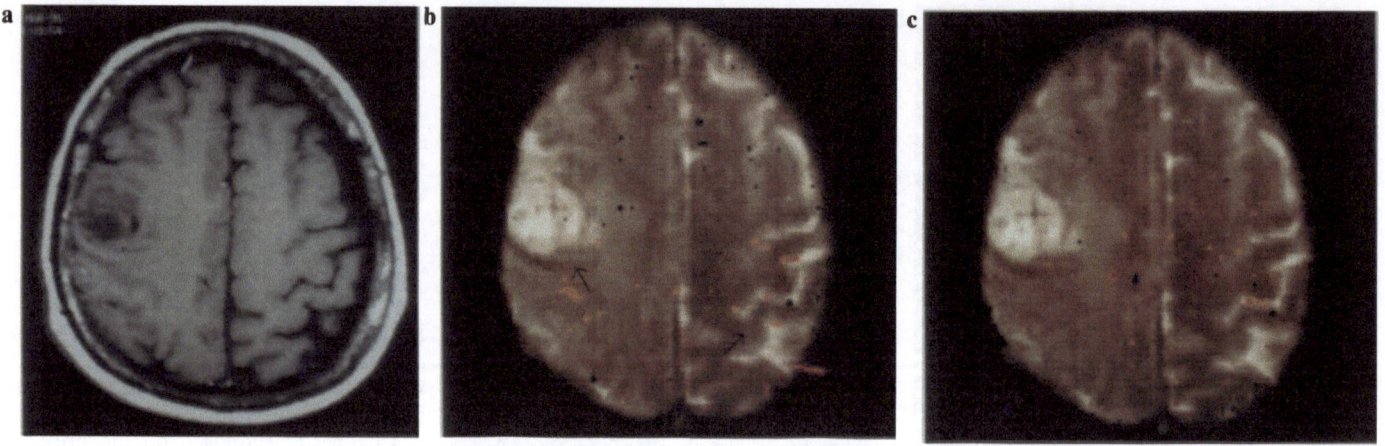

Fig. 4a-c. *Patient bearing posterior right frontal glioblastoma with no upper limb motor deficit (# 10 in Table 1).* **a** An axial unenhanced T1-weighted scan, showing part of the tumor and the mass effect with gyral effacement due to diffuse vasogenic edema. **b** and **c** Activation maps for the left and right hand tasks, respectively, are superimposed on the corresponding T2*-weighted section: the *arrow* points out the only area of significant signal increase present in the right hemisphere apparently located outside the tumor mass, but within edematous parenchyma. During ipsilateral hand task some small activated areas were visible close to central sulcus on the left side in **b** (*arrow*). The presence of ipsilateral activation signal can be due to minimal contralateral hand muscle contractions or to physiologic bilateral partial motor control

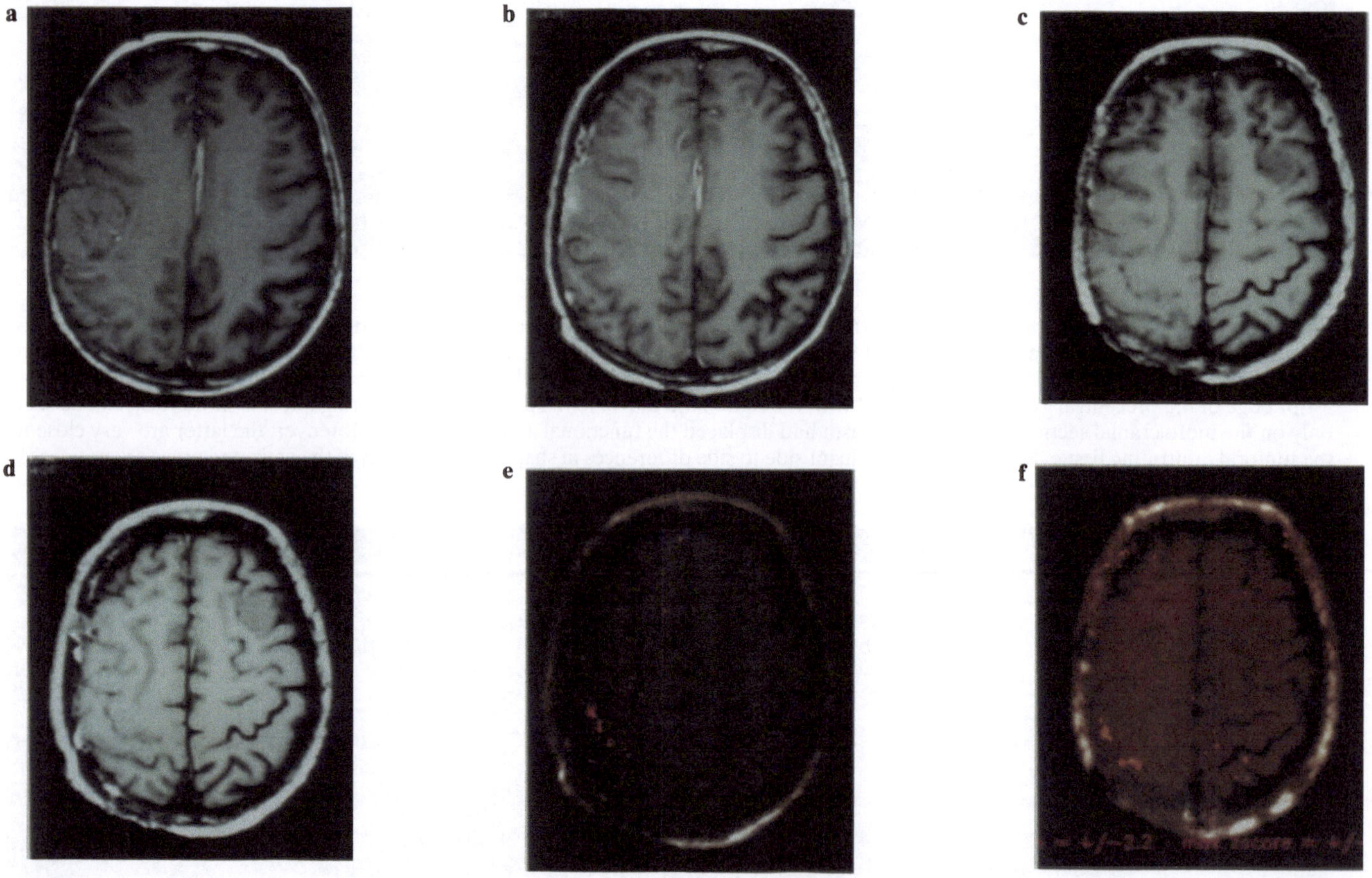

Fig. 5a-f. *Patient with right frontal posterior meningioma (# 1 in Table 1).* **a** T1-weighted scan depicting the tumor and the associated mass effect with posterior shifting of pararolandic sulci. **b** An analogous section acquired ten days after surgery. Some postsurgical bleeding and a clear reduction of the mass effect can be noticed. Some intracerebral edema is still present. **c** From the presurgical study, a section cranial to the one in **a**. The mass effect with narrowing of the sulci is clearly visible; an additional small left frontal meningioma is detectable at this level. **d** Section analogous to **c**, is acquired in the postsurgical study: a reduction of the mass effect on the sulci is visible. **e** The left hand activation map from the presurgical study is superimposed on the section visible in **c**. **f** The left hand activation map from the postsurgical study is reported on **d** section. The significantly activated areas in **e** have a slightly different shape with respect to **f**. Moreover, after surgery **f** the activated areas are shifted forward to the expected anatomical location

tion maps reported in the literature [11], in our cases the extension of the activated areas in both affected and healthy hemispheres was generally smaller. The smaller flip angle we used (10°) can partially explain the difference, since it would have produced less inflow effect and a smaller large veins-dependent signal.

Recently, in a hand motor task fMRI study of six tumor patients, Yousry et al. [6] reported that the activated areas on the tumor side appeared to be, in most of the cases, broader than in normal volunteers. The authors hypothesized that a mass effect-driven plastic cortical reorganization of hand motor area could have been the cause of such changes. We compared activated areas in the lesioned and healthy hemispheres within the same subject and did not observe substantial differences in shape between the two sides. Only in one patient was the activated area in the tumor side clearly larger than that in the contralateral one. Part of the discrepancy may have arisen from the different flip angle we used. The data of Yousry et al. [6] were obtained with a larger flip angle and may therefore have had a significant contribution from the signal associated with major veins. A neoplasm and the consequent edema can remarkably alter local vascular bed geometry, which can lead to pial veins congestion. This extraparenchymal factor may cause changes in shape and extension of activated areas. In our protocol we used a smaller flip angle (10° versus 40°), which produces a smaller large veins-associated signal. This could partly explain the lack of striking differences between the activated areas in the two sides in our study. However, the results of the two studies are not easily comparable, because differences in tumor size, location and amount of mass effect between the two populations might have been associated with quantitatively different functional alterations.

We did not observe any significant activated pixels within the tumor mass. This could be because in most cases the neoplasm did not invade the precentral gyrus, as can be supported also by the lack of significant contralateral hand motor impairment. However, the presence of activated normal parenchyma within a neoplasm can be difficult to demonstrate by fMRI, because slight differences in T2-weighted signal within the tumor can yield sharp pseudo-activation signal increases when minimal motion occurs during the task execution.

When most of the mass effect was removed by tumor excision, the activated areas shifted back to the usual position of the precentral gyrus. This was observed in two meningioma-bearing patients who were free from postsurgical motor deficits. These subjects had no direct brain parenchyma tumor invasion and the eloquent cortical areas were compressed but not directly damaged. Because of the exiguous number of subjects studied after surgery it is not possible to evaluate the effect of tumor removal on the extension of motor areas. Moreover, it is likely that, as in our cases, when no differences

in motor performance before and after surgery are noticeable, no significant motor areas extension changes can be found as well.

When patients are scanned after surgery, the presence of magnetic susceptibility artifacts associated with large hemosiderin deposits seriously complicates activated areas localization. This will be an important limitation for fMRI studies in the postsurgery setting. Functional MRI techniques, which are not based on blood magnetic susceptibility variations but on longitudinal relaxation mechanisms [12], might overcome this limitation.

The main limitation of our fMRI study is probably represented by the restricted brain volume that could be scanned with a single slice technique. Even if the measurements were repeated at least two different contiguous levels, some activated areas might not have been detected as a consequence of this technical limitation. The introduction of echo planar multislice sequences or of three-dimensional (3D) data acquisition techniques might provide a solution [13].

References

1. Kwong KK, Belliveau JW, Chesier DA et al (1992) Dynamic magnetic resonance imaging of human brain activity during primary sensory stimulation. Proc Natl Acad Sci USA 89: 5675-5679
2. Ogawa S, Tank D, Menon R, Ellermann J, Kim S, Markle H, Ugurbil K (1992) Intrinsic signal changes accompanying sensory stimulation: functional brain mapping with magnetic resonance imaging. Proc Natl Acad Sci USA 89: 5951 -5955
3. Rao S, Binder JR, Bandettini BS et al (1993) Functional magnetic resonance imaging of complex human movements. Neurology 43: 2311-2318
4. Tyszka J, Grafton S, Chew W, Woods R, Colletti P (1994) Parceling of mesial frontal motor areas during ideation and movement using functional magnetic resonance imaging at 1.5 Tesla. Ann Neurol 35: 746-749
5. Daniels DL, Yetkin ZF, Mark LP, Haughton VM (1994) Comparison of Functional MR Imaging and Anatomic Methods for Locating the Sensorymotor Cortex. Radiology 193: 186
6. Yousry T, Schmid U, Jassoy A et al (1995) Topography of the cortical motor hand area: prospective study with functional MR imaging and direct motor mapping at surgery. Radiology 195: 23-29
7. Jack C, Thompson RM, Butts RK et al (1994) Sensory motor cortex: correlation of presurgical mapping with functional MR imaging and invasive cortical mapping. Radiology 190: 85-92
8. Howard R, Alsop D, Detre J, Listerud J et al (1994) Functional MRI of Regional Brain Activity in Patients with Intracerebral Gliomas and AVMs prior to Surgical or Endovascular Therapy. [Abstract] Society of Magnetic Resonance 2nd meeting, August, 701
9. Frahm J, Merboldt K, Haenicke W, Kleinschmidt A, Boecker H (1994) Brain or vein-oxygenation or flow? On signal physiology in functional MRI of human brain activation. NMR Biomed 7: 45-53
10. Righini A, Pierpaoli C, Barnett AS, Waks E, Alger JR (1995) Blue blood or black blood: R_1 effects in gradient echo echo planar functional neuroimaging. Magn Reson Imag 13:

124   A. Righini, O. Divitiis, A. Prinster, D. Spagnoli, I. Appollonio, L. Bello, P. Scifo, G. Tomei, R. Villani, F. Fazio, M. Leonardi

369-378

11. Constable R, McCarthy G, Allison T, Anderson A, Gore J (1993) Functional brain imaging at 1.5 T using conventional gradient echo MR imaging techniques. Magn Reson Imag 11: 451-459

12. Edelman R, Siewert B, Darby D, Thangaraj V, Nobre A, Mesulam M, Warach S (1994) Qualitative mapping of cerebral blood flow and functional localization with echo planar MR imaging and signal targeting with alternating radio-frequency. Radiology 192: 513-520

13. Duyn J, Mattay V, Sexton R, Sobering G, Barrios F, Liu G, Frank J, Weinberger D, Moonen C (1994) 3-Dimensional functional imaging of human brain using echo-shifted FLASH MRI. Magn Reson Med 32: 150-155

FUNCTIONAL EVALUATION OF PARENCHYMAL ORGANS AND THE HEART WITH MRI

Functional MRI of the Kidneys

G.P. Krestin, R.A. Huch Böni

Department of Medical Radiology, University Hospital Zürich, 8091 Zürich, Switzerland

Introduction

Pathologic alterations of the kidneys include not only morphologic changes, but also functional disorders. Some diseases such as glomerular and tubulointerstitial disorders or vascular insufficiency can even lead to substantial dysfunction without visibly altered morphology. Renal angiography as well as radionuclide renography can be employed for the study of perfusion and excretory function of the kidneys. MRI, however, has the advantage to provide both information on morphology and on renal function.

MR Imaging Technique in Functional Disorders

To evaluate patients with excretory disorders, dynamic studies using a gradient recalled echo (GRE) sequence with simultaneous T1- and T2-weighting (GRASS; FFE; FLASH without spoiling gradients) should be favored. For this purpose, the rapid repetition of 16-32 single scans in the same position with a repetition time (TR) = 20-30 ms, an echo time (TE) = 8-16 ms, a flip angle of 45°-70° and a reduced matrix allows the reduction of acquisition times to 4-6 s per slice followed by a breathing period of 4-5 s. This protocol results in a temporal resolution of 8 to 10 s (Fig. 1) [1, 2].

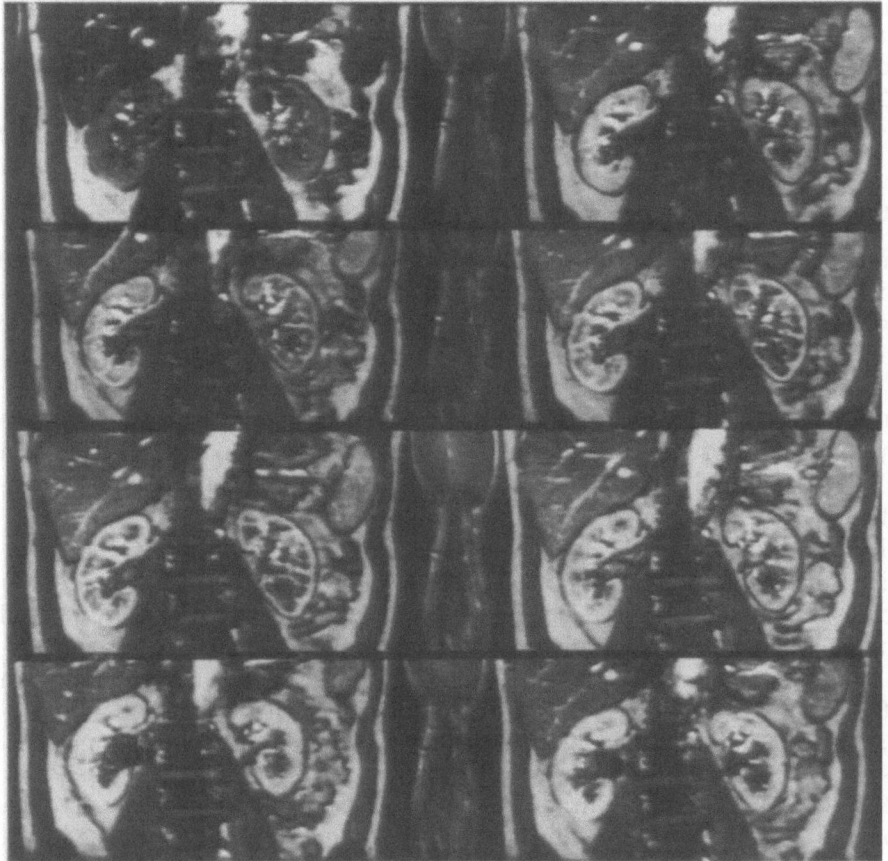

Fig. 1. *Dynamic gradient echo MRI of normal excretory function.* From left to right and top to bottom: precontrast image, and 20, 30, 40, 50, 60, 70 and 120 s following bolus injection of 0.1 mmol/kg Gd-DTPA shows cortical enhancement and concentration of contrast agent in the medulla with signal intensity decrease beginning 30 s after injection

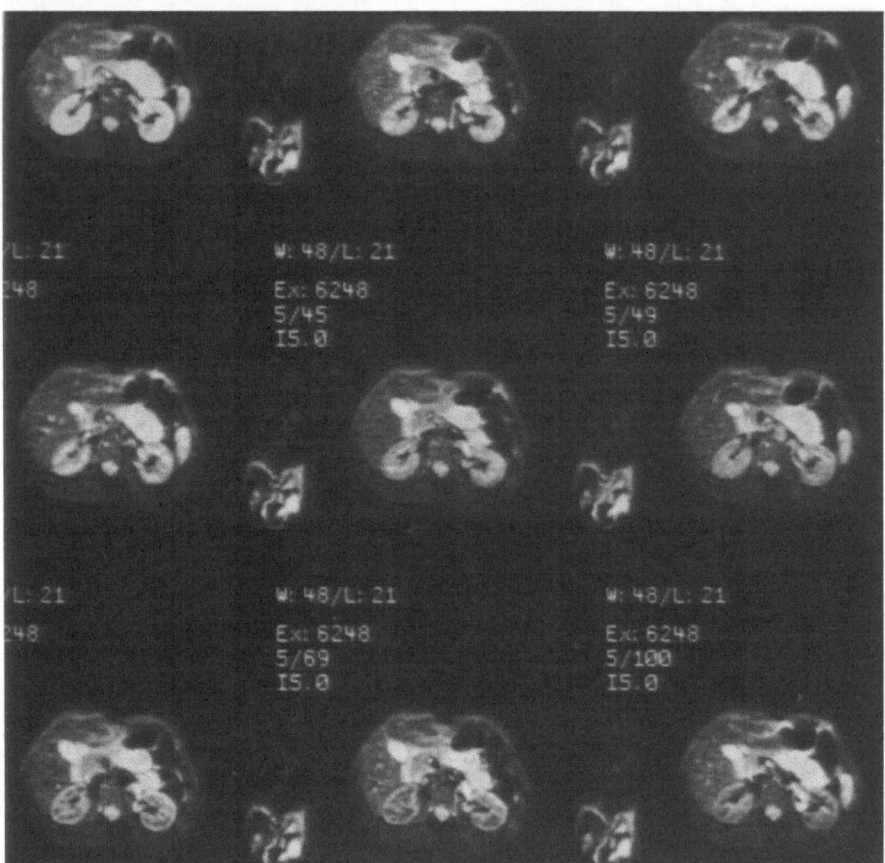

Fig. 2. *Dynamic echo-planar MRI.* Normally functioning kidneys (from left to right and top to bottom) show migration of a dark contrast material band from the renal cortex throughout the medulla

Alternatively, T2-weighted echo planar imaging (EPI) may be used for functional evaluation and might even better demonstrate the excretion of paramagnetic contrast agent (e.g. Gd-DTPA or Gd-DOTA) into the collecting ducts (Fig. 2) [3].

Evaluation of Renal Excretory Function

Depending on the arterial perfusion, an increase of the signal intensity in the renal cortex can be observed just 10-20 s after bolus injection. A maximum value is reached about 20-30 s after the first signs of perfusion, followed by a slow, constant fall of the signal intensity. This finding is due to the pronounced arterial perfusion of the renal cortex that leads to an early appearance of the contrast agent in this region. The T1 shortening effects of gadolinium produce a significant increase in signal intensity; the onset of glomerular filtration and the dilution in the extravascular space manifest themselves as a slow subsequent signal intensity decrease (Fig. 1).

Signal changes are different in the medulla and reflect water reabsorption in the tubuli and collecting ducts. Medullary signal increase occurs 10-20 s later than cortical enhancement, and reaches a maximum after 20-30 s with similar signal values as in the cortex. On unspoiled GRE images (FFE, FISP, GRASS) 30-40 s after the first visible signs of cortical perfusion, the signal intensity in the medulla decreases steeply to a minimum

which is comparable to the initial value on the precontrast image. Only when the contrast agent passes into the calyces and is diluted with non-contrasted glomerular filtrate does the medullary signal intensity increase to a level similar to that of the cortex. Excretion into the calyces usually may be demonstrated at this point and is characterized by a signal intensity decrease and susceptibility artifacts in the region of the renal pelvis [1, 4-7].

These changes of signal intensity must be interpreted with reference to the effects of the paramagnetic gadolinium compounds on the relaxation times of tissues. Since the medulla accounts for only about 1%-6.5% of the entire renal blood supply, it is understandable that the visible perfusion of medullary structures is delayed in comparison with the cortex. The onset of glomerular filtration of the contrast agent and water reabsorption in the proximal convoluted tubule, in the loop of Henle and particularly in the collecting ducts results in a marked concentration of Gd-DTPA or Gd-DOTA (50-100 fold concentration). Depending on the sequence used, contrast reversal occurs because of the now predominant T2-shortening effects of gadolinium. Therefore, the signal intensity drop in the medullary pyramids visible on unspoiled GRE images is an effect of the high concentration of the paramagnetic contrast agent [5, 6].

Ultrafast EPI provides similar characteristic time-dependent signal changes. On T2-weighted images with a TR of 2000 ms, which can be repeated every 2 s, spin dephasing as well as susceptibility effects of the contrast agent are visible in the renal cortex (Fig. 2). A "dark band" can be observed migrating centripetally from the cortex through the outer medulla and finally into the inner medulla as progressively concentrated gadolinium traverses the renal tubular system from the cortex to the papilla [3].

The described alterations of signal intensity in renal cortex, medulla and calyces are characteristic of undisturbed renal function and can be evaluated using signal versus time plots. On the other hand, an excellent delineation of the corticomedullary junction is possible in the early perfusion phase (10-20 s after injection) and in the early excretory phase (50-90 s after injection) allowing accurate detection of internal structural derangements of the kidney [8].

Functional disorders

1. Urinary Tract Obstruction/Hydronephrosis

Using dynamic contrast-enhanced MRI, patients with acute obstruction generally show the same enhancement patterns of renal cortex and medulla as healthy volunteers with the characteristic medullary signal intensity drop indicating preserved concentration ability of the kidney. In patients with chronic hydronephrosis and impaired renal function, excretion and thus signal intensity increase in the medulla are delayed and the signal intensity drop is less pronounced. In cases of severe hydronephrosis, the characteristic contrast reversal in the medulla can be missed completely. This lack of medullary signal intensity loss can be interpreted as a direct sign of decreased concentrating ability of the kidney in patients with impaired renal function [1, 6].

2. Renal Insufficiency

Contrast-enhanced dynamic studies may be used for semiquantitative evaluation of renal excretory function. In contrast to the use of iodinated agents in computed tomography (CT), administration of gadolinium compounds is not contraindicated in patients with impaired renal function. Therefore, dynamic contrast-enhanced MRI may be performed even in patients with bilateral renal insufficiency. Only in patients with severely impaired excretory function (creatinine clearance < 20 ml/min) might hemodialysis be considered to shorten elimination time. In patients with a creatinine clearance between 50 and 80 ml/min, a 10-20 s delay of medullar signal intensity decrease can be demonstrated compared to that of healthy subjects. In patients with a clearance below 30 ml/min, no signal decrease is seen anymore indicating the loss of the concentration ability of the kidney (Fig. 3) [8, 9].

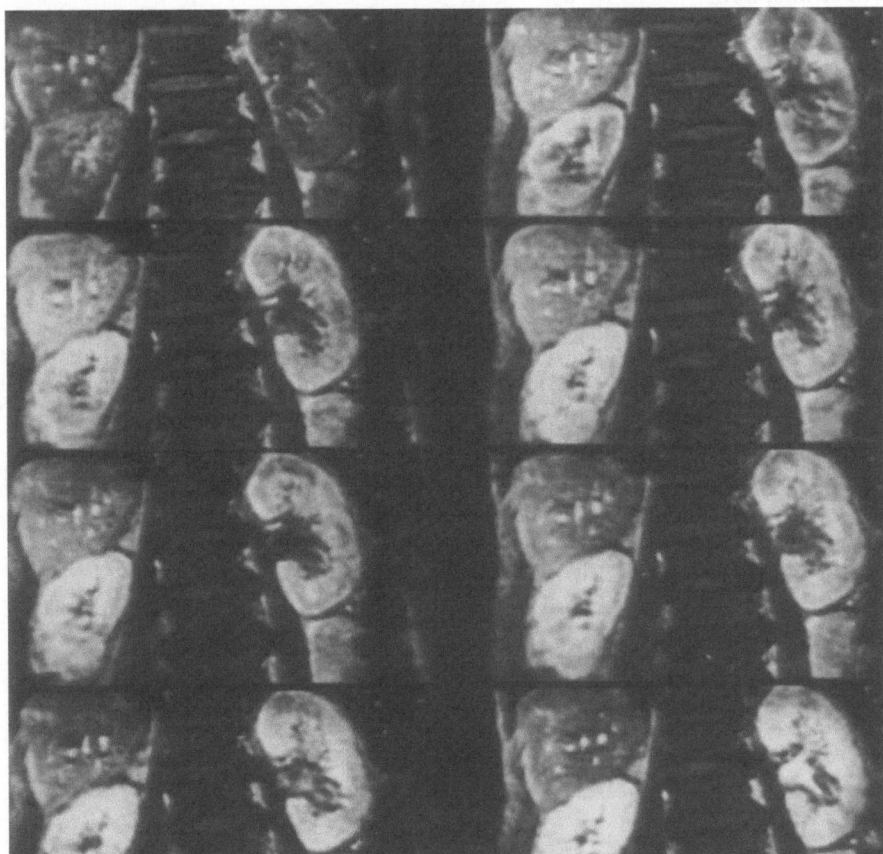

Fig. 3. *Dynamic gradient-echo MRI.* In a patient with renal insufficiency (creatinine clearance of 20 ml/min) there is cortical enhancement but loss of concentrating ability in the medulla

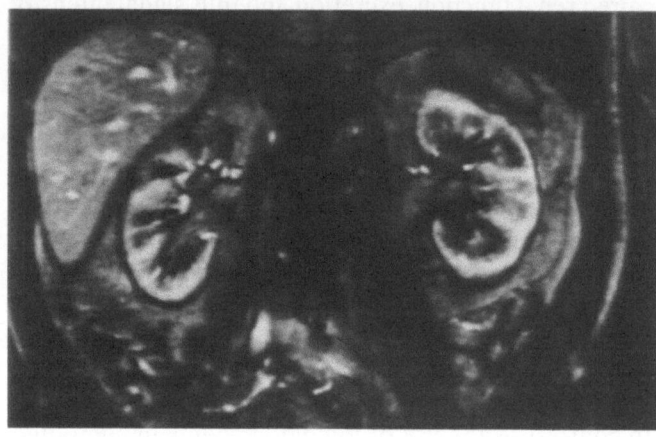

Fig. 4. *Post-ESWL contrast enhanced images.* 60 s after bolus-injection of Gd-DTPA in a patient with a calyceal stone of the left kidney treated with shock waves show segmental damage with loss of concentrating ability in the medulla at the mid-third of the left kidney

3. Adverse Reactions After Extracorporeal Shock Wave Lithotripsy

MRI proves to be an effective method for demonstrating morphologic and functional disturbance following extracorporeal shock wave lithotripsy (ESWL). Renal alterations detected by MRI are a loss of cortico-medullary differentiation present in up to 63% of cases, small subcapsular or perinephric fluid collections, hemorrhage into renal cysts and focal areas of increased or decreased signal intensities [10].

Contrast-enhanced dynamic MRI using gradient echo sequences allows detection of global and even segmental functional impairment. Following ESWL approximately 25% of patients showed regional reduction of concentration ability at the sites of shock wave application. These alterations may be visualized on dynamic MRI by the absence of the characteristic medullary signal intensity loss (contrast reversal) in the affected areas (Fig. 4) [11, 12].

Conclusions

Experimental studies demonstrate that contrast-enhanced dynamyc MRI provides at least semiquantitative

assessment of renal excretory function. Thus, MRI is the only imaging modality available providing morphologic information with a high spatial resolution while simultaneoulsy rendering functional data. Further studies are needed to define the potential of functional MRI in a clinical setting.

References

1. Krestin GP (1990) Morphologic and functional MRI of the kidneys and adrenal glands. Field & Wood, Philadelphia
2. Krestin GP (1994) Magnetic resonance imaging of the kidneys: current status. Magn Reson Q 19:2-21
3. Sartoretti-Schefer S, Marincek B, von Weymann C, Krestin GP (1994) Contrast-enhanced abdominal echo planar imaging: dynamic signal intensity changes following intravenous injection of gadolinium-DOTA. MAGMA 2:113-120
4. Carvlin MJC, Arger PH, Kundel HL, Axel L, Dougherty L, Kassab E, Moore B (1989) Use of Gd-DTPA and fast gradient-echo and spin-echo MR imaging to demonstrate renal function in the rabbit. Radiology 170:705-711
5. Choyke PL, Frank JA, Girton ME, Inscoe SW, Carvlin MJ, Black JL, Austin HA, Dwyer AJ (1989) Dynamic Gd-DTPA-enhanced MR imaging of the kidney: experimental results. Radiology 170:713-720
6. Kikinis R, von Schulthess GK, Jäger P, Dürr R, Bino M. Kuoni W, Kübler L (1987) Normal and hydronephrotic kidney: evaluation of renal function with contrast-enhanced MR imaging. Radiology 165:837-842
7. Carvlin MJ, Arger PH, Kunder HL, Axel L, Dougherty L, Kassab EA, Moore B (1987) Acute tubular necrosis: use of gadolinium-DTPA and fast MR imaging to evaluate renal function in the rabbit. J Comput Assist Tomogr 11:488-495
8. Krestin GP, Schuhmann-Giampieri G, Haustein J et al (1992) Functional dynamic MR imaging, pharmacokinetics and safety of Gadolinium-DTPA in patients with impaired renal function. Eur Radiol 2:16-23
9. Schumann-Giampieri G, Krestin GP (1991) Pharmacokinetic of Gd-DTPA in patients with chronic renal failure. Invest Radiol 26:975-979
10. Baumgartner BR, Dickey KW, Ambrose SS, Walton KN, Nelson RC, Bernardino ME (1987) Kidney changes after extracorporal shock wave lithotripsy: appearance on MR imaging. Radiology 163:531-534
11. Krestin GP, Fischbach R, Vorreuther R, von Schulthess GK (1993) Alterations in renal morphology and function after ESWL therapy: evaluation with dynamic contrast-enhanced MRI. Eur Radiol 2:227-233
12. Neuerburg J, Daus HJ, Recker F, Bohndorf K, Bex A, Guenther R, Hofstaedter F (1989) Effects of lithotripsy on rat kidney: evaluation with MR imaging, histology, and electron microscopy. J Comput Assist Tomogr 13:82-89

Magnetic Resonance Angiography in the Abdomen and Pelvis

G.P. Krestin and J.F. Debatin

Department of Medical Radiology, University Hospital Zürich, 8091 Zürich, Switzerland

Introduction

The magnetic resonance (MR) experiment is exquisitely sensitive to flow. Motion affects both T1 and T2 relaxations; the former is referred to as "time-of-flight" and the latter as "spin phase" effects. While these motion phenomena can cause considerable artifacts in conventional MR imaging, they can be exploited to form the basis of what is generally referred to as MR-angiography (MRA). Due to motion-induced signal modulation, vessels with flowing blood acquire a signal that can be differentiated from surrounding stationary tissues. MRA techniques use this signal contrast between vessels and stationary tissues for the non-invasive assessment of both vascular morphology and function.

According to which one of the underlying motion effects is exploited, two main MRA techniques are differentiated: "time-of-flight" (TOF) and "phase contrast" (PC) MRA.

Aorta

TOF-MRA is ideally suited for imaging the abdominal aorta. Aneurysms can be fully evaluated with regard to size, involvement of the renal arterial origins and containment of thrombotic regions. Furthermore, abdominal aortic dissections can be thoroughly evaluated with MRA. Inflammatory diseases affecting the aortic wall, such as Ormond's disease (idiopathic retroperitoneal fibrosis), can be readily diagnosed. Disease severity might be assessed by the degree of contrast enhancement in the aortic wall itself [1].

Renal Arteries

Renovascular disease (RVD) is implicated as the cause of hypertension in 2%-4% of patients with elevated blood pressure. It is also estimated to be the underlying cause of renal insufficiency in as many as 15% of patients on dialysis. A non-invasive screening strategy is thus highly desirable.

MRA of the renal arteries is best accomplished with the PC technique. The directional component of the phase images permits easy differentiation of arteries from veins, thus eliminating a potential source of error. Both two- and three-dimensional techniques have been successfully employed. Morphologic assessment of the renal arteries with MRA is however still handicapped by the inability to adequately visualize distal artery segments and small accessory vessels. Nevertheless, even today MRA can be employed to rule out proximal atherosclerotic renal artery stenosis in patients in whom there are relative or absolute contraindications to invasive contrast angiography [2].

While conventional angiography, the accepted gold standard, is highly sensitive in the detection of renovascular disease, it is merely 50%-80% specific. Cine-PC-based functional blood flow analysis, which is capable of measuring renal flow may overcome some of these limitations. Variable results have been reported regarding the correlation of cine-PC-based renal arterial flow measurements and PAH-clearance-based determinations of renal blood flow. This discrepancy reflects to a large extent the effect of respiratory motion on renal arterial PC analysis. Renal arteries move between 5 and 15 mm in a cranio-caudad direction depending on the exact measurement location. This motion, which occurs during the cine-PC measurement interval, causes blurring of the renal arterial margins and thus results in a artificial enlargement of the apparent vessel region of interest (ROI). A breathheld PC-imaging strategy is therefore essential for accurate PC-based blood flow quantification. With breath held PC acquisition strategies, encouraging results have been reported [2, 3].

Portal Venous System

The portal venous system can be well evaluated with breathheld TOF imaging in both the coronal and the ax-

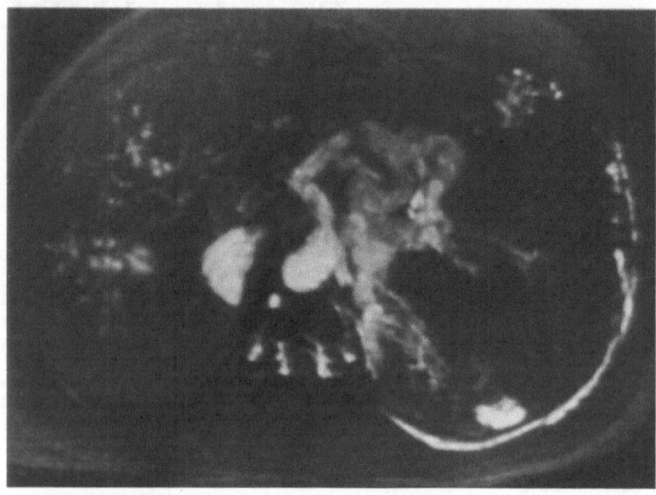

Fig. 1. *Portal vein thrombosis.* Axial MIP collapse image of the acquisition volume shows no flow in the portal vein and multiple perisplenic collaterals

ial planes. Thin sections (5-6 mm) and a moderate flip angle (30°) to reduce in-plane dephasing render excellent results and permit the diagnostic assessment of the splenic vein, the superior mesenteric vein (SMV), and the portal vein. The hepatic veins can also be displayed; their relationship to the portal veins is important especially for planning transjugular intrahepatic portosystemic shunts (TIPSS). The extent of collateral pathways can be estimated and individual spontaneous portosystemic shunts can be identified (Fig. 1).

Several studies have focused on the quantitative analysis of portal venous flow. The technique allows the easy differentiation of patients with portal hypertension into those with hyperdynamic flow and those with reduced flow. Collateral circulation may be assessed by quantifying the azygos vein. Measuring flow in these collateral vessels prior to and following therapeutic intervention allows assessment of the therapeutic efficacy. Furthermore, these flow parameters may aid in predicting which patient will suffer from variceal hemorrhage [4, 5].

Superior Mesenteric Artery

Mesenteric ischemia remains a frequently perplexing diagnostic dilemma. Cine-PC-based flow measurements may be useful in identifying patients with significant stenoses of the superior mesenteric artery (SMA). To avoid respiratory motion, flow measurements of the SMA should be performed close to the vessel's origin. For maximal diagnostic efficacy, measurements should be made both in the fasting state and following a meal. Postprandial flow in the SMA increases over 100% in normal volunteers. This postprandial hyperemia appears to be significantly smaller in patients with high-grade (> 50%) stenosis.

Renal Veins/Inferior Vena Cava

MR angiography has evolved into the method of choice for the diagnostic exploration of the inferior vena cava (IVC) and renal veins. Anatomic variations of the IVC, such as duplications, are depicted, as is anomalous course of the left renal vein. The presence of bland thrombus in the renal veins or in the IVC is seen, as is an extension of tumor thrombus into the venous system. The differentiation of benign from malignant thrombus is possible with dynamic contrast enhanced techniques. MRA has thus assumed an important role in the staging of renal cell carcinomas and is particularly well suited for the evaluation of patients with suspected renal vein thrombosis [6-9] (Fig. 2).

Acute and Chronic Venous Thrombosis and Post-thrombotic Syndrome

Deep venous thrombosis (DVT) is the third most common cardiovascular pathology following myocardial infarction and cerebrovascular stroke. The accurate diagnosis of acute DVT allows for optimal treatment, thereby reducing the risk of subsequent complications associated with DVT and with a needless anticoagulation therapy. MRA is a reliable, accurate and noninvasive method for diagnosing DVT in the femoropopliteal and pelvic regions. MRA allows simultaneous visualization of the veins of both lower extremities and of pelvic vessels bilateraly. Signs of thrombosis in MRA are:

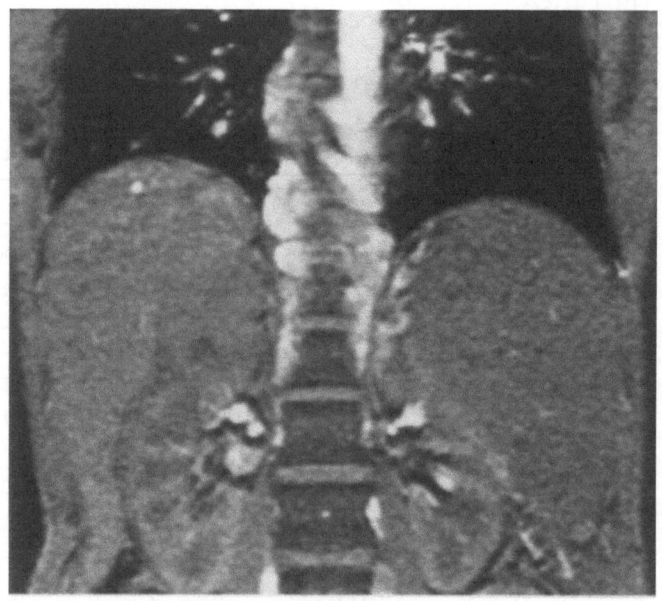

Fig. 2. *Thrombosis of the inferior vena cava.* Coronal gradient echo TOF image reveals paravertebral collateral flow in the azygos and hemiazygos system

- Complete lack of high signal flowing blood in a venous trunk
- Irregularly shaped flow void
- Eccentric filling defects with smooth margins in venous structures (on axial images)
- Demonstration of collateral vessels in chronic thrombosis.

Post-thrombotic syndrome and venous compressions manifest themselves by:
- Inconsistant diameter of vessels with smooth contours
- Successive decrease or complete loss of signal intensity in the vessel lumen and signal increase distally
- Pronounced collateral circulation (Fig. 3).

Several reports in the literature of the last 5 years describe the value of MRI and MRA in the detection of DVT. Even spin echo (SE) sequences provide high sensitivity and specificity (90% and 100% respectively). The results are similar with gradient recalled echo (GRE) sequences (sensitivity of 100% and specificity of 93% described by Spitzer et al. [10]). In a direct comparison, however, GRE images proved to be clearly superior to SE sequences [10-13].

One of the most important alterations diagnosable only with MRA is thrombosis of the internal iliac veins and their branches. Some authors describe such clinically unsuspected findings in 20%-25% of examined cases. Gehl et al. [7] used MRA to detect involvement of the inferior vena cava in 25% of patients, and they found clinically unapparent thrombosis of the opposite vein in 7 of 32 evaluated patients. Evaluation of lower extremity and pelvic veins was performed using axial slices in the majority of the published reports. Interpretation limited to maximum intensity projection (MIP) reconstructions is not reliable in the diagnosis of DVT. MRA

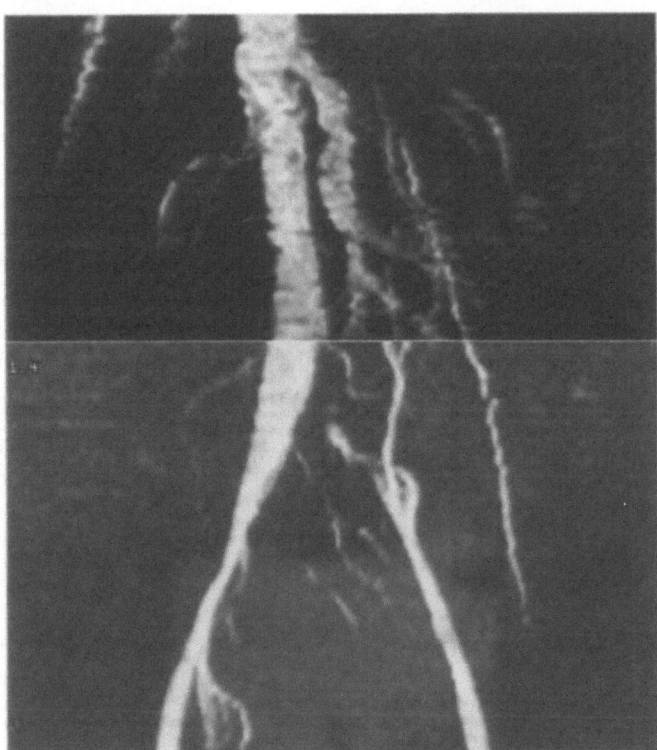

Fig. 4. *Septic ovarian vein thrombosis.* MIP image of two aquisition volumes in the pelvis and abdomen reveals occlusion of the right ovarian vein, patent left ovarian vein and occlusion of the left common iliac vein

can be used for monitoring anticoagulant and fibrinolytic therapy; it can serve as the definitive exam when results of screening are unsatisfactory, and can be useful even as a first line exam in suspected pelvic thrombosis [10, 11, 14-16].

Chronic disease, post-thrombotic syndrome and venous compressions can be reliably detected. All collateral vessels with sufficient flow are seen despite their drainage or connection to deep or superficial vessels. This represents a clear advantage compared to contrast venography in which such collaterals may be poorly opacified or even completely missed. In many cases MRI provides information on the underlying cause of a venous compression by directly visualizing space-occupying lesions and their relationship to surrounding structures [17].

Ovarian Vein Thrombosis

Septic puerperal ovarian vein thrombosis (SPOVT) is a potentially life-threatening condition in the postpartum period that may have fatal consequences without adequate treatment. This syndrome usually presents with fever, lower abdominal or flank pain, and occasionally a palpable tender linear-shaped mass. The best imaging method for diagnosis of SPOVT before the era of MRA

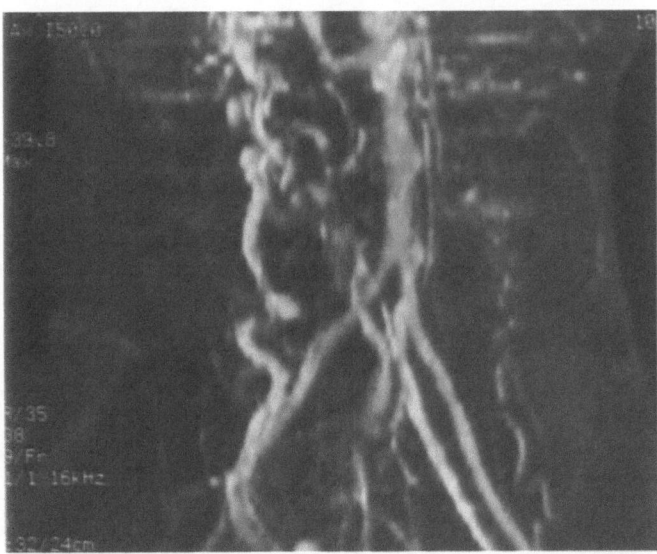

Fig. 3. *Chronic occlusion of the inferior vena cava.* MIP projection image shows occlusion of the IVC with paravertebral collaterals and patent aorto-iliac arteries

was contrast-enhanced computed tomography (CT).

MRA is an accurate method for evaluation of the postpartal ovarian veins. Due to the increased diameter during pregnancy and after delivery, these vessels are constantly depicted on two-dimensional TOF MRA. In a prospective comparative study, MRA proved to be superior to CT and duplex-Doppler ultrasound (US). Among 25 patients with septic fever in the postpartum period, SPOVT was detected with MRA in 8 cases. US detected only 4 cases of SPOVT, while contrast-enhanced CT provided two false negative and one false positive diagnoses. MRA also showed additional unsuspected thromboses of pelvic vessels (common and external iliac veins) in three patients [18, 19] (Fig. 4).

References

1. Chang J-M, Friese K, Caputo GR, Kondo C, Higgins CB (1991) MR measurement of blood flow in the true and false channel in chronic aortic dissection. J Comput Assist Tomogr 15:418-423
2. Debatin JF, Spritzer CE, Grist TM, Beam C, Svetkey L, Newman GE, Sostman HD (1991) Renovascular Disease: The role of MR-Angiography. AJR 157:981-990
3. Roubidoux MA, Dunnick NR, Knelson M, Debatin JF (1993) Renal Revascularisation: Indications and Results. Urol Radiology 14:18-23
4. Finn PJ, Kane RA, Edelman RR, Jenkins RL, Lewis WD, Muller M, Longmaid HE (1993) Imaging of the Portal Venous System in Patients with Cirrhosis: MR Angiography vs Duplex Doppler Sonography. AJR 161-989-994
5. Burkart DJ, Johnson CD, Morton MJ, Wolf RL, Ehman RL (1993) Volumetric flow rates in the portal venous system: measurement with cine phase-contrast MR imaging. AJR 160:1113-1118
6. Mohiaddin RH, Wann SL, Underwood R, Firmin DN, Rees S, Longmore DB (1990) Vena Caval Flow: Assessment with Cine MR Velocity Mapping. Radiology 177:537-541
7. Gehl H-B, Bohndorf K, Klose K-C, Günther RW (1990) Two-dimensional MR Angiography in the evaluation of abdominal veins with gradient refocused sequences. J Comput Assist Tomogr 14:619-624
8. Finn JP, Zisk JHS, Edelman RR, Wallner BK, Hartnell GG, Stokes KR, Longmaid HE (1993) Central venous occlusion: MR angiography. Radiology 187:245-251
9. Friedland GW, deVries PA, Nino-Murcia M, King BF, Leder RA, Stevens S (1992) Congenital anomalies of the inferior vena cava: embryogenesis and MR features. Urol Radiol 13:237-248
10. Spritzer CE, Sostman HD, Wilkes DC, Coleman RE (1990) Deep venous thrombosis: Experience with gradient-echo MR imaging in 66 patients. Radiology 177:235-241
11. Tavares NJ, Auffermann W, Brown JJ, Gilbert TJ, Sommerhoff C, Higgins CB (1989) Detection of thrombus by using phase-image MR scans: ROC curve analysis. AJR 153:173-178
12. Marchal G, Bosmans H, Van Hecke P et al (1990) MR angiography with gadopentetate-dimeglumine polylysine: evaluation in rabbits. AJR 155:407-411
13. Lanzer P, Gross GM, Keller FS, Pohost GM (1991) Sequential 2D inflow venography: initial clinical observations. Magn Reson Med 19:470-476
14. Erdmann WA, Weinreb JC, Cohen JM, Buja LM, Chaney C, Peshock RM (1986) Venous thrombosis: clinical and experimental MR imaging. Radiology 161:233-238
15. Evans AJ, Sostman HD, Knelson MH, Spritzer CE, Newman GE, Paine SS, Beam CA (1993) Detection of deep venous thrombosis. Prospective comparison of MR imaging with contrast venography. AJR 161:131-139
16. Sostman HD, Debatin JF, Spritzer CE, Coleman RE, Grist TM, MacFall JR (1993) MRI in venous thromboembolic disease. Eur Radiol 3:53-61
17. Richter CS, Duewell S, Krestin GP, Vesti B, Franzeck UK, Bollinger A, von Schulthess GK, Fuchs WA (1993) Dreidimensionale Darstellung der Beckenvenen mit Magnetresonanz-Angiographie. Fortschr Röntgenstr 159:161-166
18. Mintz MC, Levy DW, Axel L, Kressel HY, Arger PH, Coleman BG, Mennuti M (1987) Puerperal ovarian vein thrombosis: MR diagnosis. AJR 149:1273-1274
19. Salvader SJ, Ottero RR, Salvader BR (1988) Puerperal ovarian vein thrombosis: Evaluation with CT, US, and MR Imaging. Radiology 167:637-639

Regional Motion Analysis with Tagged MRI

L. Axel

Radiology Department, Hospital of the University of Pennsylvania, 3400 Spruce St., Philadelphia, PA 19104, USA

Introduction

Heart disease is a major cause of mortality and morbidity in the western world. Methods to evaluate cardiac function are valuable for diagnosis and management of heart disease. However, conventional cardiac function evaluation methods have many limitations. Tagged magnetic resonance imaging (MRI) provides a new imaging method that has the potential to significantly improve our ability to evaluate cardiac function.

Conventional cardiac imaging methods can provide projection images of the ventricular cavity or tomographic images of the heart wall (e.g., with conventional MRI) at different phases of the cardiac cycle. These can permit calculation of global measures of cardiac function, such as stroke volume or ejection fraction. They can also provide some information on regional function, such as radial wall motion or wall thickening in the plane of a tomographic image. However, the possibility of motion of the curved heart wall through the plane of the image can cause these measures to be inaccurate. There is also some uncertainty as to what frame of reference to use with respect to which to analyze the motion, e.g., a fixed or "floating" centroid of the ventricle. In addition, the relative paucity of identifiable landmarks in the heart wall makes it essentially impossible to analyze any non-radial components of motion or to study the patterns of motion within the wall. While fixed markers, such as tantalum screws, can be imbedded in the heart wall to permit tracking of specific material points, these methods are too invasive for routine clinical use.

The inherent motion sensitivity of MRI, through magnetization tagging or phase shifts, provides new noninvasive tools for the study of regional cardiac function. In particular, we shall be considering the use of tagging methods here. Sensitization to velocity-induced phase shifts can provide an alternative method for noninvasive motion studies.

Tagged MRI

In MRI tagging studies, we take advantage of the fact that a locally produced perturbation of the tissue magnetization will move with the underlying tissue. As the perturbed magnetization will cause a visible change in the intensity of the corresponding MR image, we have effectively created a noninvasive tissue tag whose motion as shown with MRI will reflect the underlying tissue motion. As the relaxation times of the heart wall are of the same order as the cardiac cycle time, we can use MR tags to study regional heart wall motion by creating tags in the heart wall at one phase of the cardiac cycle, e.g., at end diastole, and imaging their subsequent motions through the cardiac cycle.

MR tags are most commonly created by saturating the magnetization in a plane perpendicular to the imaging plane prior to acquiring the image data. The intersection of the tagged and imaging planes will be seen as a dark line in the subsequent image; any motion between the times of tagging and imaging will be seen as a corresponding motion of the tags in the image. The tagged plane can be created by selective saturation of the desired plane, similarly to conventional selective slice excitation [1]. However, it is generally more efficient to nonselectively create a whole family of tagging planes simultaneously with the use of spatial modulation of magnetization (SPAMM) [2]. In the SPAMM technique for tag production, we use alternating nonselective radiofrequency (RF) pulses and an intervening magnetic field gradient along the direction orthogonal to the desired tags. The strength and duration of the gradient pulses determine the spacing of the tags. By suitable choices of the relative amplitudes of the RF pulses, we can optimize the resulting tag stripe profiles. Producing two orthogonal families of tag lines results in a tagging grid [3]. The tagging process can be combined with essentially any desired imaging technique, as it is a "preconditioning" pulse sequence, like an inversion pulse used for inversion-recovery imaging. However, the use of tagging in conjunction with breathhold imaging has improved the quality of the analysis by removing the image degrading effects of respiratory motion. The tagging process has been validated by MR imaging of the motion of tags in deformable phantoms whose motion patterns have been independently calibrated [4].

Tag Tracking

While much qualitative information on regional function can be gained from simple visual inspection of tagged images of the heart, particularly with dynamic motion displays, quantitative motion analysis requires the extraction of the sequential positions of the tags from the images. The tag positions, or positions of the intersections of a tagging grid, can be tracked manually. However, the large number of tags that can easily be produced in a cardiac study makes manual tracking too time-consuming to be clinically practical. Therefore, various approaches have been pursued to make the tracking process more automated. These include "matched filter"-type approaches to recognize grid intersections [5, 6] and "edge tracking"-type approaches to trace out the tag lines [7, 8].

We have found active contours ("snakes") [9] to be useful in implementing semiautomatic tag tracking methods. In the snakes approach, the tracked tag position is determined by a combination of three "forces": (1) the image forces (e.g., attracted to lower intensities), (2) an adjustable stiffness and rigidity of the fitted tags (making the fitting less vulnerable to image artifacts causing irregularity or gaps in the tag images) and (3) a user-supplied interactive force (e.g., to move the tracking away from undesired image features). In general, there will always be a need for some user interaction to guide the automated tracking.

Regional Motion Analysis

The analysis of regional motion from the tag data can go beyond the simple measures of wall motion provided by the tomographic images of the wall alone. The motion of a given region of the wall can be considered as a combination of rigid body motion (displacement and rotation) and deformation (or strain). The strain values reflect the fractional change in length of a small segment of the wall along a given direction. Displacement is a vector quantity (having magnitude and direction at a given location), and reflects motion of a point within the wall. Strain is a higher order quantity, a tensor (depending on orientation), and reflects the motion within a small neighborhood of a point. The strain can be conveniently represented by the principal strains, or eigenvalues and eigenvectors, representing the directions and amounts of the greatest and least final lengths resulting from the motion. An advantage of strain as a measure of wall motion is that it is independent of the choice of external reference system, unlike displacement.

The motion data we have extracted from the tagged images permit us to calculate the motion of the heart wall between the tags. One approach is to assume that the deformation is homogeneous between the intersections of a tagging grid. If we can then also neglect the effects of through-plane motion, we can use the tracked two-dimensional image locations of the corners of a set of triangles constructed from the grid intersections to calculate both the rigid body motion and the strain within the triangles [10]. Even with through-plane motion, if the initial tagging planes are created orthogonal to the imaging plane, we know the within-plane components of the initial position of a grid intersection at any subsequent time.

An alternative approach to calculating the deformation patterns and strain within the wall is to use finite element modeling methods to fit the motion in the wall between the tags. This can be readily extended to create a full three-dimensional (3D) model of the heart wall by combining the tag motion data from two orthogonal sets of tagged images [11]. This approach also allows us to avoid the need to assume homogeneous deformation between the tags. The fineness of the grid determines the order of the fitting functions we can use to represent the motion. Current imaging resolution still limits us to a linear function for the variation in motion across the normal left ventricular wall, while the normal right ventricle is too thin to model any variation across the wall. Motion of the subject between acquisition of the orthogonal image sets can lead to registration problems. However, as long as each image set is well registered within itself, we can bring the two image sets into registration with each other in order to enable the full 3D modeling.

A related but distinct approach to analyzing the wall motion from tagged images is to model the wall motion with a set of parametric functions that can combine global and regional motion characterizations [12]. Such a set of parametric functions can represent more intuitive aspects of cardiac motion, such as radial and long axis contractions and twist about the long axis. The fitting of these parameter functions from the tag motion data can be carried out using a physics-based model of image forces.

Regional Motion Display

The display of the regional motion data derived from tagged MRI poses a challenging problem in data visualization. The heart wall is a thick walled 3D shell that changes in time. The motion variables to be represented are not just scalar quantities, but also vectors and tensors. Scalar quantities, such as distance moved or angle of rotation, can be represented with a pseudocolor mapping. Vector quantities, such as displacement, including magnitude and direction, can be represented with a field of proportional length arrows. Tensor quantities are even harder to display. The eigenvectors can be represented with a trihedral display as a field of two- or three-axis icons with corresponding lengths and orientations. Alternatively, the corresponding eigenvalues can be displayed as scalars. In three-dimensional motion analysis, the availability of computer workstations permits creating interactive displays that can be interactively rotated and otherwise manipulated by the viewer to facilitate the understanding of the regional variations. As with the viewing of the initial tagged images, the availability of dynamic displays is valuable to show the time evolution of the motion variables.

Applications

As the methods for the acquisition and analysis of tagged images of the heart are still undergoing active development, there is still only limited experience with the clinical application of regional cardiac motion analysis. Initial work has largely focused on defining the normal regional patterns of heart wall motion in the left ventricle and exploring how they are affected in animal models of disease and in limited series of human patients [e.g., 13-15]. The analysis methods are being extended to the right ventricle as well [16]. While it is still too early to say how useful these new methods will be for studying regional cardiac motion, as the speed and quality of the acquisition and analysis are both still improving, it seems likely that we will at least gain new insights into the normal and abnormal function of the ventricles. There is the possibility that tagged MRI could become a valuable tool for the diagnosis and management of heart disease, particularly in combination with the other evolving capabilities of MRI for evaluation of the heart.

References

1. Zerhouni E, Parrish D, Rogers W, Yang A, Shapiro E (1988) Human heart: Tagging with MR imaging-A method for noninvasive assessment of myocardial motion. Radiology 168: 59

2. Axel L, Dougherty L (1989) MR imaging of motion with spatial modulation of magnetization. Radiology 171: 841
3. Axel L, Dougherty L (1989) Heart wall motion: Improved method of spatial modulation of magnetization for MR imaging. Radiology 172: 349
4. Young AA, Axel L, Dougherty L, Bogen D, Parenteau CS (1993) Validation of tagging with MR imaging to estimate material deformation. Radiology 188: 101
5. Fisher D (1990) Automated tracking of cardiac wall motion using magnetic resonance markers. PhD dissertation, Univ of Iowa, Iowa City
6. Kraitchman DL, Young AA, Chang C-N, Axel L (1995) Semi-automatic tracking of myocardial motion in MR tagged images. IEEE Trans Med Imag 14: 422
7. Prince JL, McVeigh ER (1992) Motion estimation from tagged MR image sequences. IEEE Trans Med Imag 11: 238
8. Young AA, Kraitchman DL, Dougherty L, Axel L (1995) Tracking and finite element analysis of stripe deformation in magnetic resonance imaging. IEEE Trans Med Imag 14: 413
9. Kass M, Witkin A, Terzopoulos D (1988) Snakes: Active contour models. Int J Comp Vision 1: 321
10. Axel L, Gonçalves RC, Bloomgarden DC (1992) Regional heart wall motion: Two-dimensional analysis and functional imaging of regional heart wall motion with magnetic resonance imaging. Radiology 183: 745
11. Young AA, Axel L (1992) Three-dimensional motion and deformation of the heart wall. Radiology 185: 241
12. Park J, Metaxis D, Axel L (1995) Volumetric deformable models with parametric functions: A new approach to the 3D analysis of the LV from MRI-SPAMM. Proc 5th Intl Conf on Computer Vision (ICCV), Cambridge, MA, June 1995, 700
13. Clark NR, Reichek N, Bergey P, Hofman EA, Brownson D, Palmon L, Axel L (1991) Circumferential myocardial shortening in the normal human left ventricle: Assessment by magnetic resonance imaging using spatial modulation of magnetization. Circulation 84: 67
14. Young AA, Imai H, Chang C-N, Axel L (1994) Two-dimensional left ventricle motion during systole using MRI with SPAMM. Circulation 89: 740
15. Palmon LD, Reichek N, Yeon SB, Clark NR, Brownson D, Hoffman EA, Axel L (1994) Intramural myocardial shortening in hypertensive left ventricular hypertrophy with normal pump function. Circulation 89: 122
16. Young AA, Fayad ZA, Axel L (1995) Right ventricular surface deformation using MR tagging. Proc Soc Magn Reson: 1419

Ultrafast Imaging of the Cardiovascular System

J.F. Debatin

Department of Medical Radiology, University Hospital Zürich, 8091 Zürich, Switzerland

The implementation of stronger and faster gradient systems has laid the foundation for vast reductions in magnetic resonance (MR) data acquisition times. Beyond accelerating conventional sequences [1, 2], echo planar imaging (EPI), as first described by Mansfield in 1977 [3], now appears practical. Although much of the preliminary work with echo planar imaging has focused on the heart, EPI provides a unique opportunity to improve the morphologic and functional MR-based evaluation of other vascular structures.

Echo Planar Imaging: Theoretical Aspects

In contrast to conventional MR imaging techniques, which require a separate MR experiment for the acquisition of each line in k-space, echo planar imaging collects multiple k-space lines after a single radiofrequency (RF) excitation [4, 5]. Following an excitation, a gradient echo is formed by applying a gradient pulse with a positive amplitude followed by a gradient pulse with a negative amplitude. A second gradient echo can be produced with another positive amplitude gradient pulse. The process can be repeated a large number of times. The series of odd and even echoes may be referred to as a train of gradient echoes. With EPI, each of the gradient echoes is used to collect one separate line of MR imaging data. The actual line selected is determined by the phase-encoding gradient waveform. A small blip gradient placed between each gradient echo causes the data collection to proceed from line to line. Data for a complete image can hence be obtained following a single excitation pulse. Since data for EPI images are collected over a free induction decay, data lines acquired much beyond the tissue T2* decay time will contain little signal. The resulting compromise in the high spatial frequency image information leads to poor edge definition, resulting in the inability to visualize small vessels and delineate rapidly moving structures such as the myocardium [6].

The short T2* decay time of blood limits achievable image resolution if all k-lines are collected after a single RF pulse. T2* is not solely a tissue parameter, but rather reflects spatial inhomogeneity of the susceptibility of surrounding structures. Thus T2* will be even shorter at vascular edges, particularly if pulsatility causes motion of the surrounding walls, further limiting achievable image quality. Other limitations with regard to the length of the gradient echo train following an RF pulse arise from increases in flow-induced spin dephasing artifacts resulting in intravascular flow voids [5]. Particularly with regard to cardiovascular imaging, it is highly desirable to reduce the gradient echo train length and the data acquisition window by limiting the number of acquired data lines per RF pulse [7]. Beyond employing partial k-space acquisition coverage, this can be achieved most effectively by collecting the image data not singly, but in several packages referred to as shots. To avoid off-resonance ghosting, multi-shot EPI data should be collected in a k-space interleaved fashion [7, 8]. Due to the shortening of the data acquisition time, the high spatial frequency image information is now collected within the T2* time, translating into improved conspicuousness of small vascular structures.

This image improvement was confirmed in a recent study which compared the quality of transaxial cardiac images obtained in volunteers with single-shot EPI and two-shot EPI [9]. The qualitative and quantitative analysis confirmed that breaking up the echo train into two shots significantly improved image quality over the single-shot acquisition, particularly with regard to visualization of small arteries such as the internal mammary artery and the coronary arteries ($p < 0.05$). Intraventricular signal was far more homogeneous in the two-shot images ($p > 0.01$), facilitating delineation of the myocardium from intraventricular blood and surrounding structures ($p > 0.005$). The time penalty associated with this substantial increase in image quality is small. In that particular study, acquisition times for single- and two-shot EPI images were 98 ms and 108 ms, respectively. The increase in imaging time relative to single-shot EPI reflects the additionally required time to play out two instead of one slice select RF pulses. For a four-shot acquisition, this time penalty would thus amount to 30 ms; data acquisition time for an image based on eight shots would exceed that of a single-shot image by 70 ms.

Fewer k-lines per shot result in a shorter effective echo time and a shortened data acquisition window. This reduces flow-induced spin dephasing and thus also reduces signal inhomogeneities [2, 10]. In addition, the sensitivity to susceptibility differences are reduced in proportion to the number of shots employed along with signal voids arising from turbulence and field inhomogeneities [7]. Spatial misregistration of structures with an inplane velocity component [11] is also reduced by increasing the number of shots.

Multi-shot EPI essentially maintains the imaging speed advantage of single-shot EPI over conventional MR imaging techniques. The vastly superior image quality achieved with multi-shot EPI compared to single-shot EPI suggests the multi-shot approach to be the strategy of choice with regard to meeting the high image quality standards essential to any cardiovascular MR study.

Cardiovascular EPI Applications

The potential of ultrafast techniques with regard to cardiovascular MR imaging (MRI) will be demonstrated with a number of examples.

1. Cardiac Ejection Fraction Measurement

The determination of the cardiac ejection fraction (EF) and cardiac output (CO) must be considered an integral part of any complete cardiac examination. EF-measurements with conventional cine-MR are accurate but time-consuming [12]. With echo planar imaging (EPI) data acquisition can be performed much faster, potentially in a single breathold. Using a 4-shot EPI sequence, 16 frames could be acquired for a single section in merely 4 RR-intervals; 60 times shorter than the conventional cine data (256 RR-intervals).

Image quality was sufficient with both techniques to permit adequate delineation of the ventricular lumen from the myocardium. EF measurements based on EPI data correlated well with cine measurements.

2. Myocardial Perfusion

To be applicable in a routine clinical setting any ultrafast MR imaging approach would have to fulfill the following requirements:
1. Concomitant assessment of the entire myocardium
2. Sufficient spatial resolution to resolve the various myocardial layers
3. Adequate temporal resolution to characterize wash-in and wash-out kinetics

Meeting these requirements implies coverage of 8-10 contiguous 10 mm sections with an in-plane resolution of under 2×2 mm every one to two RR-intervals. To limit motion blurring the images should in addition preferably be collected in diastole lasting about 450 ms in a patient with a heart rate of 80 beats per minute.

A non-sequentially acquired two-shot EPI sequence fulfills these requirements, providing adequate spatial (1.5×1.5 mm in plane) and temporal (every other heart beat) resolution. The entire heart is imaged every two heart beats with spatial resolution sufficient to properly identify even small cardiac structures such as coronary arteries as well as individual valvular leaflets.

Both gradient echo (GRE) and spin echo (SE) based approaches have been evaluated. Gadolinium DTPA causes signal intensity (SI) reduction in the former and SI increase in the latter. In fact, the 2-shot SE EPI approach appears sufficiently T1-weighted to not require further inversion pulses.

3. Carotid Arteries

Cerebral infarction has been implicated as the third-most frequent cause of death in industrialized nations. It is most commonly a fatal complication of atherosclerotic disease of the carotid arterial system, which can be successfully treated with surgical endarterectomy [13]. Treatment, however, can reduce morbidity and mortality only if the disease process is diagnosed prior to the manifestation of permanent cerebral damage.

Conventional MR angiography (MRA) requires acquisition times ranging from 5 to 20 min [8- 10]. Beyond the monetary costs associated with such lengthy acquisition times, the technique is prone to motion artifacts induced by minimal patient motion and swallowing. The ensuing degradation of image quality might render the study non-diagnostic, or might even mimic pathologies such as fibromuscular dysplasia in areas of normal vascular morphology [14]. Therefore, a significant reduction of data acquisition time appears highly desirable; this can be achieved by applying EPI data acquisition strategies. Based on the theoretical considerations outlined previously, a multi-shot (8-shot) echo planar three-dimensional (3D) phase contrast sequence [15] was implemented. With this technique, 64 sections with a thickness of 2.5 mm and an inplane resolution of 1×1 mm (26×13 field of view (FOV), 256×28 matrix) could be acquired in merely 32 s. This compares favorably to conventional data acquisition techniques requiring 459 s to acquire the same amount of data (identical section thickness, FOV and matrix). A direct comparison of image quality between echo planar and conventional data acquisition strategies with regard to the ability to evaluate the carotid arterial system in volunteers revealed similar performances of the two techniques in the proximal portion of the carotid system (common carotid artery, carotid bifurcation as well as the proximal internal and external carotid arteries). Similarly, the proximal vertebral arterial segments were seen equally well with both techniques. Due to increased spin dephasing, induced by a slightly longer echo time, the more distal arterial segments were seen less well with the echo planar method than with the conventional imaging technique.

4. Trifurcation Arteries

Much attention has recently been centered on the performance of conventional MRA with regard to visualization of lower leg runoff vessels. MRA has actually been shown to be superior to conventional, invasive angiographic techniques in the identification of the distal runoff vessels in patients with severe proximal atherosclerotic disease [16]. One of the problems limiting the broader clinical application of MRA for evaluation of peripheral atherosclerotic disease is the lengthy acquisition times.

The implementation of the above outlined multi-shot EPI 3D phase contrast (PC) MRA technique overcomes this limitation: image acquisition time for 64 three mm sections is reduced to 19 s. Initial comparisons between conventional two-dimensional time of flight (2D TOF) and 3D EPI MRA of the trifurcation arteries in volunteers are encouraging. The EPI data were acquired following 2 min of arterial occlusion at the level of the thigh. With both techniques, proximal portions of the trifurcation vessels were fully visualized. Distal vessels, however, were visualized to a lesser extent with the EPI technique reflecting in-volume dephasing due to the longer echo time.

5. Calf Veins

Deep venous thrombosis (DVT) remains a frequent and potentially deadly disease. In the United States alone, the number of patients with DVT is estimated around 5 million per year. Regardless of its origin, DVT of the lower extremities can embolize into the pulmonary arteries and cause significant morbidity and mortality. Even among patients with DVT limited to the calf, lung scintigraphy reveals pulmonary embolism in 35% to 50% of cases [17].

In a recent study we evaluated the effects of two mechanical flow augmenting measures: valsalva maneuver for 20 s and venous occlusion for 3 min with a thigh cuff inflated to 80 mm Hg. While both augmentation procedures significantly increased venous flow, the effect was more pronounced following venous occlusion (p < 0.005). In both cases the effect was short-lived, however, decreasing to normal values within 30 s.

The short-lived effects of mechanical flow augmentation can be exploited with ultrafast EPI MR data acquisition strategies [18]. To facilitate adequate visualization of the small calf veins, data acquisition was divided into four shots. Forty contiguous 5 mm 2D TOF sections could be acquired in as little as 10 s. Since the technique

is not based on retrograde contrast filling of the venous system, even small muscle veins draining into the deep veins can be visualized. The entire examination, including patient positioning, can be performed in less than 10 min and provides coverage of both calves from the knee to the talotibial joint.

The resulting depiction of normal deep venous structures appears of sufficient quality to permit assessment of the presence of DVT. In a volunteer study, disease could be excluded in 93% of the evaluated deep venous segments based on EPI images alone [18].

Conclusion

EPI offers vast potential as a fast and robust method for the noninvasive evaluation of large portions of the cardiovascular system. At this time it remains an evolving method. Technical refinements are clearly necessary before EPI will become a routine clinical tool.

References

1. Chien D, Edelman R (1991) Ultrafast imaging using gradient echoes. Magn Reson Q 7: 31-56
2. Butts K, Riederer SJ (1992) Analysis of flow effects in echo-planar imaging. J Magn Reson Imaging 2: 285-293
3. Mansfield P (1977) Multiplanar image formation using NMR spin-echoes. J Phys C: Solid State Physics 10: L55-L58
4. Stehling MK, Turner R, Mansfield P (1991) Echo-Planar Imaging: Magnetic Resonance Imaging in a Fraction of a Second. Science 254: 43-50
5. Davis CP, McKinnon GC, Debatin JF, Wetter DR, Eichenberger AC, Duewell S, Schulthess GK (1994) EPI-Evaluation of the Heart. Radiology 191: 691-696
6. Farzaneh F, Riederer SJ, Pelc NJ (1990) Analysis of T2 limitations and off-resonance effects on spatial resolution and artifacts in echo planar imaging. Magn Reson Med 14: 123-139
7. McKinnon GC (1993) Ultrafast interleaved gradient-echo-planar imaging on a standard scanner. Magn Reson Med 30: 609-616
8. Butts K, Riederer SJ, Ehman RL, Thompson RM, Jack CR (1994) Interleaved echo planar imaging on a standard MRI system. Magn Reson Med 31: 67-72
9. Wetter DR, McKinnon GC, Debatin JF, von Schulthess GK (1995) Comparison of single and multiple shot echo planar strategies for cardiac MR imaging. Radiology 194: 765-770
10. McKinnon GC (1994) Interleaved echo planar phase contrast angiography. Magn Reson Med 31: 1-4
11. Wedeen VJ, Wedt RE, Jerosch-Herold M (1989) Motional phase artifacts in Fourier transform MRI. Magn Reson Med 11: 114-120
12. Debatin JF, Nadel SN, Paolini J et al. (1992) Cardiac ejection fracton: Phantom study comparing CINE MR Imaging, radionuclide blood pool imaging and ventriculography. J Magn Reson Imaging 2: 135-142
13. NASCET collaborators (1991) Beneficial effect of carotid endarterectomy in symptomatic patients with high-grade carotid stenosis. N Engl J Med 325: 445-453
14. Heiserman JE, Drayer BP, Fram EK, Keller PJ (1992) MR angiography of cervical fibromuscular dysplasia. AJNR 13: 1454-1457
15. Wildermuth S, Debatin JF, Huisman T, Leung DA, McKin-

non GC, von Shculthess GK (1994) 3D phase contrast EPI of the carotid arteries: initial evaluation in a volunteer study. In: Book of abstracts, Society of Magnetic Resonance. San Francisco, CA, P963

16. Owen RS, Carpenter JP, Baum RA, Perloff LJ, Cope C (1992) Magnetic resonance imaging of angiographically occult runoff vessels in peripheral arterial occlusive disease. N Engl J Med 326: 1577-1581

17. Barnes RW, Nix ML, Barnes CL (1989) Perioperative asymptomatic venous thrombosis: role of duplex scanning versus venography. J Vasc Surg 9: 251-260

18. Holtz DJ, Debatin JF, Unterweger M, Wildermuth S, Leung DA, von Schulthess GK (1994) Phase-contrast evaluation of venous flow-augmentation: effect on ultrafast MR-venography of the calf. In: Book of abstracts, Society of Magnetic Resonance, San Francisco, CA, P957

Rapid and Interactive Cardiovascular Imaging

D.N. Firmin, P.D. Gatehouse, J. Keegan, D.J. Pennell, P. Jhooti, R.H. Mohiaddin, G.Z. Yang

Imperial College, National Heart and Lung Institute, London, UK

Introduction

Recently there has been an increased interest in the development of magnetic resonance (MR) for the study of the cardiovascular system. Important aspects of this development include coronary imaging, the measurement of myocardial perfusion, and quantitative blood flow measurement. For optimised imaging of the heart and vessels there is a requirement for an interactively controlled rapid imaging system.

Methods

A modified Surrey Medical Imaging Systems (SMIS) console was used to drive a 0.5 T magnet for this study. The modification to the SMIS involved the addition of an Intel 860 processor card and associated software which enabled echo planar images to be acquired, reconstructed and displayed at a rate of greater than 10 frames per second. The software allowed interactive control of many imaging parameters. Both conventional and spiral echo planar sequences were incorporated on the system and a method of adaptive convolution was used to regrid sampling points as necessary prior to two-dimensional fast Fourier transformation (2DFFT).

Results and Discussion

One of the MR imaging tools that has been developed and has important implications for the measurement of the function of the heart and blood vessels is quantitative blood flow imaging. This method has allowed us to accurately measure volume blood flow [1, 2] as well as to study the details of flow patterns within the cardiac chambers and great vessels [3]. For clinical diagnosis this method has been used in the assessment of stenotic valves [4], to quantify cardiac shunts [5] and to help unravel complex congenital diseases [6]. Quantitative blood flow imaging also shows potential in the measurement of coronary artery blood velocity and flow patterns and in the assessment of coronary lesions [7, 8]. The clinical need to study dynamic changes in blood flow necessitates the development of MR techniques to image blood flow rapidly. The various methods of ultrafast imaging can be adapted to acquire velocity images, using time-of-flight principles or the phase mapping technique, by simple modification of the sequences [9-13].

The requirement to develop methods of echo planar imaging (EPI) flow measurement is not only to increase the speed of the above clinical applications but also to enable physiological studies on the flow response to exercise or drug administration, for example. Interleaved conventional and spiral echo planar imaging also offer advantages over the sub-second FLASH approaches to coronary flow imaging, mainly in terms of reducing motion problems by means of the shorter acquisition time. The hardware required for EPI is also useful for other rapid gradient echo techniques. For example short echo time flow imaging sequences can be developed and used to improve the accuracy of clinical blood flow measurement [14].

Early attempts to measure flow with EPI involved the use of flow related phase shifts [9, 10]. Firmin and colleagues [9] incorporated the method of phase velocity mapping into a 16 echo strip-selected EPI technique that was validated both in vitro using flow phantoms and in vivo by comparing the measurement of carotid artery flow with that measured using the conventional phase mapping approaches. The strip selection method enabled high resolution EPI to be applied on a conventional scanner, and since blood vessels are normally small, the strip could be offset and orientated to include them. Velocity compensation was included to some extent for all three gradient axes: the slice selection gradient waveform was velocity-corrected in the same way as in conventional gradient echo sequences, the phase-encoding waveform was corrected at the time of the imaging echo (centre of k-space) and the frequency-encoding gradient was corrected on every other echo. The flow sensitivity of the technique was, however, greater than that of more conventional sequences. The flow sensitivity of EPI is in part due to the relatively long duration of the sequence. As with more conventional scanning, the time from signal excitation to the echo is important in terms of the extent of flow related signal loss [14]. Flow in the phase-encoding and frequency-encoding directions is the most important: flow in the former direction will result in blurring whilst flow in the latter can result in Nyquist ghosts due to the induced phase alternation between odd and even echoes [15-17]. The echo time of the EPI sequence can be reduced by forming an asymmetric imaging echo in the phase blip direction. The disadvantage is that since some high spatial frequency information is not acquired, blurring can be seen in the phase-encoding direction. This problem can be resolved to some extent by applying the principles of conjugate symmetry to the k-space data. However, this correction is not actually valid when velocity-dependent phase shifts are being encoded on the data such as in the case of phase velocity mapping. McKinnon and colleagues [18] used this approach, however, in an interleaved echo planar technique capable of acquiring a cine flow study in just 4 s; errors were not measurable on the phantom validation studies but would perhaps be expected to be more significant in smaller vessels.

Spiral echo planar imaging allows the ultimate reduction in echo time because after slice selection the centre of k-space (the echo) is the first data set to be acquired. For this reason the technique is relatively insensitive to flow-related signal loss problems [19]. These sequences have again been combined with phase velocity mapping to produce rapid and accurate measurements of flow velocity. Figure 1 shows an example of magnitude and flow velocity images acquired using an optimised interleaved spiral sequence.

Gatehouse and colleagues [20] developed a single shot sequence that could be repeated at intervals of 50 ms allowing multiple frames to be acquired per heart cycle. The 40 ms spiral gradient waveforms enabled sampling over 32 cycles of k-space that could be reconstructed into a 64 x 64 matrix image. The main problem was the sensitivity of the technique to blurring due to field inhomogeneities, requiring that extremely careful shimming was performed. As well as making rapid measurements of cardiac function and assisting in clinical diagnosis, the technique offers great potential in the study of blood flow physiology. For example the single shot spiral has been applied to measuring real-time aortic blood flow velocity changes during an application of a Valsalva manoeuvre as well as before, during, and after a period of exercise [21]. If real-time measurements are not essential the acquisition period can again be shortened and interleaved to improve the resolution and reduce the type of errors outlined above.

Another important application of echo planar imaging is in the study of myocardial perfusion. The progression of a bolus of gadolinium contrast agent through the heart is monitored by acquiring images at a rate of one per cardiac cycle. A spin echo-echo planar sequence is used with an effective echo time of 32 ms. A pre-inversion pulse is used to nullify the myocardial signal prior to the infusion of gadolinium. Figure 2 shows representative images taken from two series of 100 images acquired during the infusion of a gadolinium bolus. The top images were acquired at rest whilst those below were acquired while the heart was stressed with adenosine.

The interactive capability of the system was of particular importance in this study because it enabled the se-

a
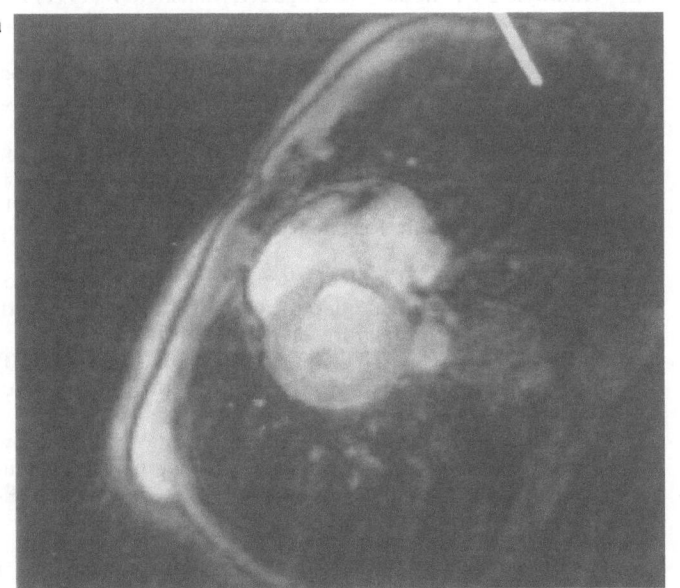

b
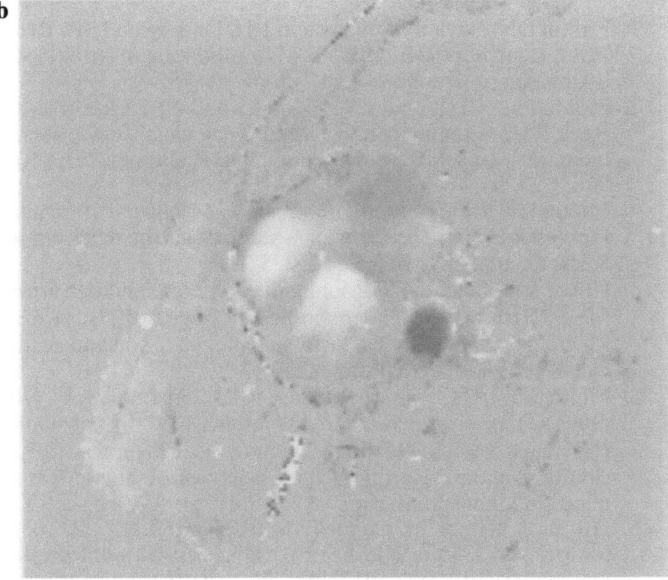

Fig. 1. a Magnitude image showing the short axis of the left ventricle acquired over 16 cardiac cycles using an interleaved spiral echo planar sequence and **b** the corresponding velocity map showing systolic flow in the ventricles and the descending aorta

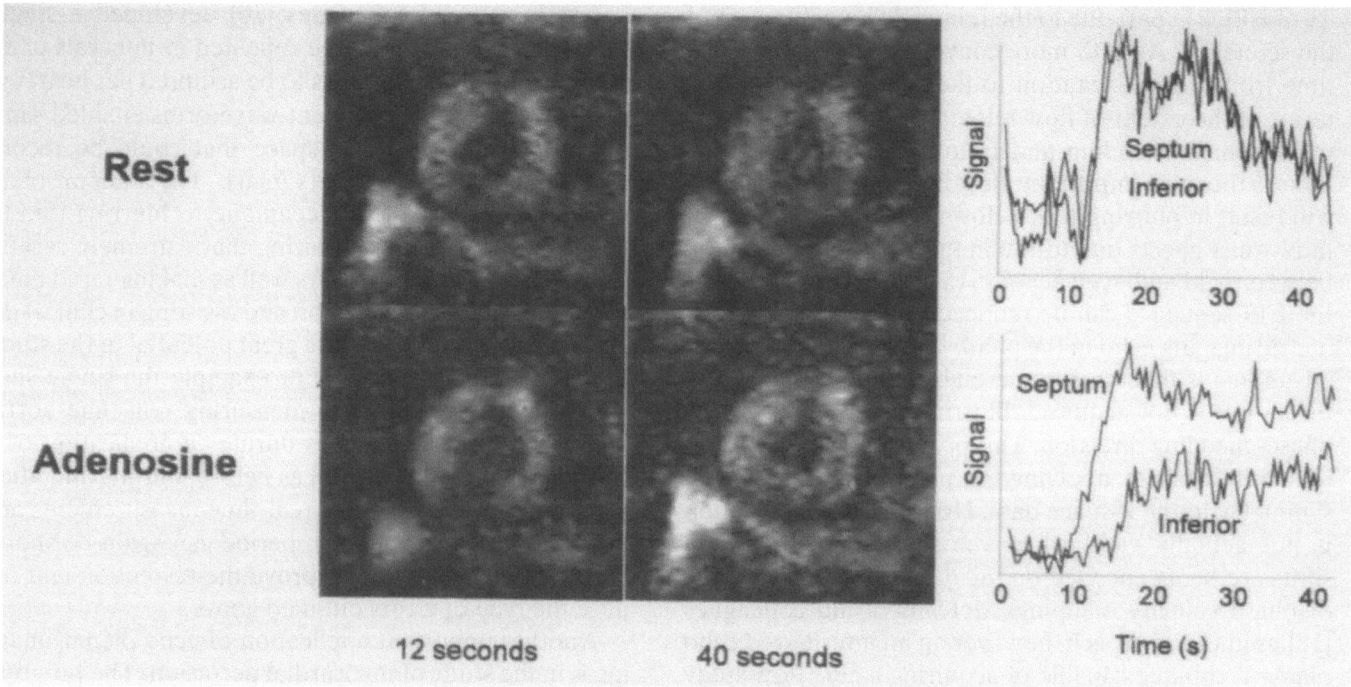

Fig. 2. *Echo-planar images taken at 12 and 40 s following a bolus injection of gadolinium contrast agent.* The images and time curve at the top show the patient at rest whilst those at the bottom show the patient stressed by use of adenosine

quence to be optimised prior to the acquisition of data and injection of the contrast agent. Particular parameters that require optimisation in this case included: the inversion time which can be affected by heart rate and residual gadolinium, slice position, and fat suppression that can be affected by shimming.

References

1. Firmin DN, Nayler GL, Klipstein RH, Underwood SR, Rees RSO, Longmore DB (1987) In vivo validation of MR velocity imaging. J Comput Assist Tomogr 11: 751-756
2. Mohiaddin RH, Wann SL, Underwood SR, Firmin DN, Rees RSO. Longmore DB (1990) Vena caval flow: assessment with cine MR velocity mapping. Radiology 177: 537-541
3. Mohiaddin RH, Bogren HG, Yang GZ, Kilner PJ, Firmin DN (1994) Magnetic resonance velocity vector mapping in aortic aneurysms. MAGMA 2: 335-338
4. Kilner PJ, Manzara CC, Mohiaddin RH, Pennell DJ, Sutton MGS, Firmin DN, Underwood SR, Longmore DB (1993) Magnetic resonance jet velocity mapping in mitral and aortic valve stenosis. Circulation 4: 1239-1248.
5. Mohiaddin RH, Kilner PJ, Rees RSO and Longmore DB (1992) Qp/Qs ratio measured non-invasively by magnetic resonance velocity mapping in patients with intracardiac shunts. Annual Meeting of the Society of Magnetic Resonance in Medicine, Berlin, vol 2. p 2519
6. Hirsch R, Kilner PJ, Connelly M. Redington AN, St. John Sutton MG, Somerville J (1994) Diagnosis in adolescents and adults with congenital heart disease: prospective assessment of individual and combined roles of magnetic resonance imaging and transesophageal echocardiography. Circulation 90:2937-2951

7. Keegan J, Firmin D, Gatehouse P, Longmore D (1994) The application of breath hold phase velocity mapping techniques to the measurement of coronary artery flood flow velocity-phantom data and initial in vivo results. Magn Reson Med 31: 526-536
8. Keegan J, Firmin DN, Gatehouse PD, Longmore DB (1994) Velocity mapping of coronary artery blood flow. MAGMA 2: 311-314
9. Firmin DN, Kiiopstein RH, Hounsfield GL, Paley MP and Longmore DB (1989) Echo-planar high resolution flow velocity mapping. Magn Reson Med 12: 316-327
10 Guilfoyle DN, Gibbs P. Ordidge RJ, Mansfield P (1991) Real-time flow measurements using echo-planar imaging. Magn Reson Med 18: 1-8
11. Butts K, Hanglandreou NJ, Riederer SJ (1993) Phase velocity mapping with a real time line scan technique. Magn Reson Med 29: 134-138
12. Firmin DN, Kilner PJ, Keegan J, Mohiaddin RH and Longmore DB (1990) The development of a subsecond flow velocity mapping technique. [Abstract] Annual Meeting of the Society of Magnetic Resonance in Medicine, New York, p 408
13. Poncelet BP, Weisskoff RM, Wedeen VJ, Brady TJ, Kantor H (1993) Time of flight quantification of coronary flow with echo-planar MRI. Magn Reson Med 30: 447-457
14. Firmin DN, Nayler GL, Kilner PJ, Longmore DB (1990) The application of phase shifts in NMR for flow measurement. Magn Reson Med 14: 230-241
15. Weisskoff RM, Crawley AP, and Wedeen V (1990) Flow sensitivity and flow compensation in instant imaging. Annual Meeting of the Society of Magnetic Resonance in Medicine, New York, vol 1, p 398
16. Duerk JL, Simonetti OP (1991) Theoretical aspects of motion sensitivity and compensation in echo-planar imaging. J Magn Reson Imaging 1: 643-650
17. Butts K, Riederer SJ (1992) Analysis of flow effects in echo-planar imaging. J Magn Reson Imaging 3: 285-293
18. McKinnon GC, Debating JF, Wetter DR, von Schulthess

GK (1994) Interleaved echo planar flow quantitation. Magn Reson Med 32: 263-267

19. Firmin DN, Gatehouse PD, and Longmore DB (1992) Comparison of snap-shot quantitative flow imaging techniques. Annual Meeting of the Society of Magnetic Resonance in Medicine, Berlin, vol 2, p 2915

20. Gatehouse PD, Firmin DN, Collins S, Longmore DB (1994) Real time blood flow imaging by spiral scan phase velocity mapping. Magn Reson Med 31: 504-512

21. Mohiaddiun RH, Gatehouse PD, Firmin DN (1995) Exercise related changes in aortic flow measured by spiral echo-planar velocity mapping. J Magn Reson Imaging 5: 159-163

Stunned Myocardium: Functional and Perfusion MR Imaging

D.H. Szolar[1], M. Saeed[2], M. Wendland[2], H. Sakuma[2], M.A. Stiskal[2], T.P.L. Roberts[2], C.B. Higgins[2]

[1] Department of Radiology, University Hospital and Karl-Franzens Medical School Graz, 8036 Graz, Austria and [2]Department of Radiology, University of California, San Francisco, CA 94143, USA

Introduction

Stunned myocardium refers to a fully reversible postischemic mechanical dysfunction that persists after reperfusion despite the absence of irreversible damage [1, 2]. Currently, diagnostic modalities applied to identify reversibly injured myocardium prospectively are based on assessment of regional myocardial function [3], myocardial perfusion [4], metabolism [5], and cell membrane integrity [6]. However, among these techniques used to image reperfused injured myocardium, none have the potential for combined evaluation of abnormal regional perfusion and function. Magnetic resonance (MR) imaging has the capability to simultaneous evaluate regional perfusion and contractile function [7, 8].

Accordingly, the present study was designed to characterize stunned myocardium by functional and perfusion MR measurements in a canine model. An important feature of the study was the combined assessment of regional myocardial function, using fast cine-MR imaging, and regional perfusion, using fast dynamic contrast-enhanced MR imaging in the same animal.

Methods

1. Animal Model

Eight dogs (10 ± 4 kg) were anesthesized (30 mg sodium pentobarbital/kg body weight), intubated and mechanically ventilated (Harvard Apparatus Co. Inc., South Natick, MA) with room air and positive end-expiratory pressure (5 cm water). In an open-chest dog model, Doppler blood flow probes (Transonic Systems Inc., Ithaca, NY) were positioned around both left anterior descending (LAD) and left circumflex (LCX) coronary artery for measuring coronary blood flow (ml/min). A reversible snare occluder was placed loosely around the LCX artery proximal to the flow probe; a snare was fashioned with polyethylene tubing and was used to produce regional ischemia (15 min occlusion) and reperfusion. The left saphenous vein was cannulated, employing a 21-gauge polyvinyl catheter, and used for MR contrast media injection.

2. MR Imaging Techniques

All images were acquired using a 1.5 T MR system (Signa, General Electric Medical Systems, Milwaukee, WI), employing a quadrature transmit and receive head coil. After the coordinates for the short axis plane of the left ventricle (LV) were determined, the following imaging sequences were acquired: First, k-space segmented cine-MR images (repetition time (TR) = 6.9 ms, echo time (TE) = 2.3 ms, flip angle = 15°, single slice = 10 mm thickness, data matrix = 256 × 128, field of view (FOV) = 24 cm) was performed to evaluate myocardial wall thickening during the cardiac cycle. Second, sixty sequential fast inversion recovery (IR) prepared gradient recalled echo (GRE) (TR = 10.2 ms, TE = 4.2 ms, inversion time (TI) = 700 ms and flip angle = 5°) images were acquired to monitor the first pass of the contrast medium (Omniscan, gadodiamide, Nycomed, Oslo) at 0.03 mmol/kg body weight.

3. Experimental Protocol

Once the animal was placed in the magnet, baseline heart rate and flow indices of the LCX and LAD were obtained. All dogs were subjected to 15 min LCX occlusion followed by at least 30 min of reperfusion. This canine model of brief coronary occlusion produces myocardial "stunning", characterized by reversible myocardial dysfunction [1, 9]. Five sets of each sequence as described above were obtained to demonstrate the presence of regional myocardial stunning at the following states: basal, occlusive, and reperfused (at 1, 10, and 30 min of reperfusion). Myocardial blood flow indices were continuously recorded except during the acquisition of MR images.

Upon completion of the imaging protocol, each animal was sacrificed by injecting a lethal dose of sodium pentobarbital intravenously. The LCX coronary artery was reoccluded at the same location as before by tightening the snare. A dual dye (2% triphenyltetrazolium chloride and

2% phthalocyanine blue) perfusion technique was used to confirm the absence of myocardial infarction.

4. MR Image Analysis

Image analysis was performed on a Sparc 10 workstation (Sun Microsystems, Mountain View, CA) operating an MR image analysis program (MRvision Co, Stanford, CA).

4.1. Wall Thickness Measurements. Short-axis images were displayed in a movie (cine) format to yield qualitative impressions of regional contraction throughout the cardiac cycle. End diastole was defined as the image with the largest luminal diameter, and end systole was defined as the image with the smallest luminal area. Endocardial and epicardial contours of the end-diastolic and end-systolic images were manually traced, carefully excluding papillary muscles, trabeculae, and epicardial fat.

In each image, the internal anterior junction of the right ventricular wall with the interventricular septum was designated as the starting point, followed by clockwise tracing. In each image, a mid-myocardial trace was synthesized between the endocardial and epicardial traces, corresponding to the center between the endocardium and epicardium. Based on this trace, 26 equally spaced circumferential "chords" were constructed perpendicular to the mid-myocardial trace synthesized between the end diastolic and end systolic contours.

Six adjacent "chords" were also obtained from the center of predetermined ischemic (LCX perfusion bed) and nonischemic (LAD perfusion bed) myocardium. This type of measurement was used to minimize the effects of coincidental abnormalities in the circumferential pixel measurement. Wall thickening was expressed as the percent systolic wall thickening according to the formula: percent systolic wall thickening = [(end-systolic wall thickening – end-diastolic wall thickening)/ end-diastolic wall thickening] × 100%. At separate "chords", percent systolic wall thickening during LCX occlusion was considered abnormal when the change was below/above the mean value at baseline state minus two times the correponding SD.

4.2. Signal Intensity Measurements. Circumferential signal intensity (SI) measurements were obtained in a similar fashion to that employed for calculating the wall thickness. In case of the basal state, the image with peak myocardial enhancement was chosen, while during occlusion and reperfusion, images which best defined the ischemic region in terms of image contrast were used for measuring the circumferential signal intensity.

Regional SI (presented as arbitrary units) was measured in each set of images using regions of interest (ROI's) (number of pixels = 14-24, pixel size = 10.3 mm^2 - 18.7 mm^2) in the center of the left ventricular chamber (blood), in the antero-lateral wall of the left ventricle (non-ischemic area), and in the center of the ischemic region (posterior wall). Care was taken to avoid pixels in the subendocardium or subepicardium that might have been altered by chamber blood or epicardial fat. Signal intensity-time curves during transit of the Omniscan were generated.

5. Data Analysis

All values are expressed as mean ± standard error of mean (SEM). Two observers blinded to the results of each other measured the SI and wall thickness of normal and stunned myocardium using the interactive analysis software program. Interobserver reproducibility was expressed as percent variability and standard deviation (SD). Percent variability was determined as the absolute value of the difference between the two measurements divided by the mean of the two measurements. Differences in signal intensity and relative wall thickening between normal and stunned myocardium were calculated using the paired Student's t-test. For two-tailed evaluation, a p value < 0.05 was considered to be significant.

Results

1. Hemodynamics

Complete LCX occlusion during the course of 15 min was confirmed by the cessation of blood flow using a Doppler flowmeter (Table 1). LCX coronary artery occlusion reduced the flow from 16.0 ± 1.4 to 0.2 ± 0.1 ml/min ($p < 0.05$), while the flow in the LAD coronary artery remained unchanged (from 12.1 ± 0.9 to 12.6 ± 0.9 ml/min). Immediately after reperfusion of the LCX coronary artery, flow in the reperfused region significantly increased to 82.7 ± 10.7 ml/min followed by a gradual decrease during the course of 30 min reperfusion (18.2 ± 1.5 ml/min). Again, there were no significant changes in LAD flow during LCX reperfusion.

2. Cine-MR Imaging

Prior to LCX occlusion, end-diastolic wall thickness and percent systolic wall thickening were uniform across the

Table 1. Hemodynamic response to coronary artery occlusion and reperfusion of the left circumflex (LCX) coronary artery

State (n = 8)	LCX Flow (ml/min)	LAD Flow (ml/min)
Basal state	16.0 ± 1.4	12.1 ± 0.9
Coronary occlusion	0.2 ± 0.1*	12.6 ± 0.9
Coronary reperfusion (1 min)	82.7 ± 10.7*†	15.4 ± 4.8
Coronary reperfusion (10 min)	38.6 ± 9.5*†	12.6 ± 2.3
Coronary reperfusion (30 min)	18.2 ± 1.5†	10.3 ± 0.9

* $P < 0.05$ compared to baseline values. † $P < 0.05$ compared to the occlusion state.

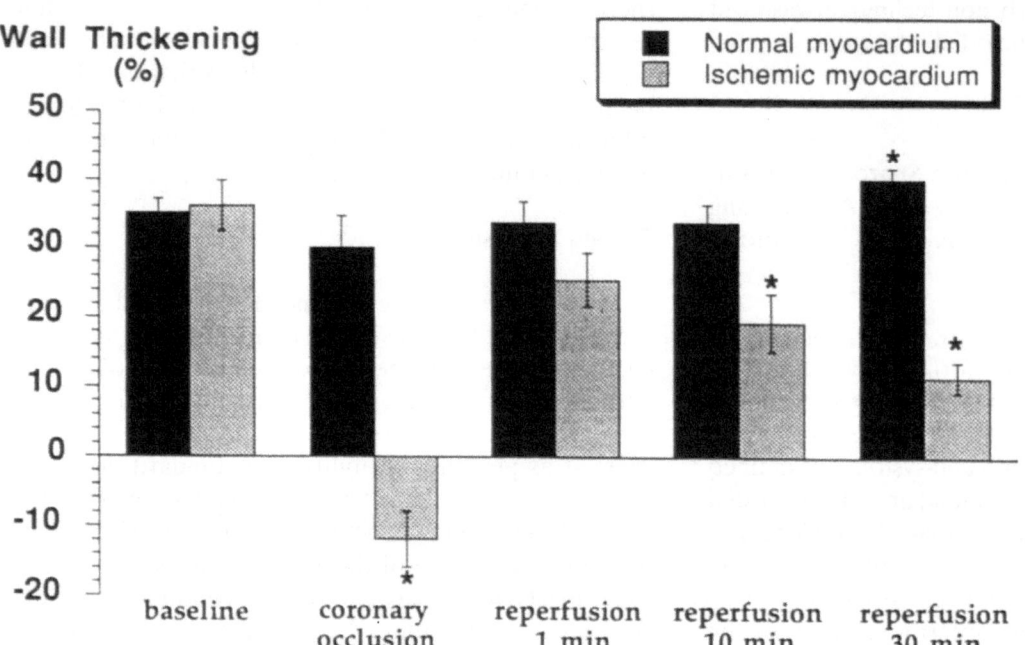

Fig. 1. *Bar graph showing changes in regional percent systolic wall thickening of normal and ischemic myocardium at baseline, during coronary occlusion and during reperfusion. *P < .05 compared to baseline value*

left ventricular wall: 7.0 ± 0.2 mm and $35 \pm 2\%$ at the anterior wall and 7.4 ± 0.2 mm and $36 \pm 4\%$ at the posterior wall, respectively (Figs. 1, 2). During coronary occlusion, wall thickening at the ischemic zone declined from $36 \pm 4\%$ to $-12 \pm 4\%$ as a result of paradoxical wall thinning (dyskinesis) (Figs. 1, 2). Immediately following reperfusion, all dogs demonstrated complete, but tran-

sient recovery in wall thickening at the reperfused zone ($26 \pm 4\%$), coinciding with the reactive hyperemic response (Figs. 1, 2). Wall thickening of normal myocardium showed no changes during LCX occlusion ($30 \pm 5\%$) nor during reperfusion at 1 min of reflow ($34 \pm 3\%$) compared to that at basal state. At later times, significant decline in wall thickening at the reperfused region

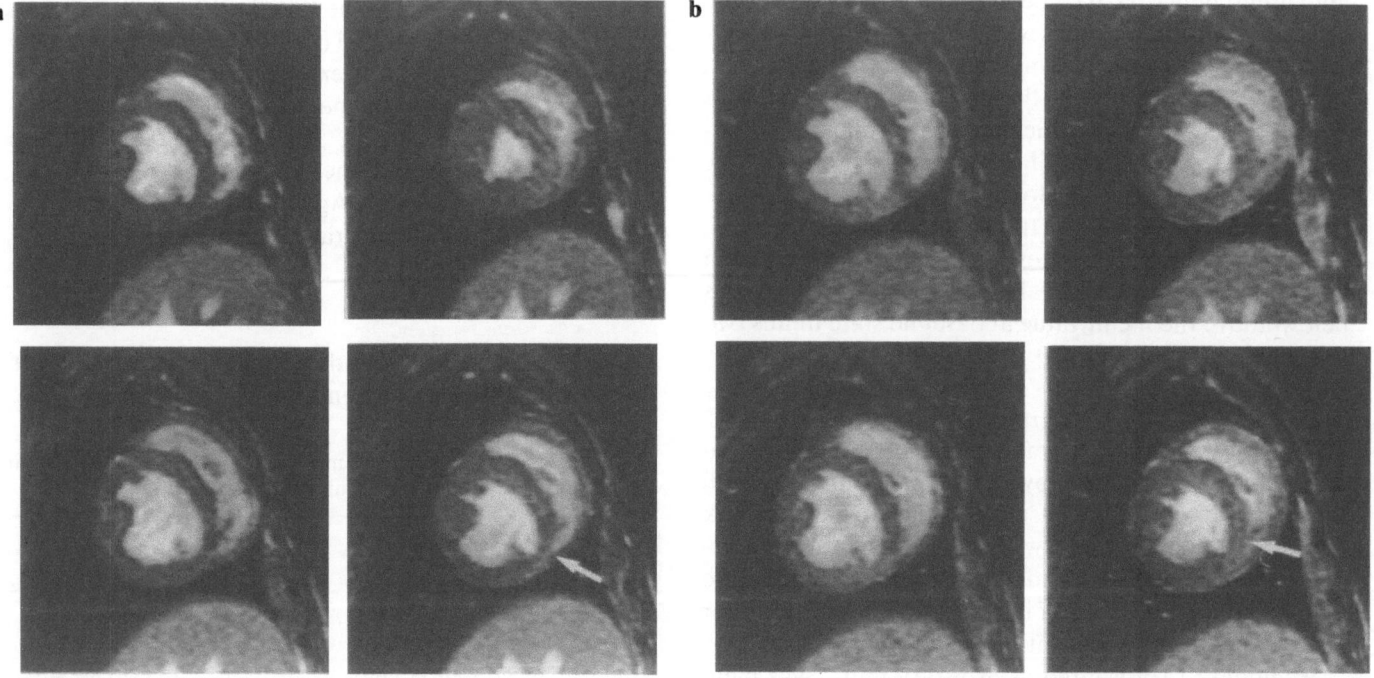

Fig. 2a-b. *Representative set of images from one animal.* **a** baseline (*upper row*) during LCX occlusion (*lower row*), and **b** at early (*upper row*) and after 30 min of reflow (*lower row*). In each row, the panels show images at end-diastole and end-systole obtained using fast cine-MR imaging for wall thickness measurement. Note the thinning of the posterior wall at end-systole evident in all images during LCX occlusion, and to a lesser degree at 30 min of reflow (*arrows*)

Signal Intensity (arbitrary units)

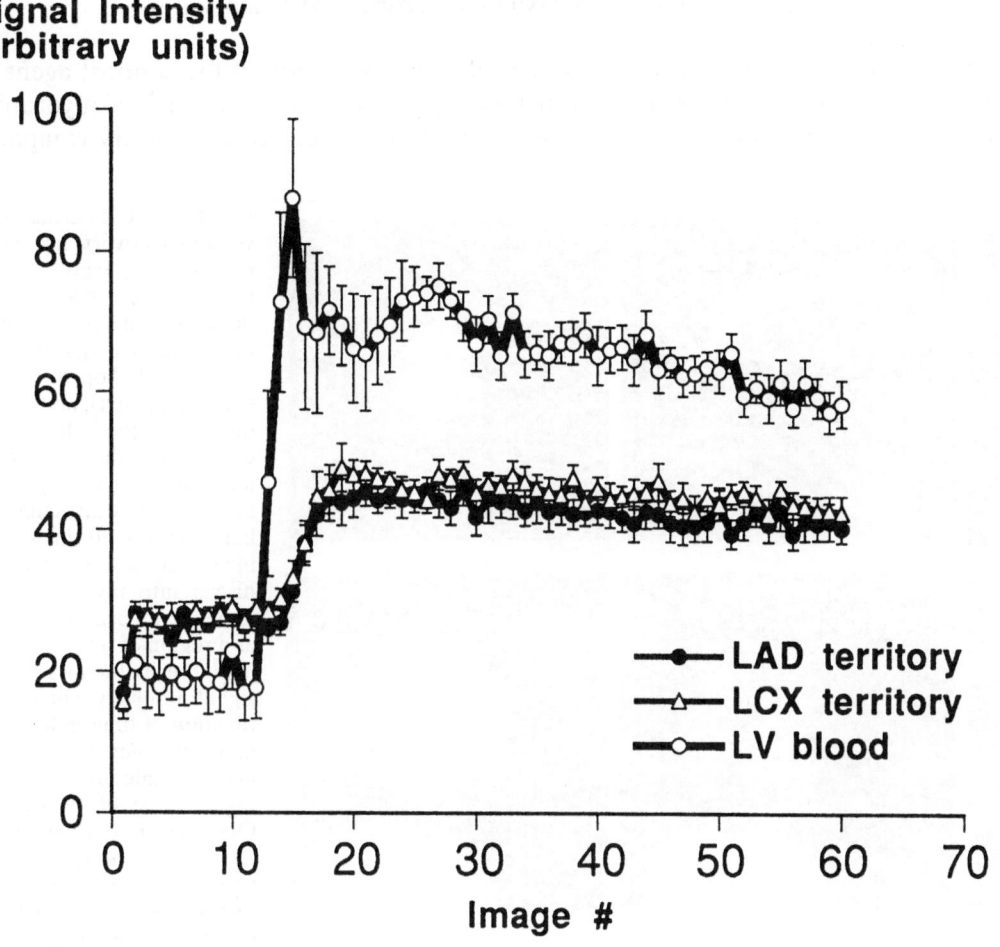

a

Fig. 3. a Basal state: Plot of temporal myocardial signal intesity changes in LV blood, LAD and LCX perfusion beds during the transit of Omniscan on inversion recovery gradient-recalled echo images (TR/TE/TI = 6.9/2.3/700 ms). Note the similarity in the profile of enhancement in both myocardial territories. Bars represent SEM. **b** Thirty minutes of reperfusion: Plot of time course changes in signal intensities of left ventricular chamber blood, normal and reperfused ischemic myocardium during passage of the contrast medium. After 30 min of reflow, there were no significant differences in the magnitude of enhancements between normal and reperfused ischemic myocardium

Signal Intensity (arbitrary units)

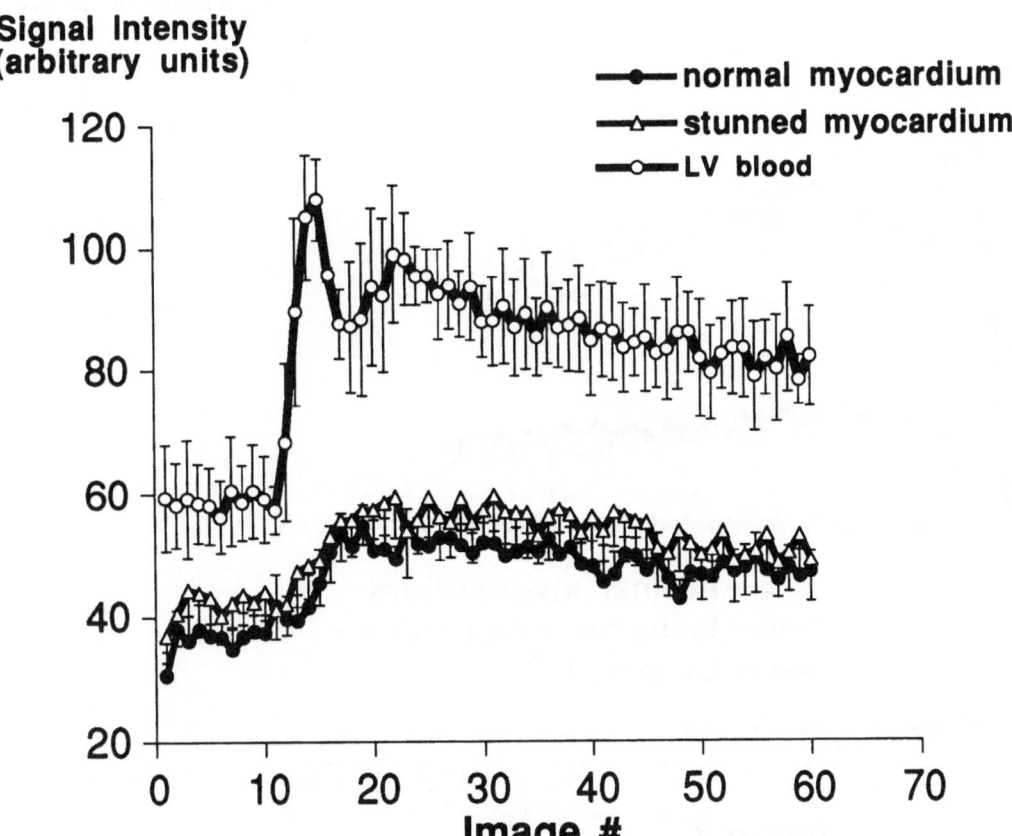

b

was observed: 19 ± 4% at 10 min and 12 ± 2% at 30 min (Figs. 1, 2). Reduced wall thickening after 15 min coronary occlusion is consistent with the definition of myocardial stunning [1, 2]. Interobserver variability for wall thickness measurements analysis was 7.0 ± 1.8%.

3. Dynamic Perfusion MR Imaging

Prior to the administration of the contrast agent there were no significant differences in regional myocardial SI between the territory of occluded artery compared to

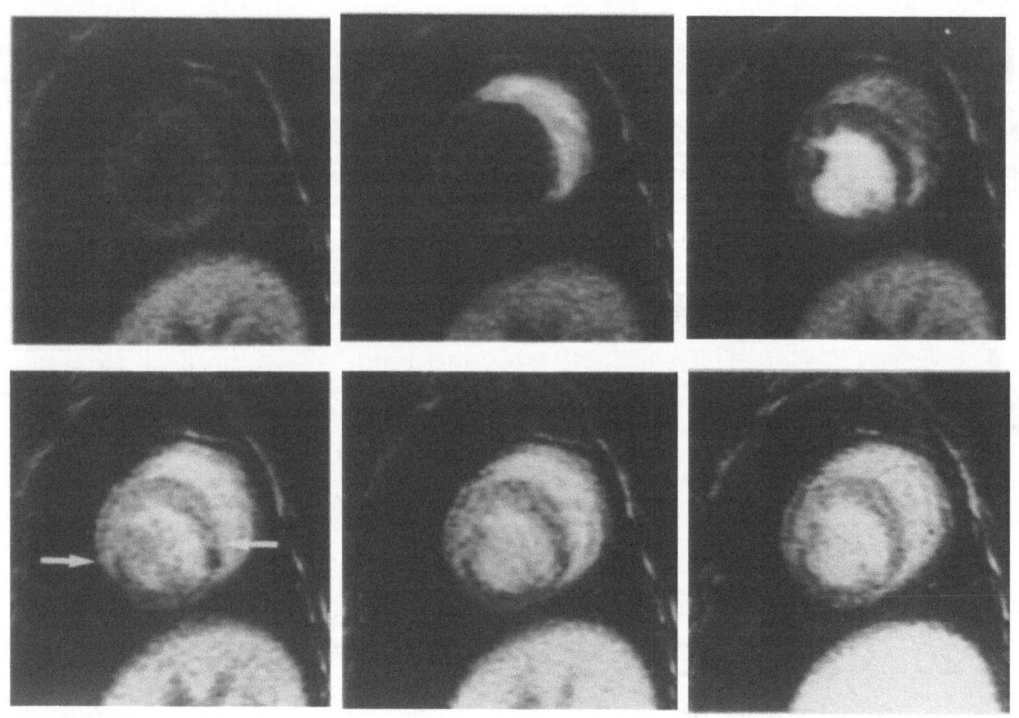

Fig. 4a-b. *LCX occlusion.* **a** Inversion recovery fast gradient recalled echo images (TR/TE/TI = 6.9/2.3/700 ms) during passage of 0.03 mmol/kg Omniscan through the heart of one animal. Top row: precontrast image (*left*), after the leading edge of the bolus of Omniscan entered the right ventricular chamber (*center*) and then into the left ventricular chamber (*right*). Bottom row: these images show the entry of Omniscan into myocardium. The ischemic myocardium is shown as a region of relatively low signal intensity (*arrows*). **b** Plot of signal intensity changes as a function of time in left ventricular chamber blood, normal and ischemic myocardium during passage of 0.03 mmol/kg Omniscan in dogs subjected to 15 min LCX occlusion. The entry of the bolus caused sharp effect on the signal of LV chamber blood and normally perfused myocardium but not in the territory of the occluded vessel

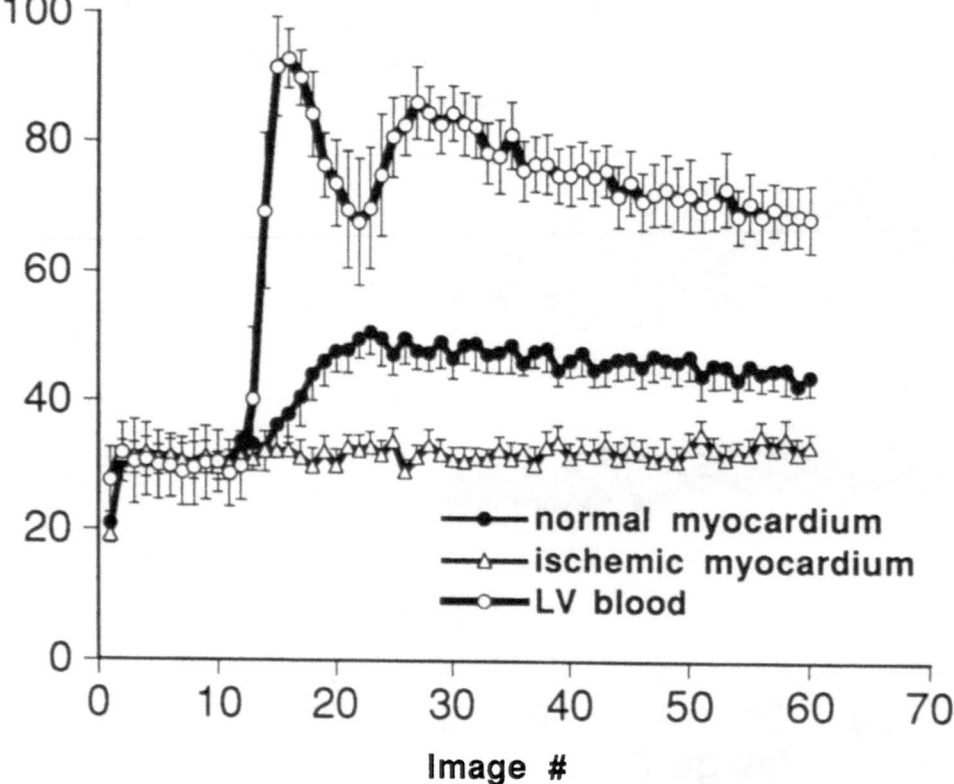

normally perfused myocardium. Before LCX occlusion, homogeneous enhancement in the LCX territory (49 ± 2 arbitrary units) and LAD territory (47 ± 2) was observed during transit of Omniscan, as demonstrated by similar circumferential SI (Fig. 3). Wash-out of the contrast medium from both areas, as reflected by a decline in SI, occurred simultaneously. All animals demonstrat-

ed a perfusion deficit in the territory of the occluded vessel (31 ± 2 vs. 51 ± 3 of non-ischemic myocardium). The ischemic region was visualized as a zone of low SI following the administration of Omniscan (Fig.4). During early (1 min) reperfusion, Omniscan caused greater increase in SI of previously ischemic compared to normal myocardium (Fig. 5). SI of the reperfused ischemic

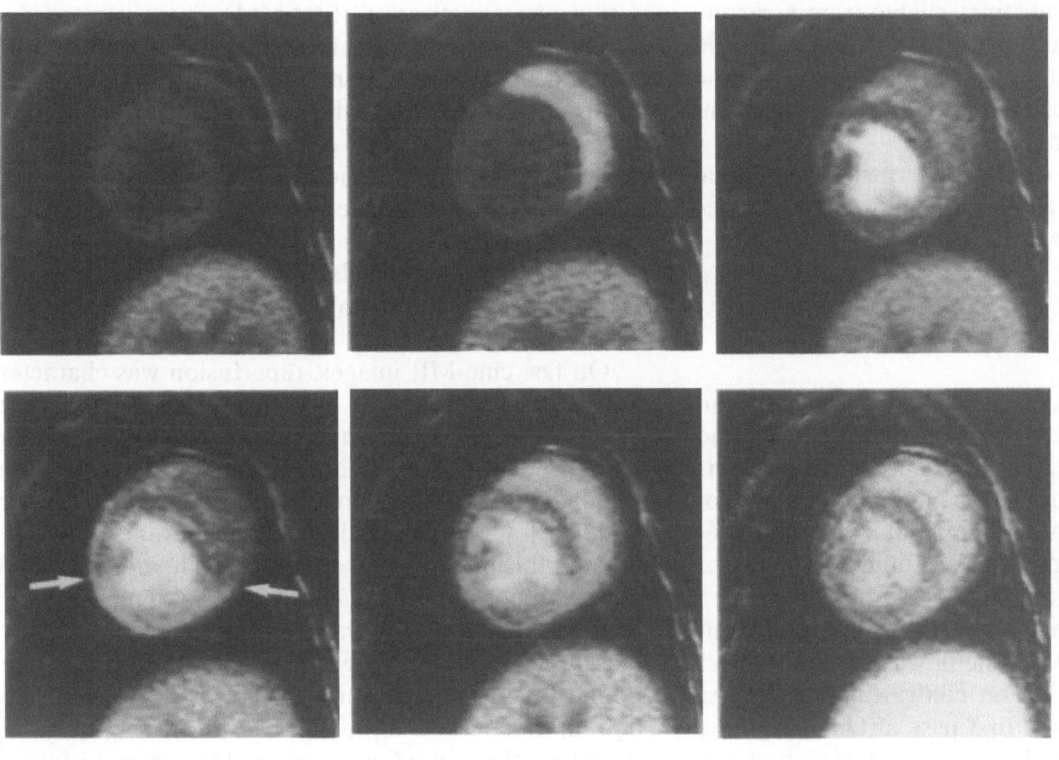

Fig. 5a-b. *Early (< 1 min) reflow.* **a** Inversion recovery fast gradient recalled echo images (TR/TE/TI = 6.9/2.3/ 700 ms) during passage of 0.03 mmol/kg Omniscan through the heart of one animal. Top row: precontrast image (*left*), after the leading edge of the bolus of Omniscan entered the right ventricular chamber (*center*) and then into the left ventricular chamber (*right*). Bottom row: these images show the entry of Omniscan into myocardium. The reperfused myocardium is shown as a region of relatively high signal intensity (*arrows*). **b** Plot of profile of signal changes in left ventricular chamber blood, normal myocardium, and reperfused ischemic myocardium (1 min of reflow). Changes in signal intensity of reperfused myocardium occurred earlier (6 -10 s) than in normal myocardium. The reperfused ischemic myocardium was demonstrated as a region of increased signal intensity for at least 1 min after the injection of the contrast medium

area increased from 33 ± 3 to 69 ± 3 arbitrary units following the administration of Omniscan ($p < 0.05$). The reperfused ischemic region was depicted as a region of high SI compared to non-ischemic myocardium (42 ± 3). At 10 min of reperfusion, the magnitude of enhancement was significantly less than that observed at 1 min of reflow. At 30 min of reperfusion, when LCX flow returned to baseline values, reperfused ischemic myocardium (59 ± 6) was indistinguishable from normally perfused (51 ± 5) myocardium (Fig. 3). The changes in signal intensity correlated well ($r = 0.73$) with the changes in flow. Interobserver variability for signal intensity measurements was $3.3 \pm 0.6\%$.

At postmortem, the dual-dye perfusion technique was used successfully in all dogs to confirm the absence of irreversible myocardial injury.

Discussion

In an experimental model of coronary occlusion and reperfusion, we have demonstrated that cine-MR and perfusion fast MR techniques can be used to characterize stunned myocardium. The complementary use of both techniques provides an incremental value for prediction of the extent of myocardial stunning. The major findings of the current study are:

1. MR perfusion imaging demonstrates the redistribution of regional blood volume/flow at the times of occlusion and reperfusion on contrast-enhanced fast MR images. During the first pass of Omniscan, the ischemic area was clearly defined as a region of low signal intensity, while on reperfusion images as a region of high signal intensity.

2. The bright reperfused region persisted for at least 10 min of reperfusion after repeated administrations of Omniscan and correlated well with the reflow hyperemia.

3. In an area corresponding to the perfusion deficit, fast cine-MR imaging demonstrated systolic wall bulging during occlusion and reduced wall thickening during reperfusion, consistent with the definition of myocardial stunning. Initial but transient recovery in regional wall thickening after reperfusion was associated with an increase in regional blood volume or flow as reflected by greater enhancement of the reperfused compared to normal myocardium on contrast-enhanced fast MR images. Reperfusion for 30 min produced progressive decline in wall thickening with restoration of normal levels at regional blood flow.

1. Myocardial Function

Only few data are available on functional MR imaging of stunned myocardium. Pettigrew et al. [10] have quantitatively validated hypoperfused myocardium in dogs

using isoproterenol stress cine-MR imaging and compared the cine-MR findings with those obtained using ultrasonic crystals. They found severe regional dysfunction with minimal to no measurable systolic wall thickening, which reversed in response to isoproterenol stress with an increase in systolic wall thickening, identifying these regions as stunned rather than acutely infarcted. Kramer et al. [11], using MR imaging with spatial modulation of magnetization (SPAMM), demonstrated dysfunction of adjacent noninfarcted myocardium during left ventricular remodeling in sheep with anteroapical infarctions. Wall thickening was increased in adjacent and remote regions at 1 week after infarction. Kerber et al. [12] measured wall motion with echocardiographic techniques and simultaneously determined myocardial blood flow with microspheres in dogs. Reduction in myocardial blood flow correlated significantly with changes in wall velocity and systolic excursion during coronary occlusion.

On fast cine-MR images, reperfusion was characterized by early recovery in systolic wall thickening, coinciding with the reactive hyperemic response, which has been previously described as a reflex of the increase in regional blood flow/volume during postischemic hyperemia [13]. Our findings derived during reperfusion are comparable with those reported by Heyndrickx et al. [13], who used intramyocardial crystals to measure myocardial function in a canine model of stunned myocardium. Reperfusion was characterized by early rebound in systolic wall thickening. After this initial rebound, there was a trend for wall thickening to be reduced in the reperfused region. During reperfusion, LCX flow increased more than four-fold. Such increase in flow is associated with an increase of approximately 40%-60% in blood volume [14]. Iwamoto et al. [15]. observed that the increase in coronary flow, with or without increases in perfusion pressure, increased regional contractile force, systolic stiffness, and oxygen consumption. Another factor for the early rebound of function is that stunned myocardium exhibits increased responsiveness to calcium as a result of postischemic hyperemia [16]. First, when stunned myocardium is challenged with inotropic stimuli, it exhibits normal or near-normal contractile function. Second, the apparent sensitivity of stunned myocardium to intracoronary calcium infusion is not decreased. The increase in intracellular calcium is postulated to be a brief phenomenon immediately after reperfusion, following which there may be either a normalization of intracellular transient or a relative calcium deficiency [16].

2. Myocardial Perfusion

Fast contrast-enhanced MR imaging revealed striking temporal changes in spatial distribution of perfusion in stunned myocardium. Perfusion MR imaging has the potential to demonstrate the differential contrast between normal, ischemic, reperfused myocardium. This contrast is generally short-lived after reperfusion depending on the increase in regional flow. Warltier et al. [17] found a several fold increase above baseline in blood flow measured by radiolabelled microspheres shortly after reperfusion. Ambrosio et al. [18] observed progressive decline in regional perfusion in stunned myocardium. Bolli et al. [19] observed in dogs after a single 15 min coronary occlusion that the vascular resistance was significantly increased in stunned compared to normal myocardium. Other studies, using radioactive micospheres, have reported gradual attenuation of postischemic hyperemia as a result of increased coronary vascular resistance [13]. However, Bolli et al. [19] found no correlation between the impairment in wall thickening and the increase in vascular resistance of stunned myocardium, suggesting that it may be an independent phenomenon. As shown in Fig. 4, during the first pass of the contrast medium through the heart the increase in signal of previously ischemic myocardium was substantially greater than that of normally perfused myocardium. This difference can be attributed to the relative blood flow/volume in both regions and/or greater extravasation of the contrast medium in stunned myocardium. It has been suggested that a metabolic byproduct (i.e. adenosine) from the previously ischemic zone may alter the extravasation rate of blood constituents. Canty et al. [20] found in a canine model that the extraction of low-molecular weight radiographic contrast agents into the myocardial extravascular space was significantly higher in the ischemic area than in normal myocardium during pharmacologic vasodilatation. As a result of diffusion of the contrast medium across the capillary wall, the whole population of nuclear spins (intra- and extravascular spins) will exhibit both spin-lattice and phase relaxation enhancement.

3. Limitations

An inherent limitation of this study is the use of cine-MR imaging for assessing regional ventricular function. Motion of the heart within the plane of imaging can affect the measurements of circumferential shortening. Hofmann et al. [21] have demonstrated in the mid-left ventricle that the long axis translation can be significant, ranging from 0.5 to 1.5 cm. Although the application of myocardial tagging [11, 22] or velocity-encoded cine-MR imaging [23] would be more accurate for assessing regional myocardial function, this study was designed to characterize stunned myocardium by the complementary use of functional and perfusion measurements in a single session. Under these circumstances, MR imaging with SPAMM is currently a far less practical proposition than fast cine-MR imaging because of the essentially longer acquisition time, and would not have allowed our study design. Unlike the SPAMM technique, fast cine-MR imaging is readily available and

permits multislice data acquisition covering the whole heart in 5-6 min. Several groups have demonstrated the high sensitivity of cine-MR imaging for detecting ischemic ventricular dysfunction [24].

The use of only one short-axis slice employed for quantitative functional assessment may represent a potential for sampling error. However, we had two reasons to use only one level: multislice acquisition of perfusion was not possible at the time the study was conducted, and the application of the centerline method – as initially described by van Rugge et al. [24] – without any need for correcting for in-plane translational motion.

Another limitation of the fast GRE technique is the relatively long acquisition time (300 ms-1000 ms), which covers a large fraction of one cardiac cycle. Preliminary studies have demonstrated the feasibility of echo planar imaging (EPI) for evaluation of real-time myocardial perfusion by reducing imaging times to as short as 50 ms-100 ms [25].

In conclusion, the complementary use of perfusion and functional fast MR imaging techniques allows the detection and characterization of myocardial stunning. This method may be useful in patients undergoing reperfusion to define microvasculature patency in ischemic regions.

References

1. Heyndrickx GR, Millard RW, McRitchie RJ, Maroko PR, Vatner SF (1975) Regional myocardial functional and electrophysiological alterations after brief coronary artery occlusion in conscious dogs. J Clin Invest 56: 978-985
2. Braunwald E, Kloner RA (1982) The stunned myocardium: Prolonged, postischemic ventricular dysfunction. Circulation 66: 1146-1149
3. Nixon JV, Brown CN, Smitherman TC (1982) Identification of transient and persistent segmental wall motion abnormalities in patients with unstable angina by two-dimensional echocardiography. Circulation 65: 1497-1503
4. Bonow RO, Dilsizian V, Cuocolo A, Bacharach SL (1991) Identification of viable myocardium in patients with coronary artery disease and left ventricular dysfunction: Comparison of thallium scintigraphy with reinjection and PET imaging with ^{18}F-fluorodeoxyglucose. Circulation 83: 26-37
5. Perrone-Filardi P, Bacharach SL, Dilsizian V, Maurea S, Marin-Neto JA, Arrighi JA, Frank JA, Bonow RO (1992) Metabolic evidence of viable myocardium in regions with reduced wall thickness and absent wall thickening in patients with chronic left ventricular dysfunction. J Am Coll Cardiol 20: 161-168
6. Gould KI, Yoshida K, Hess MJ, Haynie M, Mullani N, Smalling RW (1991) Myocardial metabolism of fluorodeoxyglucose compared to cell membrane integrity for the potassium analogue rubidium-82 for assessing infarct size in man by PET. J Nucl Med 32: 1-9
7. Hartnell G, Cerel A, Kamalesh M, Finn JP, Hill T, Cohen M, Tello R, Lewis S (1994) Detection of myocardial ischemia: value of combined myocardial perfusion and cineangiographic MR imaging. AJR 163: 1061-1067
8. Yeon SB, Reichek N, Tallant BA, et al (1991) Imaging function and perfusion defects in myocardial infarction using magnetic resonance tagging and iron oxide contrast [Ab-

stract]. In: Proc Soc Magn Reson, San Francisco, CA, p 371

9. Sinusas AJ, Shi QX, Vitols PJ, Fetterman RC, Maniawski P, Zaret BL, Wackers FJTh (1993) Impact of regional ventricular function, geometry, and dobutamine stress on quantitative ^{99m}Tc-sestamibi defect size. Circulation 38: 2224-2234

10. Pettigrew RI, Marin S, Eisner R, Leyendecker M, Schmarkey S, Patterson R (1991) Detection of partial coronary artery stenosis with isoprotenerol stress cine-MRI in dogs: validation by on-line ultrasonic crystals and flow probes [Abstract]. In: Book of Abstracts, Proc Soc Magn Reson, New York, p. 243

11. Kramer CM, Lima JAC, Reichek N, Ferrari VA, Llaneras MR, Palmon LC, Yeh I, Tallant B, Axel L (1993) Regional differences in function within noninfarcted myocardium during left ventricular remodeling. Circulation 88: 1279-1288

12. Kerber RE, Marcus ML, Ehrhardt J, Wilson R, Abboud FM (1975) Correlation between echocardiographically demonstrated segmental dyskinesis and regional myocardial function. Circulation 52: 1097

13. Heyndrickx GR, Wijns W, Vogelaers D, Degrieck J, Bol A, Vandeplassche G, Melin JA (1993) Recovery of regional contractile function and oxidative metabolism in stunned myocardium induced by 1-hour circumflex coronary artery stenosis in chronically instrumented dogs. Circulation Research 72: 901-913

14. Balaban RS, Taylor JF, Turner R (1994) Effect of cardiac flow on gradient recalled echo images of the canine heart. NMR Biomed 7: 89-95

15. Iwamoto T, Bai X-J, Downey HF (1994) Coronary reperfusion related changes in myocardial contractile force and systolic ventricular stiffness. Cardiovasc Res 28: 1331-1336

16. Ito BR, Tate H, Kobayashi M, Schaper W (1987) Reversibly injured, postischemic canine myocardium retains normal contractile reserve. Circulation 61: 834-846

17. Warltier DC, Gross GJ, Brooks HL, Preuss KC (1988) Improvement of postischemic contractile function by the calcium channel blocking agent nitrendipine in conscious dogs. J Cardiovasc Pharmacol 12 (Suppl 4): S120-S124

18. Ambrosio G, Weisman HF, Mannisi JA, Becker LC (1989) Progressive impairment of regional myocardial perfusion after initial restoration of postischemic blood flow. Circulation 80: 1846-1861

19. Bolli R, Zhu WX, Thornby JI, O'Neill PG, Roberts R (1988) Time course and determinants of recovery of function after reversible ischemia in conscious dogs. Heart Circ. Physiol 23: H102-H114

20. Canty JM, Judd RM, Brady AS, Klocke FJ (1991) First pass entry of nonionic contrast agent into the myocardial extravascular space: effect on radiographic estimates of transit time and blood volume. Circulation, 84: 2071-2078

21. Hoffmann EA, Rumberger J, Dougherty L, Reichek N, Axel L (1989) A geometric view of cardiac 'efficiency' [Abstract]. J Am Coll Cardiol 13: 86A

22. Axel L, Dougherty L (1989) Heart wall motion: Improved method of spatial modulation of magnetization for MR imaging. Radiology 172: 349-350

23. Karwatowski SP, Mohiaddin RH, Yang GZ, Firmin DN, Sutton MSJ, Underwood RS, Longmore DB (1994) Assessment of regional left ventricular long-axis motion with MR velocity mapping in healthy subjects. J Magn Reson Imaging 4: 151-155

24. Van Rugge FP, Van der Wall EE, Spanjersberg SJ, De Roos A, Matheijssen NAA, Zwinderman AH, Dijkman PRM, Reiber JHC, Bruschke AVG (1994) Magnetic resonance imaging during dobutamine stress for detection and localization of coronary artery disease. Quantitative wall motion analysis using a modification of the centerline method. Circulation 90: 127-138

25. Edelman RR, Li W (1994) Contrast enhanced echo-planar MR imaging of myocardial perfusion: preliminary study in humans. Radiology 190: 771-777

Stress-Strain Modeling with MRI

L. Axel, D.C. Bloomgarden

Radiology Department, Hospital of the University of Pennsylvania, 3400 Spruce St., Philadelphia, PA 19104 USA

Introduction

An important index of myocardial function is myocardial stress, reflecting the distribution of forces within the heart wall. Increased stress has been associated with increased oxygen demand [1], increased blood flow requirement [2], and ventricular remodeling in hypertrophy and post-infarction [3, 4]. It is a function of both ventricular geometry and cavity pressures. However, currently, there is no reliable way to directly measure stress. Invasive methods for determining stress are unreliable, due to the perturbing effects of the invasive devices used, such as implanted force transducers. Attempts to model the stress distribution within the heart wall have been limited by a lack of sufficient data on the geometry and properties of the heart wall and by the sensitivity of the calculated results to the particular corresponding assumptions made for the values of the missing data.

The development of cardiac magnetic resonance imaging (MRI) has provided a valuable technique to study the three-dimensional (3D) geometry of the heart wall during the cardiac cycle. Furthermore, the development of tagged MRI methods has now made it possible to noninvasively study the distribution of the regional strain (or deformation) throughout the heart wall for the first time. While we still cannot directly image the pressure within the ventricular cavity or the mechanical properties of the wall material with MRI, the availability of this new data on geometry and regional strain should make it possible to improve the quality of our stress models, particularly in combination with data on wall properties derived from other studies. Other potential uses of MRI include the possibility of estimating the intraventricular pressure from measurements of the velocity of atrioventricular valvular regurgitation (commonly seen in trace amounts even in normal subjects), using the simplified Bernoulli equation, as is frequently done in echocardiography. Fluid mechanical modeling of blood flow patterns measurable with MRI may also provide a means to estimate pressure differences. This approach to the study of cardiac stress is still at a very early stage and much development work remains to be done. However, it should lead to much more insight into the stress-strain relationships in the normal and abnormal heart wall, and may ultimately become clinically useful.

Heart Wall Geometry

One immediately useful contribution of MRI to the study of stress-strain relations is its excellent depiction of the 3D geometry of the heart wall, without the need for contrast injections, ionizing radiation, or any simplifying assumptions about the wall geometry. This data is a necessary component of any approach to realistic stress calculations. The heart wall contours can be extracted from a set of spatially registered tomographic images (e.g., in stacked parallel planes) to provide a set of samples of the heart wall contour, spaced by the separation of the image planes. The contours are best defined when the image plane is approximately perpendicular to the local wall surface, so that nonparallel image planes or supplementary images may be needed to optimally define the rounded heart wall. In our case, we use a set of parallel short axis images in combination with a set of rotating plane long axis images. A currently unresolved issue is the level of spatial resolution that will be needed to define the heart wall. The necessary resolution will depend on the purpose of the data and how much of the rough surface characteristics and papillary muscles one wants to include in the model. The normal right ventricular wall can also be measured, though it is much thinner and rougher than the left, so it is less well defined with conventional MRI resolution.

A 3D model of the heart wall can be reconstructed from the sampled wall contour points. From this 3D model we can calculate local wall thickness and wall curvature. The curvature can be calculated for the outer and inner walls (at some level of reconstructed detail), as well as at some calculated representative midwall surface. These wall curvatures, together with the cavity pressure, would permit the calculation of a simplified measure of wall stress, namely using Laplace's law, which assumes that the heart is made from concentric thin-walled surfaces.

Heart Wall Strain

While other imaging methods, such as high speed X-ray computed tomography, can also give us tomographic heart wall geometry data, MRI can give us unique data on regional wall strain [5-8]. Although invasive methods, such as biplane X-ray imaging of implanted radiopaque markers, may give higher precision data on regional wall motion, they generally provide a much more limited sampling of the heart wall and may result in alteration of the motion by their invasive nature.

Tagged MRI for regional strain determination relies on the ability to noninvasively create regions of altered magnetization within the tissue, either selectively, similarly to slice selection in conventional imaging, or nonselectively, with spatial modulation of magnetization (SPAMM) [6]. Such regions will have distinct appearances on MR image, such as stripes or grids. As the magnetization of a material moves with it, any motion of the tissue between the times of tagging and imaging will be seen as a corresponding displacement of the image of the tag. We can calculate local internal wall motion, and thus strain, from tagged MRI, as described in the accompanying talk. Phase shift MRI methods can also be used to measure local wall velocity, which can, in principle, be integrated to calculate internal wall motions.

Heart Wall Properties

The relationship between the stress and the strain in the heart wall is determined by the engineering material properties of the heart wall, which are not directly measurable with conventional MRI. It may, however, be possible to correlate the MRI properties, such as the relaxation times, with other important material properties, such as wall collagen content, in conditions such as scarring after myocardial infarction. It is also possible that new MRI methods to assess tissue elasticity through observation of the response to externally driven vibrations may permit in situ estimates of myocardial stiffness [9].

However, since we want to calculate the stress in the heart, we need a way to estimate the material properties. In simple materials, such as springs, one elasticity constant relates the change in the length of the spring (strain) to changes in its tension (or stress) through Hooke's law. However, tissues such as the heart wall are more complex than this in several respects. Tissue is generally nonlinear, so that the forces required to change the length of tissue depend on the initial length of the tissue. For myocardial tissue, these forces increase in a non-linear or approximately exponential fashion as

the length of the specimen increases [10]. The heart wall is also anisotropic, so that the stiffness of the tissue depends on the direction in which it is being stretched. These directions are related to the underlying structure of the heart tissue in which the muscle fibers run in parallel in a spiraling, fashion around the heart and muscle bundles are connected to others with collagen sheet structures [10]. Although the anisotropic structure of the heart wall is not directly seen with conventional MRI, the fiber structure of the heart is quite consistent between individuals, so that historic data may be applied to new subjects. In addition, there is the possibility that methods being developed to measure the anisotropy of diffusion with MRI may permit in situ MRI measurement of structural anisotropy in the heart wall [11]. As the blood content of the heart wall may vary significantly over the cardiac cycle, it may not be reasonable to assume it is incompressible, as has been done in most engineering models. Finally, the heart wall properties change dramatically during the cardiac cycle with its periodic contraction and relaxation. It is likely that practical fitting of the myocardial material properties will include only a subset of these potential considerations.

One method for calculating myocardial stress is to use myocardial material properties derived from experimental studies of *ex vivo* wall samples. However, these experimental results are best suited for evaluating the passive stretching of diastole, and additional assumptions need to be made to account for the changing properties during systole. Also, these passive in vitro measurements may not correspond to the in vivo undisturbed conditions. Nevertheless, the use of these properties allows for the estimation of intramural stresses from the observed strains that accompany the filling of the ventricle in diastole, if we monitor the transmural pressure. However, there is the potential for MRI to provide estimates of the material properties and internal stresses in the heart wall, given an assumed parametric form of the myocardial constitutive law and the transmural pressures, through the use of iterative computer modeling of the heart wall with the constraints of the MRI-derived data on the regional geometry and strain.

Finite Element Heart Wall Modeling

In engineering applications, finite element methods are widely used to compute the stress and strain distributions within complex structures. Typically, the structure is represented as a grid or mesh of discrete material points in space, with the values of properties such as stress at locations between these points assumed to vary smoothly with the position between them. Thus, the problem of calculating the distribution of stress or strain within the structure is reduced to the simpler task of calculating the values at the grid points. For a given structure and constitutive law, the strain (and accompanying stess) distribution, resulting from the application of a given external load, can be computed by minimizing the net strain energy. These methods have been applied to modeling the heart [10]. Starting with a particular assumed form of the constitutive law for passive myocardium and initial guesses for the values of the parameters, both based on in vitro measurements, and the values of the transmural pressures, we can calculate the stress and strain distributions in the myocardium. We can then compare the calculated and observed strain distributions, and iteratively solve for the values of the constitutive parameters that minimize the discrepancies between them. This approach has been used by Moulton et al. to make initial steps toward estimating myocardial material properties from a tagged two-dimensional image set acquired in diastole [12]. The corresponding stress distributions are directly extracted from the calculations. Alternatively, we could use the observed strains to calculate the corresponding stress distribution for a particular form of the constitutive law, and again seek the values for the constitutive parameters that minimize the net strain energy. In either case, we can use the constraints of observed geometry and strain data from MRI together with pressure boundary conditions to jointly find the material properties and stress distribution.

We are currently pursuing these approaches. To validate the results, we are using data from tagged MRI of deformable phantoms subjected to known pressures to estimate the material properties. These derived values are then compared to independently measured values. We are also using multiplanar tagged MRI of animals instrumented with MR-compatible pressure monitors to start the finite element modeling of stress distributions, using a particular form of the constitutive law [10].

Future Developments

There will always be a need to make some simplifying assumptions to permit calculation of the stress distribution within the heart wall. However, the availability of accurate three dimensional data on the geometry and strain distribution within the heart wall from tagged MRI studies should allow us to avoid the need for some

of the previously necessary simplifications and *a priori* assumptions. With anticipated technical improvements in cardiac MRI, we should be able to better determine the strain distribution within the wall, particularly transmurally, in order to further improve the mechanical modeling. If some of the other potentially powerful MRI methods for noninvasive tissue characterization and pressure estimation can be developed further, we may be able to make even more realistic estimates of intramural stresses.

References

1. Sarnoff SJ, Braunwald E, Welch GH, Case RB, Stainsby WN, Macruz R (1958) Hemodynamic Determinants of Oxygen consumption of the heart with special reference to the tension-time index. Am J Physiol 192: 148-156
2. Jan KM (1985) distribution of myocardial stress and its influence on coronary blood flow. J Biomech 18: 815-820
3. Alper R (1971) Cardiac hypertrophy. Academic Press, New York
4. Pfefer MA, Braunwald E (1990) Ventricular remodeling after myocardial infarction. Experimental observations and clinical implications. Circulation 81: 1161
5. Zerhouni E, Parrish D, Rogers W, Yang A, Shapiro E (1988) Human heart: Tagging with MR imaging-A method for noninvasive assessment of myocardial motion. Radiology 168: 59
6. Axel L, Dougherty L (1989) Heart wall motion: Improved method of spatial modulation of magnetization for MR imaging. Radiology 172: 349
7. Axel L, Gonçalves RC, Bloomgarden DC (1992) Regional heart wall motion: Two-dimensional analysis and functional imaging of regional heart wall motion with magnetic resonance imaging. Radiology 183: 745
8. Young AA, Axel L (1992) Three-dimensional motion and deformation of the heart wall. Radiology 185: 241
9. Muthupillai R, Lomas DJ, Rossman PJ, Greenleaf JF, Manduca A, Ehman R (1995) Magnetic resonance elastography by direct visualization of propagating acoustic strain waves. Science 269: 1864
10. Hunter PJ, Smaill BH (1988) The analysis of cardiac function: a continuum approach. Prog Biophys Molec Biol 52: 101
11. Wedeen VJ, Reese TG, Smith RN, Rosen BR, Weisskoff RM, Dinsmore RE (1995) Mapping myocardial architecture with diffusion anisotropy MRI. Proc Soc Magn Reson: 357
12. Moulton MJ, Creswell LL, Actis RL, Myers KW, Vannier MW, Szabó BA, Pasque MK (1995) An inverse approach to determining myocardial material properties. J Biomech 28: 935

Magnetic Resonance Imaging in the Evaluation of Valvular Prosthetic Function

E. Di Cesare, A. Costanzi, C. Masciocchi, R. Maurizi Enrici

Department of Radiology, University of L'Aquila, 67100 L'Aquila, Italy

Introduction

Following patients with prosthetic valve replacement is quite difficult. Indeed, fibrosis, calcification and tearing of the leaflet are probably the fate of most bioprosthetic valves after 10 years. Separating valve dysfunction from other causes of symptoms, such as diminished left ventricular contractility, coronary arterial disease and pulmonary disease may be difficult. Catheterization is frequently different and risks are reported. Nowadays, the echo color Doppler is much more reliable even when the metallic structures in the mechanical valve cause echo reflections and shadowing which mask events distal to the struts. Therefore, detection of thrombus or vegetation around the metallic struts is not easy.

The transesophageal echocardiographic approach to the visualization of chambers posterior to the prosthesis gives good quality images of valvular and paravalvular structures because it is applied in proximity to the heart. However, artifacts and flow-masking caused by the synthetic material of the artificial valve prostheses may interfere with the diagnostic capabilities of transesophageal ultrasound analyses.

High-field magnetic resonance (MR) examinations (1.5 T) are considered safe for patients with biomedical prosthetic heart valves. In fact, in vivo evaluation of the beating heart showed that the deflection forces caused by the static magnetic field are lower than that exerted on the valve [1-10]. We considered different valve models to define: (1) the artifact entity for each type of valve; (2) the flow pattern in normo-functioning valve prostheses; (3) the pathological transvalvular or paravalvular leakage flow.

Material and Methods

Thirty-four patients (25 males and 9 females) with age ranging between 39 and 69 years (mean, 43 years) were included in our study. They had 28 aortic and 13 mitral valves replaced with 15 biological, 13 Carpentier-Edwards, 2 Hancock and 26 mechanical prostheses, which included 1 Hall-Kaster, 1 Edwards, 16 Sorin, 2 Bjork-Shiley, 3 St. Jude, 1 Duromedics and 1 Smeloff-Cutter.

A low-field MR unit (0.2 T) was used for the study, with cine-MR technique and short repetition time (TR) and echo time (TE) sequences (TR= 50 ms, TE = 15 ms, flip angle (FA) = 60°); the acquisition matrix was 160 × 256 with 35 cm field of view and slice thickness of 10 mm. The images were acquired on planes parallel and perpendicular to the valvular plane. The last 8 patients, including 5 with biological Carpentier-Edwards, 2 with Sorin and 1 with Edwards mechanical prostheses, were studied with a 0.5 T superconductive magnet with gradient echo short TR-TE sequences with cine-MR technique (TR = 15 ms, TE = 7 ms, FA = 40°).

A semiquantitative analysis with double-blind evaluation was performed by two experienced radiologists for definition of the artifact entity. Three classes were distinguished: (class 1) artifact of minimum entity, if circumscribed to the valvular structure, was considered not significant; (class 2) medium artifact, smaller than 1 cm in size in the images perpendicular to the valvular plane, allowed evaluation of valvular functionality; (class 3) significant artifact, severely impairing the evaluation of valvular functionality at cine-MR. Analysis of the flow was performed behind the valve to define normal or pathological function.

Mitral regurgitation was judged to be present when a signal void emanated from the mitral valve prosthesis into the left atrium during ventricular systole. Aortic regurgitation was identified by the appearance of a signal void extending from the aortic valve prosthesis into the left ventricular chamber during ventricular diastole. The origin, shape and extension of the signal void within the respective cardiac chamber were noted throughout the cardiac cycle. The transverse image that showed the largest signal loss was used for measurement of the signal void area. When there was more than one reflux, jet areas were added.

Transvalvular turbulent flow (evidence of signal loss) in which the jet originated from inside the valve ring was considered to be physiologic if small ($2-3$ cm^2 jet area),

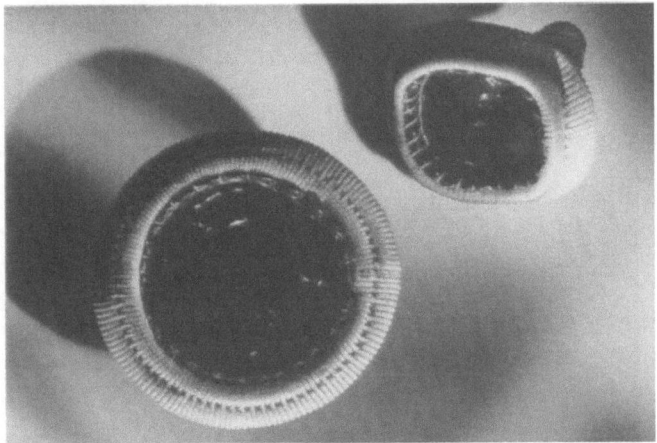
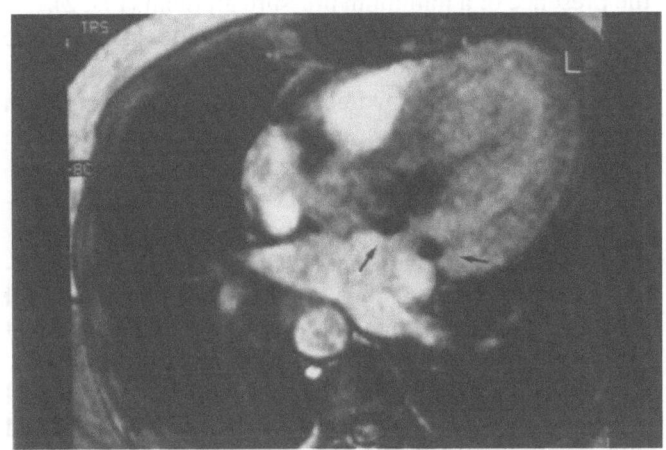

Fig. 1. a Biological prosthesis. **b** Metallic valve ring produces artifacts at the level of the annulus (arrows)

or pathologic when large (over 3 cm² jet area). Paravalvular leakage was thought to be present if the jet originated laterally from the valve; such leakage was considered a pathological finding.

Results

Our investigation showed the presence of irrelevant artifacts produced by the biological valves. In particular, the analysis performed at aortic level showed artifacts in 12 patients, limited only to the area of the valve ring which did not impair the evaluation of the valvular function. In the 2 cases with aortic Hancock prostheses, the semilunar leaflets could be well visualized on the transvalvular scan plane. In the 3 Carpentier-Edwards mitral prostheses, artifacts were observed strictly at the annulus; evaluation of normal valve function was nevertheless possible (Fig. 1).

More relevant artifacts were produced by mechanical prostheses. Disc cardiac valves in particular produced significant artifacts which did not allow adequate transvalvular evaluation of valve function. Conversely, when scan planes were acquired perpendicularly to the valves, artifacts were produced in the region of the valve ring and obturator. At the supra-aortic level, turbulence in the ejection phase was always observed and could be explained by

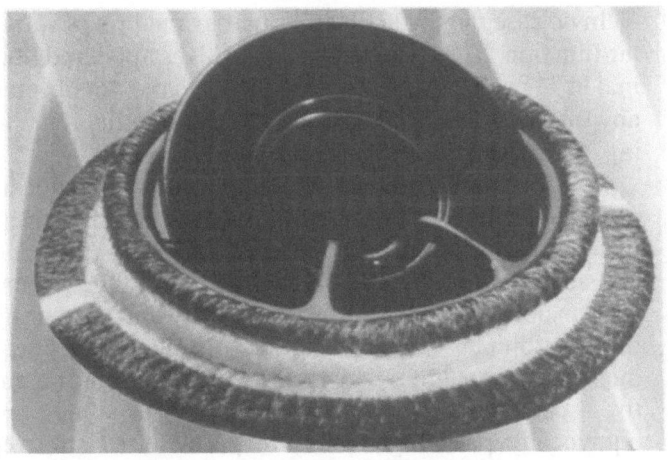
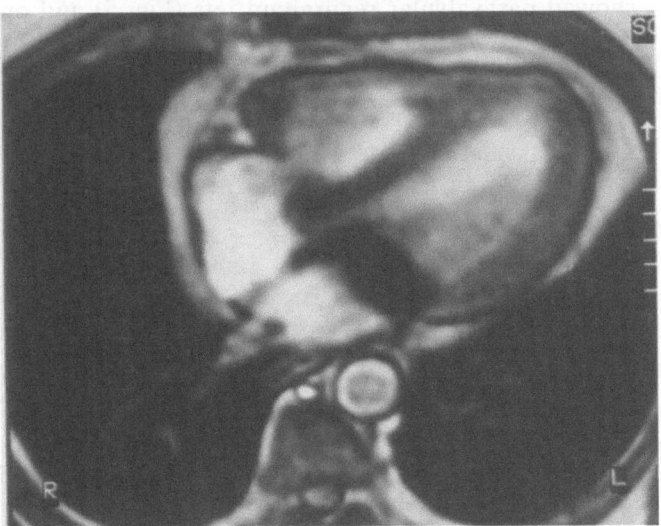
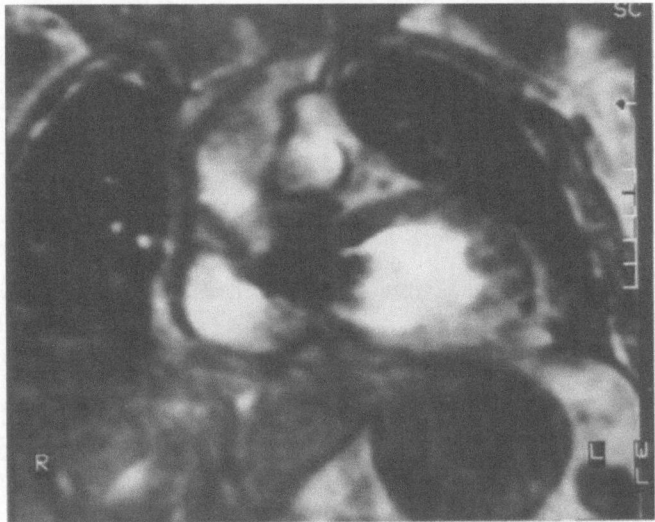

Fig. 2. a Mechanical single disc prosthesis. **b** Mechanical mitral valve. Bar artifacts are present proximal to the annulus. **c** Coronal scans show small bar artifacts at telediastolic phase

the presence of a minimum pressure gradient (Fig. 2).

Similar considerations could be made for the two bileaflet valves examined. In particular, the Sorin valve produced only small artifacts and a correct evaluation could be performed on scan planes perpendicular to the valvular plane. Transvalvular scans were excluded because they did not allow a good diagnostic and functional assessment. Phenomena of aortic supravalvular turbulence were constantly observed (Fig. 3). Extremely well-circumscribed artifacts were produced also by caged ball prostheses with non-metallic obturators, which did not represent an obstacle to diagnostic evaluation (Fig. 4).

A semiquantitative analysis showed that biological prostheses (Edwards-Carpentier, Hancock) produced slight artifacts, classifiable under class 1. All the mechanical prostheses were considered class 2, but the bileaflet valve produced more moderate artifacts than

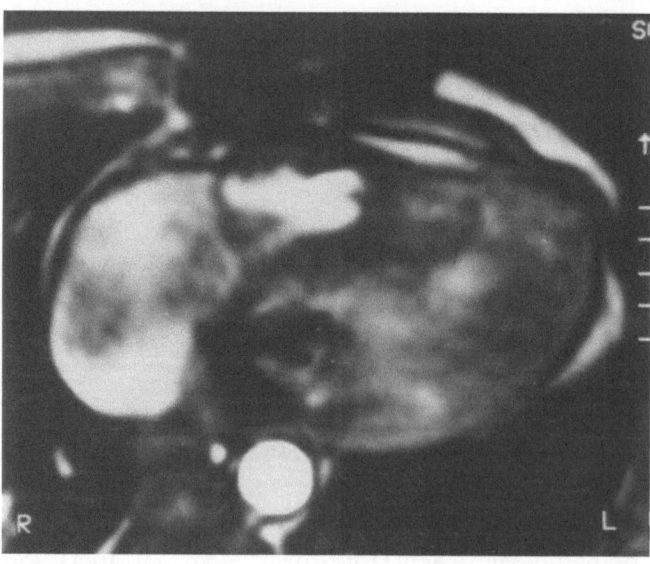

Fig. 4. *Caged ball prosthesis with metallic obturator.* Also in this case, artifacts are observed at the level of the annulus

did the other mechanical valves.

In no case did the artifacts impair evaluation of valvular function. The flow through the valves appeared normal in 34 prostheses. In 7 prostheses, we did not observe any turbulent flow through the valve and in the remaining cases it was considered normal.

Seven of 41 prostheses were clinically and echocardiographically considered to be malfunctioning. These included 3 aortic Sorin prostheses, and two mitral and two aortic Carpentier-Edwards prostheses. One patient with an aortic disc prosthesis who underwent MR during the ejection phase showed marked turbulent flow documented by signal loss which caused dimming of the entire ascending aorta. This was attributed to a high, unequivocally pathologic pressure gradient. Of the remaining 4 aortic malfunctioning prostheses, three showed paravalvular regurgitant jets (Fig. 5) and one

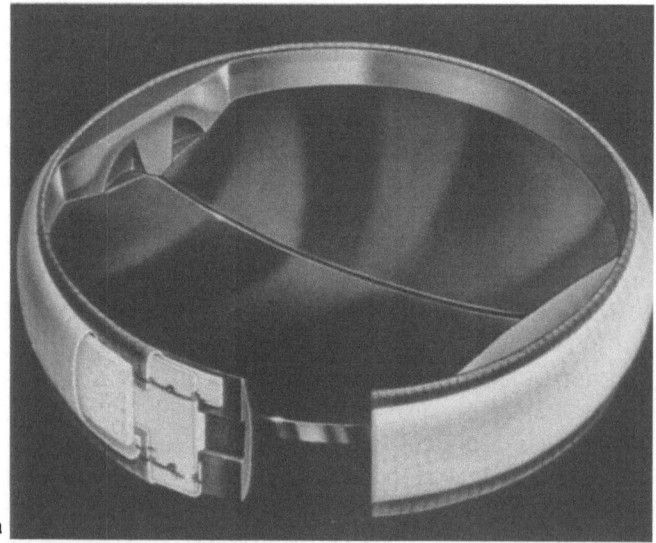

a

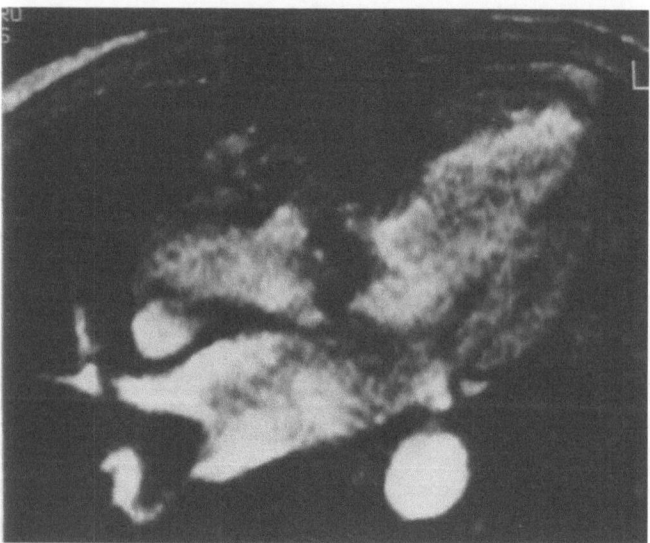

b

Fig. 3. a Mechanical bileaflet valve. **b** Long axis on aortic valve shows artifacts located at the level of the annulus

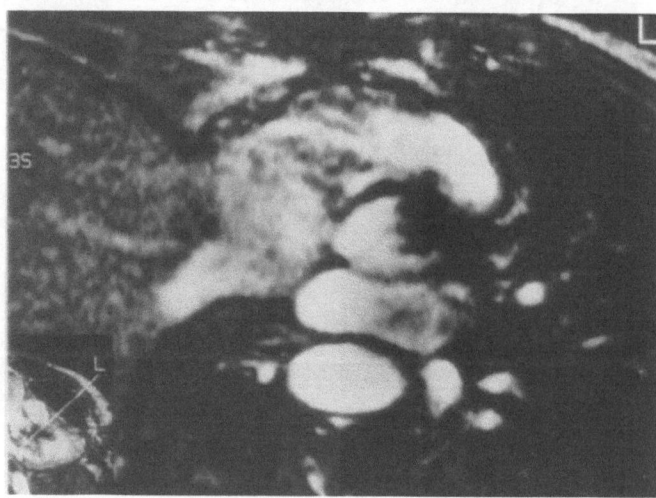

Fig. 5. *Paravalvular leakage flow in the aortic valve prosthesis*

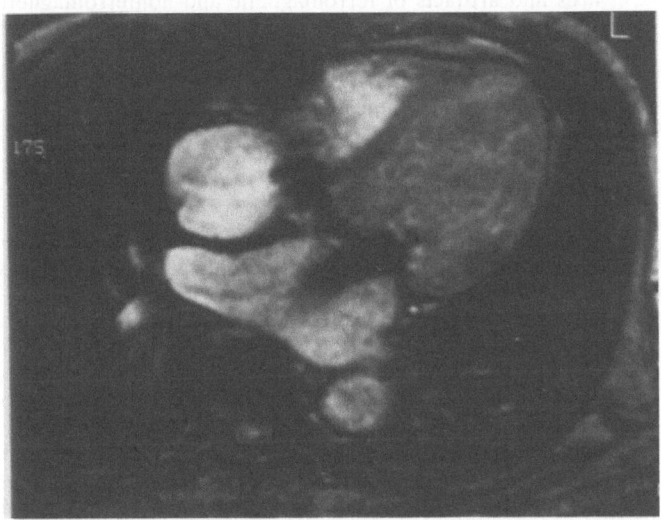

Fig. 6. *Pathologic signal loss at the level of the left atrium due to mitral Carpentier-Edwards prosthesis regurgitation*

showed transvalvular regurgitant flow. In one case, MR examination of the mitral prosthesis by Carpentier-Edwards showed a large turbulent regurgitation flow during the systolic phase characterized by left atrial signal loss (Fig. 6). This pattern was attributed to valvular insufficiency. A quantitative analysis was made through evaluation of the ratio between the turbulent flow region and left atrial region. In the other case, mitral disease was due to malposition and formation of a narrow angle between mitral plane and outflow tract. During the ejection phase, this caused aortic subvalvular turbulence. The mitral anterior leaflet producing out-flow obstruction was damaged and also caused atrial regurgitation in the systolic phase.

Discussion

According to the literature, MR can be considered a safe imaging technique for the evaluation of patients with valvular prostheses. The most alarming event conceivable is represented by dislodgement or deflection of the prosthesis. Therefore, researchers were induced to submit heart prostheses to high magnetic fields in vitro [8, 9]. These test studies showed that Bjork-Shiley and St. Jude prostheses do not deflect or dislodge by themselves, while most other prostheses showed only moderate deflection forces even when submitted to 1.5 T magnetic fields. In any case, the exerted strength was inferior to the cardiac strengths observed during contraction. The only exception was represented by the caged ball prosthesis with metallic obturator, probably due to its high ferromagnetic qualities and mass. Therefore, Starr-Edwards prostheses, model Pre 6000, were ruled out for MR studies.

On the basis of this information, it was possible to

carry out an in vivo MR evaluation of patients with heart valves. In particular, our study technique was considered safe because a low magnetic field was employed. The analysis of artifact entity provided surprising results. Biological prostheses produced minimal artifacts that allowed evaluation of part or all of the prosthetic valve leaflets. Artifacts were not significant and were circumscribed to the region of the valve ring which was composed of ferromagnetic material. Our interest was awakened by the semilunar shape of leaflets in the Hancock prosthesis after evaluation on the scan plane parallel to the valvular structure.

Similar considerations can be made also for mechanical prostheses. In the case of disc prostheses, which did not produce particularly relevant artifacts, a functional evaluation was possible on planes perpendicular to the valve. In patients with this type of prosthesis, MR examinations showed supra-aortic turbulence [11]. This was quite moderate and explainable by the presence of a minimum pressure gradient, as in patients with well-functioning heart valves. This finding can be observed with echocardiography and is explained by obturator rigidity [12]. The same considerations were made for bileaflet prostheses by Sorin, which produced smaller artifacts than did the others, also allowing partial demonstration of hemidiscs. In these regions, morphologically different supra-aortic turbulence was evident, usually not so relevant as that produced by disc prostheses. A double artifact was more frequently observed near both valvular leaflets. Also in this case, a functional analysis could be easily carried out. Similarly, the Smeloff-Cutter prosthesis, a caged ball with non-metallic obturator, produced moderate artifacts. Physiologic regurgitation was assumed when only a small area of signal void was found on MR images. The presence of multiple small reflexets was indicative of physiologic valve functioning. Severe pathologic regurgitation was demonstrated by a large area of signal loss. Pathologic transvalvular or paravalvular leakage flow in aortic valve prostheses was clearly differentiated and surgically confirmed.

The evaluation of prostheses gave interesting results whose significance rose when the technical limitations implied in echocardiographic and Doppler evaluation were considered. Indeed, difficulties in evaluating the region distal to the prosthesis depended on the inability of ultrasound beams to pass through. Moreover, the assessment of flow is oftentimes performed on planes not properly chosen for quantitative and semiquantitative analysis. This observation is important in the cases of mitral insufficiency and aortic valvular stenosis which are properly evaluated only with the transesophageal approach [13].

Over the transesophageal approach MR imaging offers the advantage of being more tolerated by the patient, but it cannot evaluate structural abnormalities of valve prostheses because the valvular structures are covered by metallic artifacts. In the case of malfunctioning heart valves, it was possible to correctly demonstrate this pathologic condition characterized by the presence of turbulence. Particularly at the mitral level, MR shows turbulence in the case of insufficiency and allows quantitative evaluation by assessing the ratio between the area of mitral regurgitation and the left atrial region. This assessment is performed using the criteria mentioned above, which allow differentiation among minimum, medium and severe insufficiency (less than 20%, between 20% and 40%, superior to 40%, respectively) [14].

In conclusion, MR allows functional evaluation of both biological and mechanical heart valves, in particular if investigations are performed with low-field units which produce small artifacts circumscribed to the annulus. The only exceptions are represented by caged ball prostheses with mechanical obturators (Starr-Edwards, Pre 6000), whose high ferromagnetic qualities increase attraction forces and implied risks. The use of MR could be of interesting value in the diagnostic evaluation of mitral regurgitation and aortic obstruction to avoid the uncomfortable application of transesophageal echocardiography. Moreover, the increasing application of velocity--encoded cine-MRI for the evaluation of flow across the valves will enhance the potential of this technique [15].

References

1. Persson BRR, Stahlberg F (1989) Health and safety of clinical NMR examinations. CRC, Boca Raton, FL
2. Budinger TF (1987) Nuclear Magnetic Resonance (NMR) in vivo studies: known thresholds for health effects. Arch Phys Med Rehabil 68: 162-164
3. Shellock FC (1989) Biological effects and safety aspects of magnetic resonance imaging. Magn Reson Q 2: 25-30
4. New PFJ, Rosen BR, Brady TJ, et al (1983) Potential hazards and artifacts of ferromagnetic and nonferromagnetic surgical and dental materials and devices in nuclear magnetic resonance imaging. Radiology 147: 139- 148
5. Laakman RW, Kaufman B, Han JS, et al (1985) MR imaging in patients with metallic implants. Radiology 157: 711-714
6. Shellock FG, Crues JV (1987) High-field MR imaging of metallic biomedical implants: an in vitro evaluation of deflection forces and temperature changes induced in large prostheses. Radiology 165-150
7. Lund G, Nelson JD, Wirtschafter JD, Williams PA (1986) Tatooing of eyelids: magnetic resonance imaging artifacts. Ophtalmic Surg 17: 550-553
8. Pusey E, Lufkin RB, Brown RKJ, et al (1986) Magnetic resonance imaging artifacts: mechanism and clinical significance. RadioGrapraphics 6: 891-911
9. Shellock FG, Crues JV (1988) High-field magnetic resonance imaging of metallic biomedical implants: an ex vivo evaluation of deflection forces. AJR Am J Roentgenol 151: 389-392
10. Randall PA, Kohman LJ, Scalzetti EM, Szeverenyi NM, Panicek DM (1988) Magnetic resonance imaging of prosthetic cardiac valves in vitro and in vivo. Am J Cardiol 62: 973-976
11. Sondergaard L, Thomsen C, Strahlberg F, Gymoese E, Lindvig K, Hildebrandt P, Henriksen O (1992) Mitral and aortic valvular flow: quantification with MR phase mapping. J Magn Reson Imaging: 295-302
12. Koppensteiner R, Moritz A, Schlick W, et al (1991) Blood rheology after cardiac valve replacement with mechanical prostheses or bioprostheses [Abstract] Radiology 180: 589
13. Khandheria BK, Oh J (1993) Transesophageal echocardiography: state-of-the-art and future directions [Abstract]. Radiology 186: 588
14. Sechtem U, Pflugfelder PW, Cassidy MM, White RD, Cheitlin MD, Schiller NB, Higgins CB (1988) Mitral or aortic regurgitation: quantification of regurgitant volumes with cine MR imaging. Radiology 167-425
15. Hartiala JJ, Mostbeck GH, Foster E, Fujita N, Matthias CD, Chazouilleres AF, Higgins CB (1993) Velocity-encoded cine MR in the evaluation of left ventricular diastolic function: measurement of mitral valve and pulmonary vein flow velocities and flow volume across the mitral valve. Am Heart J 125: 1054-1066